Child language disorders

Child language disorders

DOROTHY M. ARAM, Ph.D.

Assistant Professor, Department of Pediatrics,
Case Western Reserve University School of Medicine;
Speech Pathologist, Rainbow Babies and Childrens Hospital,
Cleveland, Ohio

JAMES E. NATION, Ph.D.

Professor and Chairman, Department of Communication Sciences,
Case Western Reserve University,
Cleveland, Ohio

Illustrated

The C. V. Mosby Company

ST. LOUIS • TORONTO • LONDON   1982

MOSBY

A TRADITION OF PUBLISHING EXCELLENCE

Editor: Julia Allen Jacobs
Assistant editor: Fawn Chapel
Manuscript editor: Lucy C. Golfin
Design: Susan Trail
Production: Jeanne A. Gulledge

The C.V. Mosby Company
11830 Westline Industrial Drive, St. Louis, Missouri 63141

Library of Congress Cataloging in Publication Data

Aram, Dorothy M., date
    Child language disorders.

    Bibliography: p.
    Includes index.
    1. Language disorders in children.   I. Nation,
James E., date. II. Title. [DNLM:
1. Language disorders—In infancy and childhood.
WL 340 A661c]
RJ496.L35A7   618.92′855   81-14063
ISBN 0-8016-0288-2   AACR2

GW/VH/VH 9 8 7 6 5 4 3 2 1   03/D/328

For
our parents:
Hazel, Wallie, and **Margaret**

Preface

Basic to the orientation of *Child Language Disorders* is that multiple types of language disorders in children exist. We suggest that these various language disorders arise from differing points of disruption in the language processing system. We also focus on the complex intrinsic and extrinsic factors that either cause these language disorders or shape their development. Rather than concentrate on description and remediation of disordered language behavior, we maintain that because of the heterogeneity seen in these children, we must draw distinctions among different disturbances in language processing.

We begin our treatment of child language disorders in Chapter 1 with a series of short case studies calling attention to the diversity of children falling into this subject area. Drawing from these case studies we offer a definition of child language disorders that serves to guide the material in the remainder of the book. Chapter 2 digresses in time to examine the historical approaches taken to child language disorders that have influenced our field's present views and practices. These past and present contributions lead to the development of our orientation to child language disorders, overviewed in Chapter 3, through the presentation and explication of the Child Language Processing Model. This model presents three principal processing segments, each with specified processing stages that may be disrupted. In turn these processing stages are tied to a child's understanding and use of the phonologic, syntactic, semantic, and pragmatic aspects of language behavior, allowing for differentiation among language disorders. Further, language-disordered children are seen to vary one from another in terms of the environment in which they mature and the various lines of intrinsic development occurring, including development of the peripheral sensory and motor systems, behavioral control, neurologic organization for language, and neurologic stability. Causal factors responsible for disordered language processing are examined in Chapter 4, and, in particular, complex interactions among causal factors are traced.

The remainder of the book is organized around segments of the Child Language Processing Model. Chapter 5 summarizes research directed toward transductions of speech to language in language-impaired children, concentrating on difficulties in auditory attention, discrimination, rate, memory, and sequencing. Language to thought to language processing is the subject of Chapter 6, where research directed toward language disordered children's comprehension, integration, formulation, and repetition is reviewed. Language to speech transductions, primarily motor programming disorders or developmental verbal apraxia, compose the subject area examined in Chapter 7. Chapter 8 summarizes assessment tools available for evaluation of each of the processing segments and reviews our view of diagnosis of child language disorders. The book concludes with Chapter 9, a reinterpretation and organization of existing treatment approaches around a language-processing framework. The position taken is that many effective therapy approaches exist, and the need is not simply to develop new alternatives; rather what is needed is a means by which an approach may be discriminately selected and applied to the individual processing problems present.

Child Language Disorders therefore provides an approach for viewing the diversity and complexity of children, research findings, assessment tools, and treatment approaches. Our aim has been to provide a perspective toward an area of study that is as applicable to current research and clinical practices as to knowledge and practice that will emerge in the next several years.

We have been supported in the preparation of this manuscript by many persons. Certainly, chief inspiration has been derived from the countless children and their families with whom we have worked and learned. In addi-

tion, several individuals have provided more immediate but nonetheless immeasurable support in this undertaking. Meg Guncik, who typed the entire manuscript in its various drafts and attended to other never-ending details, deserves special thanks, not only for all the pages she turned out but especially for her ability to remain good-natured. Barbara Ekelman added cheer and tracked down details when time was running short. Samuel J. Horwitz, Division Chief of Pediatric Neurology, not only encouraged the completion of this text but made possible divisional support. Mr. Alex Johnson provided remarkable insights as a reader of the manuscript, and his support helped along the way. We also wish to thank Anne Van Kleeck for the detailed and most helpful suggestions that she made in reviewing an early draft of this manuscript. And finally, John, Bethany, and Jonathan Aram provided comic and loving diversion that allowed one half of this team to recharge her energy when it ran low.

Dorothy M. Aram
James E. Nation

Contents

Child language disorders

chapter 1

Real kids with real problems

A DIVERSE COLLECTION OF CHILDREN

Language disorders appear in children of various ages and in countless behavioral manifestations. They stem from a range of biologic and environmental causes. These children demonstrate all the developmental variety seen in other children with the additional impact on development prompted by their language disorder. Each child is unique. Each represents the special dynamic interactions that evolve over time among his biologic and psychologic mechanisms and the environment in which he interacts.

What the child with a language disorder presents at any given time during development is a culmination of these complex interactions over his life span. Understanding the language disordered child as a result of the interactions between himself and his environment allows the speech-language pathologist to retain yet unravel the diversity and distinctiveness encompassed by this group of children. Fig. 1-1 provides a schematic representation of the language disordered child as a result of these complex and dynamic biologic, psychologic, behavioral, and environmental interactions over time.

A major theme of this book is that child language disorders encompass a heterogeneous group of children. Language disordered children present as many dissimilarities as similarities among themselves. We maintain that study of this diverse group of children requires an orientation which recognizes these essential differences. In the following chapters our aim is to provide a comprehensive view of child language disorders that provides a cohesive perspective yet requires speech-language pathologists to differentiate among the children they meet.

Snapshot case studies

As a backdrop to a definition of child language disorders and the contents of this book, a series of short case studies follows. The intent here is to illustrate the diverse biologic and psychologic equipment that language disordered children bring to the task of language learning and the range of environmental stimulation and support available to them. Each summary is taken from a case history of a real child. Each presents a real problem for the child, the family, and involved professionals. These short descriptions demonstrate the broad range of children included within the scope of child language disorders and once again reveal that few human problems are simple. Rarely will simple explanations or solutions explain or solve human

1

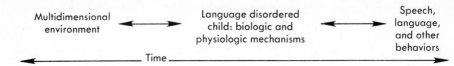

FIG. 1-1. Child language disorders are complex interactions that take place over time.

problems of which one, child language disorders, is the concern of this book.

Stanley

Compared to the other children in the classroom for the trainable mentally retarded, Stanley differs in the apparent attention that he pays, his ability to stick with long, complex directions, and his tendency to correct himself when he makes an error. His classmates are superior in their use of expressive language, but 10-year-old Stanley is using only 25 different words, many of which sound very similar. Although he produces only single consonant + vowel combinations and does not join words together, he gets his major points across through highly expressive pantomime. For example, when he was shown a picture of a chicken, he put his hands under his armpits and flapped his elbows.

The product of a complicated pregnancy and delivery, Stanley is clearly a retarded child with no skill area reaching an 8-year level. Yet educational placement has been an unresolved issue since his preschool days. In many ways his understanding and learning are greater than that expected of a trainable mentally retarded child. Yet his complete lack of expressive language until a year ago limited his ability to demonstrate even what he did know on verbal intelligence tests that were used to determine his educational placement.

The strain of having an exceptional child was only one of the many problems leading to the separation and ultimate divorce of Stanley's parents several years ago. Although Stanley has stayed with his mother, both parents continue to show active care and concern for their only child.

Danelle

Sitting passively in a corner of her crib, Danelle looked every bit the waif she was. This 18-month-old girl recovering from meningitis vocalized in very soft, mewing sounds at times; however, it was doubtful that she used any words meaningfully.

After the meningitis her hearing ability had been questioned, yet both her middle ear reflexes and responses to pure tone audiometry had been found to be normal. What she understood was difficult to determine, because she generally retreated from attempts at interaction. Although she did not give indication that she recognized any of her body parts or was able to identify any pictures, one wondered if her steely black eyes took in and understood more than she would reveal. Although Danelle showed visual alertness by waiting for the return of the vanished in a game of peekaboo, attempts to get her to play pat-a-cake or any imitative game met with a lack of interaction.

Having contracted meningitis three weeks earlier, Danelle seemed to have completely recovered physically and the intravenous feedings had long since been removed. However, her quietness among the floor of demanding babies was striking. While some of the staff attributed the meningitis and three-week hospitalization to her current behavior, others pointed out the discrepancy between her behavior and other post-meningitic children. They felt that Danelle's behavioral responses stemmed most probably from a long-standing developmental problem. The history from the foster mother was sparse and its reliability questionable. What was known was that Danelle had been removed from her "mentally ill" natural mother at 8 months old and since had lived with the same foster mother, who very adequately provided for Danelle's physical well-being, yet seemed to provide only a minimally stimulating environment.

Ruth

Ruth was not the brightest student but was managing to hold her own in school and soon would be promoted to the second grade. Then her congenital heart disorder again flared up, and the cardiologists decided a cardiac catheterization was in order. The risks were presented as minimal, and since Ruth's shortness of breath and dizziness seemed to be increasing, the parents agreed to the procedure. But what started out as a relatively low-risk procedure ended with a devastating effect on Ruth.

Several hours after the catheterization, she complained of an excruciating headache, vomited, and not long afterward experienced difficulty moving the right side of her body. Then she stopped talking and for weeks remained mute. Through persistence her father taught her to signal "yes" by one squeeze on his hand and "no" by two squeezes. Slowly over several months she began talking again, first in single, very unclear words and then in short, telegraphic sentences. After several more months she began walking.

Two years later she continued to have a gait problem and dysarthric speech. The stroke had an even greater impact on her learning. At first she was placed in a learning disabilities class, but after it became apparent that she had pronounced difficulty understanding as well as speaking, she was moved to a class for the retarded. Here she has again begun to do elementary reading and mathematics and is seen three times a week for speech and language therapy. Two years have passed since her stroke. Progress is slow, and it is doubtful that Ruth will ever regain her premorbid level of ability.

Arnold

Arnold spent most of his seven years traveling from city to city with his three younger siblings and his unmarried parents who ran a concession stand with a midwestern carnival company. Except for occasional periods when all four children were dropped off at the paternal aunt's home for several days, at which time they were "cleaned up, fed, and taken to the doctor if they were sick," Arnold, in the aunt's words, "lived a life worse than an animal." According to court testimony in which the aunt was granted custody of the children, Arnold spent most of his days uncared for in dingy motel rooms, rarely receiving adequate food or medical attention, much less parental attention, but frequently receiving physical abuse, especially from his father. Until placed with the aunt, Arnold usually was dressed in girls' clothing, since that was what was available. Arnold's mildly retarded mother was described as the father's "pawn," who propagated children to increase the size of their welfare check. Habitually moving from city to city, Arnold had never attended school.

When first seen for a comprehensive developmental assessment, Arnold had been in the custody of the aunt for three months and had recently begun attending first grade. Because of his complete inability to function socially or educationally in the classroom, Arnold was referred for further testing. The psychologist who was the first of the team members to meet with Arnold commented that "he is the closest I've seen to a modern day feral child." Although he placed in the low educable mentally retarded (EMR) range on intelligence

testing, any formal testing could not be considered a reliable prognosticator of intellectual ability because of the severe emotional, physical, and experiential deprivation to which he had been subjected. Although he spoke in connected speech, Arnold's speech was completely unintelligible. A mild conductive hearing loss was discovered that apparently resulted from longstanding, chronic middle ear infections.

Arnold scored no higher than a three-year level on any tests of language comprehension, and observations of spontaneous behavior further indicated no higher language ability in any sphere. How much of this deficient speech and language behavior could be attributed to the extreme environmental conditions, to the chronic hearing loss, to emotional factors, or to a possible genetically based mental retardation were questions that remained to be unraveled through ongoing diagnosis and treatment.

Bill

Bill was affectionately referred to as "Little Bug" by his clinician. It is a nickname that captured his physical petiteness and the manner in which he so rapidly darted around the room. Early on, Bill attended only briefly to tasks and showed only minimal organization in his play activities. Such observations led his pediatrician to view him as a moderately retarded child. He urged the mother to place Bill in a preschool for the retarded and to seek speech and language therapy.

At 3 years old Bill was only beginning to use single words. Although it was initially thought that a difficulty with learned movements of his articulators (apraxia of speech) complicated his language disorder, Bill responded so rapidly to a naturalistic-cognitive approach to therapy that in nine months he was using three- and four-word phrases with an extensive, intelligible vocabulary. Apraxia of speech no longer seemed a component of his problem.

After a year of treatment Bill's attention and level of play activity had improved markedly. His comprehension of syntax and semantics were age appropriate, and his nonverbal intelligence measured in the high average range. At 4 years old, although having made significant progress in many spheres, Bill continues to present an expressive language deficit, especially in syntax.

Both parents drifted from social drinking into alcoholism, which for Bill's mother persisted throughout her pregnancy with Bill. Since shortly after Bill's birth, however, the mother has maintained abstinence and has channeled her guilt into very effective stimulation and support for her son. The father continues his drinking, yet has managed to hold a top level management position in a major company. Marital problems abound, and Bill is cared for solely by his mother.

Alan

As a second grader, 8-year-old Alan shines in math, where he clearly is the best pupil in his class. His teacher wonders if Alan's physician father encourages prowess with numbers and calculations. Alan's handwriting is poor, and although he participates in gym, his performance exposes his mild right hemiplegia. While Alan's reading and language arts do not stand out as deficient when compared to his classmates, in reference to his own abilities these areas are weak. Alan received articulation therapy for two years and now evidences no difficulty with speech production.

Language deficits had never been questioned and were documented only when Alan was included in a research study comparing the language ability of left and right hemiplegic children. Through this testing he was found to have a vocabulary comprehension level more than two years below his chronologic age, and his comprehension and use of syntax were at the 10th percentile on the Northwestern Syntax Screening Test (Lee, 1969). His performance on the Token Test (De-Renzi and Vignolo, 1962) fell off markedly from the 100% correct on the parts requiring comprehension and retention of two and three bits of information to 10% on the sections requiring the longest retention of information. Although Alan presents semantic and syntactic language deficits in both comprehension and formulation, apparently his outstanding ability in other areas has allowed him to compensate for these problems.

Many of Alan's problems arose from an acute infection at 8 weeks old that resulted in a right hemiparesis. A current CAT (computerized axial tomography) scan revealed a large area of porencephaly involving much of the left frontal lobe, extending to the left parietal region with hemiatrophy of the left cerebral hemisphere. Bilingualism also complicates the picture. Alan was born in France and speaks French at home with his family. He has lived in the United States for most of his life and speaks English at school and with his friends.

CHILD LANGUAGE DISORDERS: A DEFINITION ENCOMPASSING DIVERSITY

Stanley, Danelle, Ruth, Arnold, Bill, and Alan all have language disorders. They are "real kids with real problems." Each is distinct from the others, and each represents the complexity and diversity found in children with language disorders. Differences are readily apparent in their ages, in the nature and severity of their language disorders, in the number and type of associated problems, in the potential factors causing their problems, and in the amount and quality of their environmental experiences.

If child language disorders includes such a diverse group of children with widely varying disorders, what commonality holds this area of study together? We submit that child language disorders can be generalized as:

The study of children with disordered language behaviors related to language processing dysfunctions that appear as variable patterns of performance and are shaped by the developmental content in which they occur.

In Chapter 3 we will examine this working definition in detail. For now we want to apply this definition to the brief case histories just summarized, demonstrating our perspective toward child language disorders.

First, the topic of study addressed here concerns *children*. Yet childhood may encompass a large age range. Age undeniably is a crucial variable in understanding the normalcy or abnormalcy of any behavior, as well as in designing and selecting appropriate diagnostic and treatment procedures. Prognosis or long-term outlook as well depends on the child's age in conjunction with other factors. Eighteen-month-old Danelle presents very different language behavior, requiring different assessment and intervention tools than, for example, 10-year-old Stanley or even 4-year-old Bill. Furthermore, although child language disorders reside in children, the disorder may be present throughout development (as with Alan and several of the others described) or it may be acquired after a period of normal development (as with Ruth).

Second, the group of children studied all present observable *disordered language behavior;* none is normal in this regard. The language disorder may be minimal as in Bill's case where his limitations were not recognized until tested for a study on hemiplegic children, or profound as for Stanley who at 10 years old is limited to 25 single words. Also, the disordered language may be confined to one aspect of language such as predominantly expressive syntax as seen with Bill, or include multiple aspects such as exemplified by Arnold.

Third, we see disordered language behavior arising from *language processing dysfunctions* that vary from child to child. For example, some may present sensory processing deficits as did Arnold with long-standing chronic middle ear infections. Others may have reduced cognitive processing capabilities, at least one of the processing dysfunctions contributing to Stanley's severe language disorder. Others may have demonstrable or inferred neurologic deficits impairing language comprehension or fomulation, for example, the left hemisphere lesions present since infancy in Bill and acquired during first grade by Ruth. Much of this book will be devoted to explaining these variable processing dysfunctions and their relationship to observable language behavior.

Fourth, despite major differences among children, *recurrent patterns or types of language disorders occur* in this population of children that will be detailed in Chapter 3. Although we advocate viewing children with language disorders as unique in the complex behaviors and processing dysfunctions they present, commonalities do arise. Patterns of language performance common among language disordered children may be identified depending upon the language processes disrupted and the levels of language impaired.

Finally, the form that disordered language behavior and processing dysfunctions take will be *molded by the developmental context*

in which the child grows. Factors intrinsic to the child, including concomitant physical and emotional problems, as well as extrinsic factors (notably the persons and experiences available in the environment) will aid or impede the course of growth inherent in childhood. For example, motor limitations such as with Ruth or Alan present additional handicaps with which these children must cope. Children may develop language in spite of the people or experiences they encounter as with Arnold, or conversely, in very large part, because of the positive relationships and opportunities provided, as seen for Bill.

These children are only six of the estimated 2.1 to 10 million children with language disorders (Perkins, 1977). All children will be as individual, although not always as complex, as the six children presented in this chapter. Yet each shares having disordered language behavior related to processing dysfunctions, both of which are shaped by the intrinsic and extrinsic contexts in which they develop. The mission of this book is to preserve the variability presented by language disordered children but to provide an orientation that allows for cohesive study, diagnosis, and management of this diverse group of children.

Before developing our orientation to child language disorders further in Chapter 3, Chapter 2 will trace historical approaches to its study, since we believe current practices have evolved from and have been shaped by what has gone before.

STUDY QUESTIONS

1. Are the hearing results reported on Danelle what are expected after meningitis? (See Roeser, Campbell, and Daly, 1975; Vernon, 1967.) What effect may chronic otitis media have on language and learning? (See Hanson and Ulvestad, 1979; Ventry, 1980.)
2. Is Bill's course of development typical of a child diagnosed as suffering from the fetal alcohol syndrome? (See Clarren and Smith, 1978; Streissguth, Herman, and Smith, 1978.)

3. In the following chart compile what you know or infer about each child's age, language behavior, possible language processing dysfunctions, and intrinsic or extrinsic developmental context. Although these concepts may be new to you and not fully understood, try your hand at organizing the information for each child in this manner, then reflect on the positive and negative factors you believe will influence each child's long-term outlook. Information from Stanley has been summarized in this manner as a sample.

| | Age-related variables | Disordered language behavior | Language processing dysfunction | Developmental context | |
				Intrinsic factors	Extrinsic factors
Stanley	10 years old; ? period remaining for spontaneous language development	25-word vocabulary; no connected speech; CV's only; some gestures	? neurological status; cognitive processing dysfunction	some degree of retardation	divorced yet concerned parents
Danelle					
Ruth					
Arnold					
Bill					
Alan					

chapter 2

Historical heritage of child language disorders

HISTORICAL PERSPECTIVE SHAPES THE PRESENT

Chapter 1 introduced child language disorders as a field encompassing very diverse children. A definition of child language disorders was offered based on a complex set of interactions among the child's language behavior, processing breakdowns, and the intrinsic and extrinsic developmental context in which he grows. Just as diversity is a fundamental characteristic of the children studied here, so too are the approaches taken to study these children. Part of these differences in perspective has resulted from differing trends that have emerged throughout the past 25 years.

In order to appreciate how the field has developed, an understanding of past contributions is essential. Therefore before entering into an expanded discussion of our approach toward child language disorders, Chapter 2 will summarize the major trends of the past and the contributions made to the study of child language disorders. Several reasons motivate this digression into history. First, views held today have very much evolved out of previous work and directions of earlier clinicians and investigators. Second, multiple perspectives to child language disorders have emerged throughout the history of study in this area. Some perspectives have provided fruitful directions for further work. Some have led to dead ends. Others have been suggested but not fully explored. However, each of these lines of earlier developments has in some way influenced the work we do today. Third, those of us working in the field today owe thanks to the many people and ideas that have been prominent before us. We have developed to the present level of sophistication in this field because of the very important contributions of those whose work preceded ours. Rather than ignoring these earlier workers, we maintain that their directions need to be incorporated into current perspectives. Careful study of much of this earlier work frequently reveals that "new" approaches are often not so new but have been elegantly described and applied in earlier years. Finally and most important of all, we feel that the field of child language disorders needs a broad multiperspective view. This framework not only allows the clinician and researcher to address the diversity seen in their young clients, but also allows them to incorporate the diverse approaches that have been and are being used to study, diagnose, and treat these children.

This chapter traces the early historical roots of child language disorders in the fields of medicine and education of the deaf. These origins gave rise to three pivotal individuals: Mildred McGinnis, Helmer Myklebust, and Muriel Morley, who working independently gave "birth" to the field of child language disorders by their recognition of this important area of study and through their ground-breaking contributions. Next emerged the era of etiologic typology that dominated the late 1950s and early 1960s. Most workers in this period were caught up in the concept of differential diagnosis, attempting to sort out the "true" etiologies for language disorders. With the explosion of new knowledge in linguistics, the day of linguistic and psycholinguistic explanations was ushered in. Here the consuming passion has been to provide increasingly detailed descriptions of child language development and disorders. The day of linguistic and psycholinguistic explanations is currently very much alive and can be credited with giving systematic and scientific order to the previously largely intuitive language data base. Finally, another contemporary line of study of child language disorders has emerged, one that involves searching for processing explanations for child language disorders.

HISTORICAL ROOTS: DIVERGENT SOURCES

Child language disorders as a specialty in speech-language pathology grew out of three important and divergent sources of information: (1) adult aphasiology, (2) other medical disciplines, and (3) the field of deaf education. Researchers and clinicians working within these disciplines diagnosed, described, and treated language disordered children long

before a specialty of child language disorders emerged. These professionals established the sources of information from which the pioneers in speech-language pathology developed their perspectives toward the study of child language disorders.

Roots in neurology: adult aphasia

In the 1800s, impetus for the study of the relationship between language behavior and that part of the brain responsible was sparked by the provocative work of Broca (1861 a, b) and Wernicke (1874). The discipline of "neurolinguistics" was born, dominated early by neurologists and anatomists but later joined by psychologists, linguists, and speech pathologists interested in brain-behavior relationships. The study of adult aphasia, acquired language disorders caused by brain lesions, directed attention toward the relationship between language symptoms and localization of lesions. The perspective of explaining observed behaviors in terms of neurologic processing was begun.

Various patterns of language deficits were reported in adults who had sustained known neurologic injury. These contrasts of language abilities became the focus of heightened interest. Exciting theories about language localization and processing emerged. Numerous aphasiologists, among them Goldstein (1942, 1948), Head (1926, 1963), Marie (Cole and Cole, 1971), Pick (Brown, 1973), and Weisenberg and McBride (1935, 1964) developed classification systems and an array of terminology specifying the language and neurologic disorders seen in adult aphasics.

It was only logical and a matter of time until parallels between adult aphasia and child language disorders were noted. As will be seen, the study of adult aphasia had a major impact on the early work in child language disorders; it served as both the inspiration and experience base from which the pioneers in language pathology launched their work. Today many investigators continue to look for parallels between language disorders seen in adults with acquired lesions and those presented by children with developmental disorders. A question that continues to be actively addressed is "what child language interventionists can teach adult aphasiologists or vice versa" (Leonard and Holland, 1980).

Roots in other medical disciplines

Aside from the neurologists studying adult aphasia, a handful of individuals representing various other medical disciplines, notably child neurology, psychiatry, and pediatrics, began to present descriptions of children who did not talk. Case reports appeared in the medical literature, and both physical and psychologic explanations were offered for why children did not talk (Town, 1911; Worster-Drought and Allen, 1929).

It is understandable that much of the early work in medical disciplines, with its neurological roots in adult aphasia, referred to children with language disorders as aphasic. For example, just five years after the appearance of Broca's (1961 a, b) work, Vaisse (1866, as cited in Benton, 1959) described retardation of language development in children who apparently were neither deaf nor mentally defective. He called the condition "congenital aphasia" and advanced the hypothesis that the condition was due to the same types of focal lesions that caused aphasia in adults.

Orton (1937) is perhaps one of the first neurologists to become concerned with communication disorders in children. His 1937 book, *Reading, Writing and Speech Problems in Children: A Presentation of Certain Types of Disorders in the Development of the Language Faculty,* draws heavily from information derived from adult aphasia. In Chapter 1, "Language Losses in the Adult as the Key to the Developmental Disorders in Children," Orton

provided classifications, descriptions, and treatment programs for several syndromes of child language disorders. These included developmental alexia (the reading disability), developmental agraphia (special writing disability), developmental word deafness, developmental motor aphasia (motor speech delay), developmental apraxia (abnormal clumsiness), stuttering in childhood, and a group of combined or mixed syndromes. He emphasized heredity and the role of cerebral dominance as causal factors for these disorders. In many respects, Orton sowed the seeds for much of the contemporary work in the neurologic basis of child language disorders. Other early neurologically oriented descriptions of children with developmental language disorders include those of Worster-Drought (1943), who described congenital auditory imperception and Guttman (1942), Alajouanine and Lhermitte (1963), and Basser (1962), who focused on acquired aphasia in children.

Psychiatrists, psychologists, and pediatricians were among the medically based professionals who also provided early descriptions of language disordered children emphasizing childhood aphasia, many of which appeared during the 1950s and early 1960s. Benton (1959, 1964) is often credited with providing one of the classic descriptions of childhood aphasia; however, a number of persons preceded him in providing detailed case studies as well as summary data for large groups of children considered to be aphasic.

Strauss (1954) in a paper titled "Aphasia in Children" reflected on his 30 years of experience with aphasic children. He preferred to refer to this children's disorder as "oligophasia," signifying a deficit in language or lack of language development rather than a loss of language. He identified three types of oligophasia, including a receptive oligophasia (primarily a disturbance in auditory perception), an expressive oligophasia (a disturbance recognizing and forming phonemic patterns), and a central oligophasia (a disorder of symbolization). Strauss (1954) discussed this condition from a genetic psychologic point of view. It is interesting to note that as early as 1954, Strauss discussed normal and disordered language acquisition in reference to Piaget's (1926) stages of cognitive development. Although Strauss and his co-workers (1947, 1955) are probably better known for their work directed toward a wider spectrum of brain damaged children, they offered insightful comments about language disordered children, preceding by more than twenty years recent interest in applying Piagetian principles to the study of children with disordered language (Morehead and Morehead, 1974; Muma, 1978).

Ingram and Reid (1956) described the characteristics and presumed etiology of 78 children observed in a department of child psychiatry as developmentally aphasic. For their group of 65 boys and 13 girls between the ages of 6 and 15 years, they provided summary information about family and social backgrounds, results of psychologic and educational assessments, and descriptions of behavior and personality disturbances. They also compiled information on descriptions of speech defects and receptive and expressive aphasia, twinning, and laterality (handedness, eyedness, and footedness). Of the early descriptions of aphasic children, Ingram and Reid provided the most comprehensive information based on a large number of children. Other case studies are scattered throughout the medical literature of this period. Exemplary of these is Karlin's (1951) detailed description of a 6-year-old child whom he diagnosed as having congenital verbal auditory agnosia. In his case presentation, Karlin contrasted this condition with auditory agnosia in adults.

The emphasis in much of this medically based literature was on identifying and describing conditions in children similar to those seen in adults with known central nervous system lesions. The term *aphasia* or *dysphasia* (implying a lesser disorder) was then borrowed from the adults and applied to children with the modifying words "childhood" or "developmental." The assumption underlying the use of these words was that neurologic dysfunctions, if not overt lesions, also were responsible for the disordered language seen in children.

Controversy has persisted regarding the appropriateness of the use of the term *aphasia* with language disordered children (Chappell, 1970; Hardy, 1965; Strauss, 1954). Among the important issues debated was the application of a term meaning loss of language to a group that has never acquired language (Benton, 1959). Advocates of this term maintained that modifying the term with *developmental* or *congenital* denoted that the absence of language was present throughout development. A more serious criticism was the assumption of neurologic impairment in children who for the most part were without demonstrable central nervous system lesions. Numerous investigators saw aphasia as one manifestation of presumed brain damage (Benton, 1959, 1964; Strauss, 1954), yet verified brain damage was typically absent and terms such as *brain dysfunction* or *minimal brain dysfunction* were used to suggest that neurologic dysfunction caused these disorders even though specific lesions could not be documented.

Today the terms *congenital aphasia* and *childhood aphasia* continue to be used, and the issue of their appropriateness remains unsettled. The terms are used by some speech-language pathologists, especially those working in medical settings, to reflect both the medical heritage toward diagnosis of disease entities and the assumption that neurologic dysfunction is responsible for a particular child's language disorder. Others prefer labels that refer to the disordered behavior rather than presumed etiology, using terms such as language *disordered children* or *phonologically impaired* children. Consistent with our view that language disorders arise from varied processing breakdowns, we maintain that the language disorders of some but not all children may arise from demonstrable central nervous system lesions or from assumed neurologic dysfunction, in which cases "aphasia" is an apt term. Not all language disordered children are aphasic; rather, we suggest that aphasic children represent a subset of language disordered children. Whether or not a clinician or investigator uses the term *aphasia* to refer to that subset of language disordered children depends on his or her perspective as to the importance of etiologic and processing dysfunction in language disordered children.

Roots in education of the deaf

The second major group of workers who laid foundations for child language disorders were the educators of the deaf who can be traced back even before the very important work of de l'Épée and Heinicke in Europe in the late part of the eighteenth century (Silverman, 1961). These professionals were experienced in observing and remediating children who did not talk. Therefore, it is not surprising that they were in the forefront in drawing attention to children with little or no language and in developing techniques for working with other types of language disorders.

Although a number of persons within the field of education of the deaf have contributed to the study of child language disorders, the work of Ewing (1930) was particularly notable. It drew attention to aphasic children and gave rise to one of the earliest treatments for these children. Similarly, from their years of experience with deaf children, Myklebust

(1954), McGinnis, Kleffner and Goldstein (1956), and Hardy (1965) all emerged to be important molders of the field of child language disorders. Persons such as these all arrived at the fundamental observation that some children with and without hearing impairments learned language easier than others. They provided very valuable and basic descriptions of the aphasic as opposed to the hearing impaired child. Of equal importance was their initiation of a tradition of special educational approaches to teach language to those who did not acquire it naturally. They therefore provided a heritage of behavioral description of the language abilities of disordered children coupled with the educators' experience in teaching language to the language impaired.

From the preceding brief summary, it is evident that the study of child language disorders had its roots in various professions; however, the focus was medical. Neurologists studying adult aphasia, other medical and medically based professionals adapting this work to children, and the educators of the deaf all had a major impact on theory, diagnosis, classification, and treatment of child language disorders. Theory met with practice, both offering important lines of inquiry from which the specialty of child language disorders was nurtured.

THE THREE M'S

The 1950s were ripe for a coming together of the independent lines of work in child language disorders that established it as an area of study in its own right. To demonstrate this movement, this section will discuss the important influences of three workers who provided a significant body of early literature in child language disorders and attracted attention to the needs of these children.

The three professionals, Mildred A. McGinnis, Helmer R. Myklebust, and Muriel E. Morley, although each worked independently physically and in many ways theoretically, were to be in effect the grandparents of the specialty of child language disorders. No student of child language disorders can undervalue the original contributions and insights of these three individuals. The study of child language disorders owes them an immeasurable debt.

Mildred A. McGinnis

Although McGinnis' landmark book, *Aphasic Children: Identification and Education by the Association Method,* was not published until 1963, her influence and her work, including other publications, preceded that date. Shortly after World War I, McGinnis found herself in an opportune position to juxtapose work being done with both adult aphasics and deaf children. As a teacher at the Central Institute for the Deaf in St. Louis, McGinnis' task was to improve the teaching of speech to deaf children. Included in her first class of children were an 8-year-old girl and her 6-year-old brother who failed to develop speech and learn lipreading despite having better hearing than the other children in the class. McGinnis described the brother and sister as alert and responsive children, but as being unable to learn speech through the methods used with deaf children (McGinnis, 1963).

At the same time that McGinnis was involved with this class of hearing impaired children, she also was providing speech therapy to World War I servicemen who had acquired language disorders from injuries. She commented on the striking similarity between the speech and language disorders presented by adult aphasics and the brother and sister in her class for deaf children. This observation led her to hypothesize that the children presented a congenital form of the condition observed in adults following acquired head trauma. She then modified her approach used with the adult aphasics and applied it to the two children, who were not learning language from conventional approaches for the deaf. With this new teaching method, the brother and sister surpassed their deaf classmates in speech and language learning. Their response to treatment suggested to McGinnis that these children might present problems more similar to adult aphasics than to deaf children (McGinnis, 1963).

McGinnis, along with Kleffner and Goldstein (1956), provided description, classification, and probably most notably a systematic teaching method for aphasic children. These workers defined aphasia in children as an inability to understand and/or express language resulting from a central nervous system dysfunction. From this they described two subgroups: expressive or motor aphasia and receptive or sensory aphasia. Expressive aphasia was characterized as (1) lack of expressive speech; (2) adequate understanding of speech, comparable to a normal child; (3) vocalizations consisting of patterns of sounds repeated over and over; (4) a partial or complete inability to imitate actions or positions of the tongue, lip, and jaw or of sounds and words; (5) adequate control of muscles used in speech and for other acts such as chewing or swallowing; (6) adequate hearing; and (7) adequate intelligence. Receptive aphasia was characterized as (1) a lack of understanding of speech; (2) lack of expressive speech that could fall into one of four categories (little or no vocalization; scribble speech—jabber or chatter that had considerable inflection and was usually accompanied by facial expressions and by gestures; echolalia; or appropriate use of a limited number of words or phrases); (3) adequate control of muscles used in speech and for other acts such as chewing and swallowing; (4) a discrepancy

between ability to hear and ability to understand spoken language; and (5) a discrepancy
between intelligence and ability to understand spoken language.

Probably McGinnis is better known for her
development of a teaching method for aphasic
children that she called the *association method*. This method has also been termed the
"phonetic" or "elemental" approach but is
commonly referred to as the "McGinnis method." The approach is highly structured and is
used in an invariant manner. The major principles of the Association Method were outlined by McGinnis, Kleffner, and Goldstein
(1956) and later amplified by McGinnis
(1963).

McGinnis and her co-workers provided this
field with parallels between aphasic children
and adults, defined aphasia in children, provided invaluable descriptions of these children, proposed a dichotomous classification of
receptive and expressive aphasia in children,
and contributed a major teaching method.
Their definition emphasized that childhood
aphasia must be differentiated from peripheral hearing and speech disorders, mental retardation, and severe emotional disturbances,
a theme that was to influence and dominate
the study of child language disorders for some
time to come.

Helmer R. Myklebust

As a psychologist working with hearing impaired children at Northwestern University,
Myklebust was interested in why children did
not respond to sound. Through many observations and test procedures, he brought attention to the fact that not all children who did
not respond to sound or did not develop language were hearing impaired.

In 1954 his book, *Auditory Disorders in
Children,* appeared. Here he differentiated
four groups of children with "auditory disorders" caused by (1) peripheral deafness,
(2) aphasia, (3) psychic deafness, and (4)
mental deficiency. From this evolved Myklebust's most influential legacy to child language disorders: the concept of differential
diagnosis based on presumed etiology. In fact,
his 1954 book is subtitled *A Manual for Differential Diagnosis*. Its impact resulted in
viewing these etiologic categories as mutually
exclusive. He states:

> Children who do not develop speech frequently do
> present problems of auditory responsiveness and capac-
> ity. However, many of these children do not have re-
> duced acuity. It is the responsibility of the clinician to
> determine which of the various conditions is present.
> This means that the diagnostic problem is one of differ-
> ential diagnosis. Before a diagnosis is made, the condi-
> tion must be differentiated from others which may pro-
> duce the common symptom of lack of response to sound.
> It is of genuine importance that the condition be dif-
> ferentially diagnosed early in life. The auditory disorders
> of the aphasic, mentally deficient and emotionally dis-
> turbed child should not be confused with those of the
> child who has peripheral deafness. Such confusion may
> seriously impede later development and adjustment.[*]

In the one diagnostic group, aphasia, that
he clearly defines as language disordered,
Myklebust (1954) like McGinnis based his
classification and description on the work
done with adult aphasia. He says:

> While the nature of aphasia in children is different
> from that which is sustained in adulthood, there is essen-
> tially no difference from the point of view of definition and
> classification. Aphasia is a language disorder which re-
> sults from damage to the brain. Aphasia literally means
> lack of speech but this definition is inadequate because
> aphasia is not basically a speech disorder. It is a disorder
> in symbolic functioning. It is an inability to comprehend
> the spoken language of others, an inability to speak, or an
> inability to use language internally for purposes of think-
> ing to oneself.[*]

Myklebust's (1954) classification of childhood aphasias falls into four groups, and he

---

[*]From Myklebust, H.R., *Auditory Disorders in Children:
A Manual for Differential Diagnosis*. New York: Grune &
Stratton, Inc., 144 (1954).

credits Weisenberg and McBride (1935) and Goldstein (1948) for giving rise to the typologies and the inferred neuroanatomic bases for the language disorder. His four categories are (1) predominantly expressive aphasia, (2) predominantly receptive aphasia, (3) mixed receptive-expressive aphasia, and (4) central aphasia.

☐ **How does Myklebust (1954) describe these four types of childhood aphasias? How much information is provided about the specific language characteristics? Does he present evidence for verified lesions of the central nervous system?**

Myklebust's (1955) approach to working with aphasic children stressed experience-based learning in a parallel movement to that in deaf education known as the "natural language" approach (Groht, 1958). Representational play formed the basis of much of his naturalistic language teaching. He was influenced by Piaget's (1926) work in child development and his own understanding of the role of auditory functioning in the development of language. Central to his approach was the early development of "inner language" considered as the child's awareness of happenings and meaning of experiences.

Myklebust is therefore credited with providing indirect information about child language disorders through his interest in auditory disorders in children. Although he provided information about classification, description, and treatment of aphasic children, his greatest impact on the early growth of the area of child language disorders was his emphasis on differential diagnosis based on etiologic typologies.

Muriel E. Morley

Muriel E. Morley may well be remembered as a "woman for all seasons" in the profession of speech-language pathology. Although she is credited with bringing an early and important influence to the study of child language disorders, her total work far surpasses the confines of that subject matter.

The first edition of her major work, *The Development and Disorders of Speech in Childhood,* was published in 1957, revised for the second edition in 1967, and updated for the third edition in 1972. What she has accomplished and where we feel she has been most influential is stated in the preface to her third edition.

This book was first written to place on record (a) the results of an investigation into the development of speech in a community, with comparisons between those whose speech development was considered to be within normal limits, and those who had some failure of speech development; (b) clinical information based on observation during treatment, reactions to treatment, results of treatment, and a follow-up over a number of years in order to gain greater understanding of varying types of speech disorders and their prognosis . . . (c) as the results of these investigations over a period of ten years a simple, tentative classification of speech disorders in childhood emerged and was described, with suggestions for diagnosis and the possibilities of prognosis.*

In her classification of speech disorders in childhood Morley's (1957) first category was disorders of language that she subclassified into (1) aphasia of two types, mainly receptive and mainly executive; (2) alexia; (3) agraphia; and (4) delayed development of speech associated with (a) general mental retardation, (b) mental illness, and (c) hearing deficiency. Her second category, disorders of articulation, included a subcategory termed *articulatory apraxia.*

Morley's (1957, 1967, 1972) contribution to the study of child language disorders has been extensive. Her books are filled with charts, tables, and diagrams reporting the volume

---

*From Morley, M.E., *The Development and Disorders of Speech in Childhood.* (3rd ed.) Edinburgh: Churchill Livingstone, viii (1972).

nous data she has collected. She has presented detailed historical and behavioral descriptions of children with language disorders, and she provided one of the earliest and most detailed descriptions of articulatory apraxia including its differential diagnosis from isolated developmental dysarthria and dyslalia. Her work covers definitions, classifications, and differential diagnosis for language disordered children. Unlike her American contemporaries, Muriel Morley provided for her day specific details of the language characteristics of the children she described. She did not allow her inferences to stray far from the well-recorded observations that formed her data base.

• • •

The 1940s and 1950s were dominated by these three important individuals who to a very large measure devoted their professional lives to providing extensive descriptions and developing remedial techniques for children with language disorders. Contributions common to all included their insistence that subtypes of language disordered children existed; that these language disordered children could be distinguished from other developmental problems such as deafness and mental retardation; that etiology was an important variable for understanding disordered language in children; and that special teaching approaches were required if these children were to learn language. Although each worked separately and their approaches differed radically, their joint efforts established child language disorders as a specialized field of study.

What contributions to the study of child language disorders were made by other major speech pathologists writing at about the same time? *(See Backus and Beasley, 1951; Berry and Eisenson, 1956; Van Riper, 1954; West, Kennedy and Carr, 1947.)*

ERA OF ETIOLOGIC TYPOLOGIES AND DIFFERENTIAL DIAGNOSIS

The work of the "Three M's" set the stage for the entrenchment of etiologic typologies for classification, diagnosis, and treatment of language disordered children in the 1950s and 1960s. Following Myklebust's (1954) lead, the etiologic categories used included some form of (1) deafness and hearing impairment, (2) emotional disturbance and autism, (3) mental retardation, (4) childhood aphasia and apraxia (neurologically based language disorders). Reflecting societal concerns in the early 1960s, a fifth category entered into the system, (5) cultural or social deprivation (Adler, 1964; Wood, 1964).

The tenor of the times led to an either-or approach to differential diagnosis where the primary concern was to identify the child's more global problem: was he deaf, was he aphasic, was he emotionally disturbed, was he mentally retarded? In this process of differential diagnosis the emphasis was more toward gathering information about related aspects of development (physical, emotional, social, adaptive, and intellectual) and less toward obtaining specific information about the child's language development. It appeared as if the workers of the time expected each diagnostic category to present rather homogeneous speech and language behavior representative of the etiologic typology. Table 2-1 from Myklebust (1954) exemplifies the areas of observation and summary expectations for his four etiologic categories.

Numerous writers of this era generally reflected and furthered this etiologic trend. For example, Adler (1964) in *The Non-Verbal Child* differentially diagnosed children into the categories of brain damage, mental subnormality, emotional illness, and deafness. He did so through examination and comparisons of vocalization, gestures, response to

Table 2-1. *The characteristic performance of each type on the areas evaluated in making*

Type of disorder	History	Behavioral symptomatology
Peripheral deafness	Indicates alertness in general and often consistent response to loud sounds. Not bizarre or seriously retarded genetically.	Not bizarre. Compensatory use of other sensory avenues. Integrated and use environmental clues well.
Aphasia	Indicates some retardation in development. Confusion regarding hearing. Lack of shyness but not bizarre.	Disinhibited, hyperactive and forced responsiveness. Not use other sensory avenues in compensatory way.
Psychic deafness	Began using speech, then stopped. Many anxieties. Willfulness in rejection of environment. Withdrawn and in world of their own.	Bizarre, no compensatory use of senses. Not relate to people. Poor social perception. No projective use of hearing or voice and no gesture.
Mental deficiency	Retardation in all development is most characteristic in history.	Responsive but in low genetic and concrete manner. Not bizarre.

From Myklebust, H.R., *Auditory Disorders in Children: A Manual for Differential Diagnosis.* New York: Grune *a differential diagnosis*

	Test findings				
Auditory responses	**Mental capacity**	**Social maturity**	**Motor capacity**	**Language functioning**	**Emotional adjustment**
Consistent and integrated. Good listening behavior. Use hearing projectively. Give scanning responses.	Cluster around average level. Little scatter. Integrated and consistent in performance on tests.	Good except for communication area. Average social quotient of approximately 90.	Good but balance may be disturbed. No generalized incoordination or retardation.	Good inner language. Good gesture. Use voice projectively. Behave symbolically.	Good responsiveness to people through vision. Social perception and contact with environment is good.
Inconsistent, erratic, cannot listen. Disturbed in auditory perception. Not use hearing projectively.	Inconsistent and much scatter. Perceptual disturbances improve with structuring.	Retarded in all areas but especially in communication, socialization, and motor areas. Average social quotient of approximately 75.	Slightly delayed in sitting and walking. Generalized incoordination.	Poor inner language. Little or no use of gesture. Not use voice projectively. May unexpectedly use a word. May be echolalic.	Emotional expression lacks intensity. Try to relate to people. Are not oblivious or bizarre.
Seem to willfully reject sound, give indirect responses. No projective use of hearing. Not disturbed in auditory perception. May show fear of sound.	Not perceptually disturbed. May do well on formboards. Reject the test situation in total or in part. Behavior suggests good mental ability.	Deficient in all areas but notably in socialization. Average social quotient of approximately 80.	Stereotyped activity. Rigidity and random movements. Only slight retardation in sitting and walking.	Good inner language but used only for phantasy. No use of gesture and do not use voice projectively. May be mute.	Withdrawn in own world. Lacking in relationship to people. Stereotyped and bizarre.
Respond directly or indirectly to tests which are suitable genetically. Use hearing projectively.	Marked retardation in general.	Marked generalized retardation in all areas. Average social quotient of approximately 55.	Generalized retardation with incoordination. Marked delay in sitting and walking.	Language is deficient but not seriously discrepant with mental age. Retarded in all phases of language development.	Passive, phlegmatic, infantile and deficient in animation.

Stratton, Inc., 352-353 (1954). Reprinted by permission of Grune & Stratton, Inc., and the author.

sound, sensitivity to visual and tactile clues, motor behavior, and formal intelligence tests.

Similarly but with minor modification, Wood (1964) discussed language characteristics and therapy for children whose language disorders are associated with central nervous system impairment (including aphasia, dysarthria, and apraxia), mental retardation, emotional disturbance, hearing loss, speech deprivation, and immaturity. Still in a somewhat different manner, McGrady (1968) discussed four causes that result in learning-language disorders: sensory deprivation yields hearing and visual impairments; experience deprivation results in cultural deprivation and lack of opportunity; emotional disorganization results in psychosis, neurosis, and personality disorders; and neurologic dysfunction leaves mental retardation and specific learning disability.

□ Compare Adler's (1964), McGrady's (1968), and Wood's (1964) etiologic categories for child language disorders. What similarities and differences exist? How does Adler's (1964) chart on pages 73 and 74 compare to that of Myklebust (1954)?

An etiologic typologies approach to language disordered children was not confined to the United States. A British work of this era is that of Minski and Shepperd (1970), who in an analysis of 474 noncommunicating children relate their disorders to subnormality (mental retardation), deafness, emotional disturbance, aphasia, brain damage, and psychosis. These authors' cross categorization of etiologic typologies and their recognition that many of the children's difficulties are due to a multiplicity of causes brought out a major difficulty with this approach to viewing child language disorders; namely, children in each etiologic category are not homogeneous in their language.

As the 1960s ended, several sources were voicing dissatisfaction with this approach to child language disorders (Marge and Irwin 1972):

> The common practice in the literature is to relate language disabilities to etiology so that the clinician speaks of congenital aphasia, autism, speech and language of the mentally retarded, and so forth. This practice appears to be no more than a persistent need to follow the medical model of defining disease states or types by describing the *cause* and the *sequela*. The application of this model to personal and social behaviors, such as language, has resulted in a semantic morass of confusion, in which authors have dwelled upon etiologies rather than specific characteristics of the language behavior in need of modification. The search for an etiology has been frequently unsuccessful, and if one is found, the conclusions become highly speculative . . . In view of these and other arguments, classification schemes built on etiological factors alone are not very meaningful in the management of language disabilities.[*]

After stating this position and developing it further in his discussion of language disabilities in children, it is puzzling to see that Marge and Irwin organized the remainder of the book around etiologic typologies: language disabilities of emotionally disturbed children, of hearing impaired children, of disadvantaged children, and of cognitively involved children.

Although Marge and Irwin (1972) as well as Minski and Shepperd (1970) recognized the inadequacy of an etiologic typologies approach to child language disorders, the era had not yet ended, and new trends were not sufficiently strong to break with tradition. However, they did introduce what would become a growing disenchantment with etiologic typologies.

A major unfortunate outcome of the etiologic differentiation of children was that it served

---

[*]From Marge, M., The general problem of language disabilities in children. In M. Marge and J.V. Irwin (Eds.). *Principles of Childhood Language Disabilities.* Englewood Cliffs, N.J.: Prentice-Hall, Inc. 82-83 (1972).

to divide treatment domains. The mentally retarded and emotionally disturbed were typically considered to belong to the psychologist, psychiatrist, or special educator, while children with hearing impairments became the province of educators of the deaf. Aphasic and culturally deprived children with language disorders belonged to the domain of the speech-language pathologists. Children with aphasia seemed to fall to the speech-language pathologists, because remedial/curative therapy was not available from the neurologists, the primary medical professionals responsible for these children. Since culturally deprived children's language problems were seen as modifiable by appropriate environmental change and stimulation, the speech-language pathologist readily became an important member of the compensatory education team in various poverty programs, notably preschool programs such as Project Headstart.

Inability to classify language disordered children into mutually exclusive etiologic categories, recognition of the co-occurrence of many of these etiologies, and the failure to see homogeneous language patterns related to these categories were basic reasons leading to the gradual de-emphasis on the either-or differential diagnosis of child language disorders. The premise underlying the etiologic typologies approach was that causal factors differentiated among language disordered children. Although this premise continues to be accepted by many workers in the field including ourselves, the practices of the 1950s and 1960s led to a static overemphasis on etiology without regard to the children's language behavior. As more was learned about the language of disordered children, it became increasingly clear that these broad etiologic categories would no longer serve as an exclusive approach to study, classification, or remediation of child language disorders.

DAY OF LINGUISTIC AND PSYCHOLINGUISTIC DESCRIPTIONS

Two influences were fundamental in the 1960s movement toward detailed behavioral descriptions of child language disorders. The first influence emanated from the linguistic developments ushered in by Chomsky (1957, 1965) and the interest in linguistic theory was spurred by his work. This explosion in linguistic study resulted in a second area of remarkable development that would come to have a profound influence on child language disorders: the application of linguistic theory to the psychologic processes involved in man's actual use of language, an area of study that soon came to be known as psycholinguistics.

The previous period's overemphasis on etiologic categorization typically was at the expense of specific detailed description of actual language behavior. With these new movements in linguistics and psycholinguistics leading the way, crude, impressionistic descriptions of language behavior gave way to highly detailed, precise, and powerful descriptions. Questions of what was learned in language acquisition, how language was learned and developed, what biologic and environmental factors contributed to language learning, and numerous other topics concerning man's use of language were pursued with vigor. Of the many issues studied many new findings filtered into approaches taken with language disordered children; however, probably the major impact of linguistic and psycholinguistic developments was in providing speech pathologists with a means of describing, ordering, and analyzing children's language.

Thus information in linguistics and psycholinguistics was quickly utilized by speech-language pathologists in their study of the language disordered child. As each new theory or set of data came in about normal language development, it was soon used to compare and contrast children with language disorders. The profession was eager to adopt and adapt information as it accrued. The understanding, diagnosis, assessment, and treatment of child language disorders could not wait until all the linguistic theories were worked out. Rather, as new ways of describing and understanding normal children's language were presented, these theories shaped subsequent work with the language disordered child. Normal linguistic and psycholinguistic data had and continues to have a very important impact on the study of child language disorders. The "day of linguistic and psycholinguistic description" continues to be very much alive and well.

Application of this linguistic-psycholinguistic information to child language disorders joined the literature of the mid 1960s and was eventually to address the phonologic (sound system), syntactic (grammar), semantic (meaning), and finally the pragmatic (functions and modifications of language in context) parameters of language. New methods and tools for the understanding, description, and treatment of disordered language were developed. Developmental information provided a systematic, logical, and normative guide for comparison and remediation. No longer were speech-language pathologists merely providing intuitive naturalistic experiences for the children they served, nor were they taking them through the steps of the association method. Now they were drawing and extrapolating from the normal literature and giving "method to the madness" of therapy with language disordered children.

Syntactic descriptions

Following Chomsky's lead in syntactic theory (1957, 1965), the earliest application of modern linguistic theory was to syntactic disorders. The syntactic level of language, also called grammar and sentence structure, concerned the study of word order, functional words, and inflectional endings. We learned that knowledge of word order allows the child to differentiate between the subject and object of "Marie kicked Tabby" and "The policeman was shot by the thief." As a part of syntactic learning, we became aware that children also develop use of the "little parts of speech" which develop meaning as a function of the sentence structure in which they are used. Thus "for-of," and "a-an-the" are distinctions that must be made as a part of syntactic learning. Also recognized as part of syntax were inflectional endings: markers used to indicate differences in verb number and tense (eat-eats, look-looked); pronoun number, person, and case (he-his-him, they-he); noun number, possession, and derivations (dog, dogs, dog's, doghouse); adjective comparatives (good-better-best; hot-hotter-hottest); and the like.

As the formal rules for syntax as a linguistic system were being worked out, students of child language development began applying these descriptive systems to normal children in the process of developing language. A whole body of literature developed documenting the normal stages of syntactic development that served as a normative base for persons working with language disordered children.

☐ **The student of child language disorders should have command of normal syntactic development (e.g., Brown, 1973) and is referred to Dale (1976), de Villiers and de Villiers (1978), Lee (1974), and Menyuk (1969, 1977) for refreshing and updating.**

What was known about normal language development began to be applied to children with syntactic disorders in the mid 1960s. A landmark paper by Menyuk (1964) compared the grammar of normal children to those with functionally deviant language using a generative model of grammar. Menyuk not only provided a description and comparison of these children's language; she suggested that children with deviant language did not present simply an infantile pattern of syntax. As well, she spurred research into a linguistic characterization of language disorders in children. Soon after, Lee (1966) brought together the information about normal development to outline both assessment and remediation tools for the speech-language pathologist. In 1966 her original version of Developmental Sentence Types appeared, derived largely from the early work of Brown and Fraser (1964), McNeill (1965), and others (Braine, 1963; Menyuk 1964 a, c; Miller and Ervin, 1964). The Developmental Sentence Types provided both a means for comparing normal and deviant syntactic development and a logic for guiding language therapy. Within a few short years Lee and several co-workers were instrumental in extending methods of syntactic analysis. She presented the Developmental Sentence Scoring System (1971, 1974); revised the earlier form of the Developmental Sentence Types (1974); developed the Northwestern Syntax Screening Test, one of the first and most widely used diagnostic tools comparing syntactic comprehension and expression (1969, 1970); and worked out an interactive language development teaching approach directed primarily toward syntax (1975).

Following Menyuk and Lee's lead, many others attended to disordered syntax and the literature filled with syntactic descriptions of various populations of language disordered children. Of the many contributors, Leonard (1972), Tyack and Gottsleben (1975), and Trantham and Pedersen (1976) stand out as having a particular impact on clinicians working with language disordered children. Leonard (1972) addressed the fundamental issue of "What is Deviant Language?", concluding

that the frequency of usage of particular syntactic structures best differentiates normal from deviant language rather than absolute characteristics. Tyack and Gottsleben (1975) developed a method for analyzing language samples that was to be widely adopted, and Trantham and Pederson (1976) summarized normal language development, suggesting it is "The Key to Diagnosis and Therapy for Language Disordered Children."

This important period provided a methodology for describing disordered syntax, assessment procedures designed to tap various syntactic structures, and treatment programs for facilitating syntactic development in those children whose acquisition was not normal. While syntactic description continues to be a current line of investigation, the almost sole focus on syntax and syntactic disorders in the late 1960s gave way to widespread study of other aspects of language behavior in the early 1970s.

Semantic descriptions

In part the broadening of psycholinguistic horizons was motivated by a growing awareness that a single syntactic utterance, such as "mommy sock," could have multiple meanings, depending on the context in which a child says the utterance. Furthermore, exclusive concentration on the syntactic structure was seen to miss much of what the child was saying, both insights articulated by Bloom (1970). Investigation thus turned to semantic concerns in an attempt to understand what a child meant when he spoke and how children's meanings developed over time.

The study of semantics and its application to the language disordered child received major impetus from Bloom's work. This work bridged the development of semantics and syntax. From this and work by others, notably Clark (1973), Leonard (1976), and Nelson (1973), the investigation of semantic acquisition and semantic disorders in children moved out of the realm of vocabulary testing and entered into the study of semantic features embodied in the lexicon. Semantic relations were studied as well as the social and cognitive processes contributing to semantic learning.

Meaning in language became viewed as arising from words, the lexicon itself, or the relationship that exists between words. Lexical items (words) were seen to make reference to an observable referent (object, action, relationship) or a concept (faith, intelligence, yuky). While the lexicon has dictionary meanings, for an adult and particularly for children in the process of development, meaning is largely determined by individual experience and what each person abstracts from that experience (Clark, 1973; Nelson, 1973). Although considerable agreement was seen to exist for lexical words with relatively concrete referents (chair, walking), "fuzzy zones" were recognized (cup, glass), and the meaning of more abstract lexical items were found to be more subject to individual experience and connotation (e.g., marriage, honesty, expensive).

In addition to the meaning derived from lexical items, meaning derived from word relationships also received attention. Thus for example, a 2-year-old saying "Daddy shoe" could mean "Daddy's shoe," "Daddy, put on my shoe," or "Daddy has on shoes," depending on the context and intention of the child. The meaning in such statements was seen not to arise from the words alone, since the words used in these three interpretations remain the same, but rather from the relationship between the two words. In "Daddy's shoe", the shoe is possessed by Daddy, while in "Daddy, put on my shoe", Daddy is the agent of the action, and in "Daddy has on shoes", Daddy is the experiencer.

Persons such as Morehead and Morehead (1974), MacNamara (1972), Bruner (1975),

and others studied the cognitive underpinnings of semantic learning. Nelson (1973) and Clark (1973) led the study of early lexical development, and investigators such as Leonard (1976) and Brown (1973) detailed the development of semantic relations. All these studies focusing on normal children soon shaped the study and descriptions of child language disorders.

□ **To review semantic development, the reader is referred to Bloom and Lahey (1978), Clark (1973), Leonard (1976), and Nelson (1973).**

Closely following the description of the development of semantics in normal children, several investigators began describing the semantic relations in various groups of language disordered children (Freedman and Carpenter, 1976; Leonard, Bolders, and Miller, 1976). Others applied the information for normal acquisition of semantics to the remediation of semantics in language disordered children (Leonard, 1975; MacDonald, Blott, Gordon, Spiegel and Hartmann, 1974; Miller and Yoder, 1974). The findings pertinent to semantic disorders in language disordered children will be returned to and detailed in Chapter 3. This thrust toward semantic description has provided a further means of describing the language of language disordered children, although a major stumbling block to continued study has been a well-developed theory of semantic development in children. As well, increasing importance began to be placed on the functions that language serves for a child, how children's use of language varies according to the context, and how these contextual modifications change as the child matures—concerns that became known as pragmatics.

Pragmatic descriptions

The 1970s saw a coming together of work in diverse disciplines, including sociolinguistics, philosophy, psychology, and linguistics, which addressed the pragmatics of communication. The study of pragmatics concerns the intentions of the speaker during communication or the functions that language serves, as well as how one modifies language according to contextual considerations, such as the age and relationship of the listener, the formality or informality of the situation, and so forth. Investigators in child language turned to pragmatic concerns as it became increasingly apparent that children talk for a reason or intend to accomplish something through their language. Realization grew that learning the appropriateness of language to the situation or learning the social rules of communication, termed "communicative competence" by Hymes (1971), was as important to language learning as was syntactic or semantic achievements.

Piaget (1926) presented one of the earliest and probably best known approaches to categorizing communicative interaction of young children into egocentric language (repetition, monologue, and collective monologue) and socialized language (adapted information, criticism, commands, requests and threats, and questions and answers). More recently, a number of writers have studied the functions or intentions of communication (Austin, 1962; Dore, 1974; Halliday, 1973; and Searle, 1969), each providing a somewhat different perspective toward how children use their language.

Others have directed their study to a description of the modifications that children make in their language depending on various social parameters. Bates (1976 a, b) has been in the forefront of this study of the development of language within a social context. Although she has documented a number of socially based aspects of language development (for example, development of polite form, discourse elements), her study of propositions, performatives and presuppositions, and conversational postulates has had the greatest impact on the study of both normal and disordered pragmatic development. Various other writers have studied children's language modifications depending on differing listener characteristics (for example, Gallagher, 1977; Gleason, 1973; Keenan and Schieffelin, 1976; Sachs and Devin, 1976; Shatz and Gelman, 1973).

From this lead in normal pragmatic development, application is being made to the language disordered child. Such studies are currently filling convention presentations and are beginning to find their way into publications. For example, Prutting (1979) has summarized developmental stages of pragmatic acquisition while Miller (1978) has provided a protocol for systematically observing the communicative interactions of language disordered children. It is anticipated that the next few years will result in a more thorough description of the pragmatics of language disordered children, just as semantics, phonology, and syntax have received such treatment earlier.

□ **As a review of the pragmatic level of language, the reader is referred to Bates (1976 a, b), Halliday (1973), Moerk (1977), Wood (1976), and the other references cited above.**

Phonologic descriptions

Phonetic and phonemic development and disorders have long been studied in the field of speech-language pathology, forming the basis for the classification of articulation disorders. Prior to the 1970s, children with difficulty developing the sounds of their language were generally viewed as having articulation disorders. Parallel with developments in syntax, semantics, and pragmatics, the "day of linguistic-psycholinguistic description" brought new theories about the development and use of the sound system. Questions were raised about the distinctions between phonology and articulation, phonology being considered a rule-governed, abstract system of sounds, whereas articulation was the process and mechanisms through which the sound system was produced.

Phonologic theory and investigation during the past 10 to 15 years have focused on identifying the features that distinguish one sound category from another (Cairns and Williams, 1972; Chomsky and Halle, 1968; Jakobson, 1968; Smith, 1973; among others) and the phonologic rules (Oller, 1973) or phonologic processes that account for the rule-governed selection and use of sounds in connected speech (Hodson, 1980; Ingram, 1976; Shriberg and Kwiatkowski, 1980; Stampe, 1969; Weiner, 1970). Thus, speech-language pathologists began viewing the previously recognized distinctions in manner of production of different sound classes as clusters of acoustically perceivable and motorically generated features. For example, if a child did not observe distinctions between sound such as /p-b/ or /s-z/, the feature of voicing was implicated, whereas if a child used a /b/ in place of an /f/, he would be seen as not correctly observing the voice, strident, and continuant features.

Phonologic process or rule specification led to viewing children's sound omissions, substitutions, and distortions as developmentally predictable and systematic. For example, nana/banana or bella/umbrella could be characterized as weak syllable deletion, a process found in normal development; or pupu/pudding began to be termed reduplication of syllables, again a normal process in early phonologic development. Other commonly identified phonologic processes have included the following: cluster reduction (tar/star), fronting (tuti/cookie), backing (goggie/doggie), deletion of final consonant (ca/cat), and stopping (ti/see).

□ **The study of phonology and its development and use in children should be a part of the background information of a student of child language disorders.** *(See Ingram, 1976 a and b; Shriberg and Kwiatkowski, 1980; Weiner, 1970; Hodson, 1980; and Singh, 1976, for further study in this area.)*

Speech-language pathologists were quick to apply this information to phonologic and articulation disorders. Many investigators in speech-language pathology demonstrated how linguistic analyses could be applied to phonologic errors and disorders. For example, McReynolds and Engmann (1975) and McReynolds and Huston (1971) encouraged the description of misarticulations through application of distinctive feature analysis. Although many others have applied phonologic analyses to children's sound system disorders (including among the early investigators Compton, 1970; Crocker, 1969; Oller, 1973; Pollack and Rees, 1972), Ingram (1976 a, b) perhaps has been foremost in stimulating application of phonologic principles to language disordered children, a topic we will return to later. As in semantics and pragmatics, the last few years have witnessed a burgeoning of applications of phonologic theory to clinical populations. Phonologic descriptions of children with disordered systems continue to appear (Edwards, 1980b; Oller, Jensen and Lafayette, 1978), diagnostic protocols for analyzing deviant phonologic systems have recently been developed (Compton and Hutton, 1978; Hodson, 1980; Shriberg and Kwiatkowski, 1980; Weiner, 1970), and remedial approaches based on phonologic processes are beginning to be articulated (Edwards, 1980a; Hodson, 1978; Paden, 1980). Here, too, we as a field are only entering further development and application of phonologic theory and normative findings to disordered populations. This line of our heritage will continue into the years that follow.

Generally, this period of linguistic and psycholinguistic description has contributed a detailed method of analysis and description of child language disorders from the perspective of normal language acquisition. It has provided a level of understanding and logic that to this point had been almost totally lacking. This descriptive period provided a fundamental data base on which more comprehensive views of child language disorders could be based. For example, Bloom and Lahey (1978) drew together much of this work, including their own, and presented the study of child language development and disorders as form (words and the relations between words), content (meaning or semantics), and use (the functions and contexts of messages).

An unfortunate outcome of this period has been to view language disordered children as a homogeneous group without regard to etiologic considerations. Perhaps this disregard for etiology has been in some respects an over-response or backlash to some of the nonproductive practices of the preceding era of etiologic typologies. That movement falsely assumed that children categorized by primary etiologies would present similar language behavior. Rather than developing more meaningful views toward etiology, the whole etiologic approach was abandoned and energies were channeled into description of language behavior. The emphasis in describing language was on comparison to normal acquisition leading to the "delay model," that the disorder was one of degree rather than kind. Differences between children were underplayed, leading to the assumption that what held for one group of language disordered children was true of others (Freedman and Carpenter, 1976; Leonard, 1972; Leonard, Bolders and Miller, 1976; and Morehead and Ingram, 1973).

Finally, perhaps one of the most imortant contributions of this period has been to provide a model to systematically guide speech-

language pathologists in developing treatment approaches. No longer were they "intuitive language stimulators"; rather, they became well-schooled in linguistic analysis and description of normal and disordered language behavior, using this as a road map to intervention.

The "day of linguistic-psycholinguistic description" has already had a major impact and influence on the study of child language disorders, remains currently vital, and is expected to continue exerting great influence in the future. It is the backbone of assessment and treatment in child language disorders.

SEARCH FOR PROCESSING EXPLANATIONS

Attempts to understand child language disorders in terms of processing disruptions have surfaced through the history of child language disorders, with renewed interest in this enterprise emerging in the 1970s. Depending on particular points of view, concepts of processing, and the clinical populations studied, professionals have searched for neurologic, sensory, perceptual, linguistic, and cognitive processes that account for normal and disordered language. They have proposed various theories, frameworks, models, and hypotheses as explanations for the processing events underlying language behavior.

From this work, two major trends stand out in the child language disorders literature: (1) viewing child language disorders as stemming from auditory processing breakdowns and (2) tying language breakdown to higher order stages within the language processing system. These trends reflect the search for the underlying physical mechanisms that when disrupted result in faulty processing of linguistic information. These faulty processes in turn result in disordered language behavior. In short, processing explanations attempted to understand the interface among anatomy, processing, and behavior.

Auditory processing explanations

Implicit in the writing of McGinnis (1963) and Myklebust (1954), whose work grew out of their involvement with hearing impaired children, was the assumption that many child language disorders arose from auditory disorders. However, they simply noted that auditory disorders may cause language disorders but did not attempt to elaborate on the underlying auditory processing dysfunction.

Following the work of McGinnis and Myklebust, the subject of childhood aphasia became a focus of study for other professionals. These workers began to consider the underlying processing deficit responsible for the difficulties in comprehension and use of language encountered by these children. Thus, they advanced some of the first process-based distinctions among language disordered children. They began to explore and acknowledge auditory processing as having a primary role in language learning and language disorders—a theme that continued to remain central to the study of child language disorders. Exemplary of the auditory processing explanations advanced are those of Hardy (1965) and Eisenson (1968, 1972). Although Hardy made a wide range of contributions to the study and treatment of aphasic children, one of his major contributions was the specification of a series of processes involved in receiving auditory information. Hardy proposed a model of the central nervous system processes intervening between the acoustic stimuli and a psychomotor response. Although he included storage and motor output components, the receptor system received the most detailed treatment. He presented this model as a means of conceptualizing points at which the language disordered child may encounter difficulty processing auditory information.

Eisenson, long noted for his work with aphasia in adults (1954, 1957, a, b, c), carried this emphasis to even greater extremes. In his unitary concept, auditory processing disorders were seen by him to be *the* point of breakdown for childhood aphasia. He states: "With only rare exceptions, we regard the child with developmental aphasia as one with basic auditory perceptual impairments." Eisenson (1968, 1972) considered children's expressive disturbances to be a manifestation of that child's perceptual disorder, that is, to be a secondary effect of the decoding impairment. Eisenson's unitary concept of auditory processing disorders as the basis of childhood aphasia had a major influence on the broader field of child language disorders. In the 1970s, a significant focus of writing, research, and remediation for child language disorders centered on auditory processing, a topic addressed in detail in Chapter 5.

Multistage processing explanations

Unlike Eisenson (1978) and to a lesser degree Hardy, other writers in speech-language pathology took a more encompassing view of the multiple stages of processing that underlie language and language disorders in children. Their work had a broader influence since its focus was across child language disorders rather than primarily childhood aphasia. Although numerous model makers have contributed to a processing perspective in speech-language pathology, we have chosen to exemplify the trend by summarizing several approaches specifically directed to child language disorders.

Morley, in her extensive 1967 revision of *The Development of Disorders of Speech in Childhood,* became one of the early processing modelmakers. Fig. 2-1 is her diagrammatic

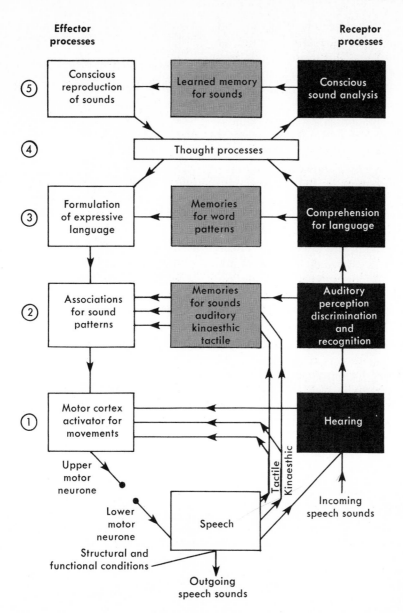

FIG. 2-1. Some processes involved in speech. *Level I:* Basic sensation and movements. *Level II:* Receptor-effector processes for articulate sounds. Basic articulation. *Level III:* Receptor-effector processes for integration of articulation with language. *Level IV:* Mental processes associated with the reception and expression of thought through spoken language. *Level V:* Conscious sound analysis and synthesis. (From Morley, M.E., *The Development and Disorders of Speech in Childhood.* [3rd ed.] London, Churchill Livingstone [1972].)

representation of the effector, receptor, and thought processes for the development of speech and language. The model also serves to indicate where breakdowns can occur in these processes that might account for various speech and language disorders. Morley viewed this presentation as a major modification of her approach to and understanding of child language disorders.

Bangs (1968), whose interest was language and learning disorders of the preacademic child, enumerated a series of "avenues of learning" relevant to the acquisition of language, including sensation, perception, memory retrieval, attention, and integration. These avenues of learning essentially formed a multistage processing orientation to child language disorders, and Bangs herself used these processing concepts in assessing and treating language disordered children.

In 1969 Berry presented one of the most comprehensive discussions of the neural and psychologic bases for language processing in children. She emphasized the continual, unitary, interdependent nature of language processing, stressing that dysfunction of one aspect of the system would affect the entire system. She viewed her approach as transactional and described it in the following way:

> In the transactional view the message undergoes constant modification and elaboration from receptor to response, in which process a vast company of neuronal assemblies "with collaterals unlimited" mediate and modify the code. The transaction begins in the peripheral receptive systems where the code first may be altered; and it continues in classical sensory-motor routes, in multisensory convergences upon polyvalent neurones of reticular, limbic, subcortical and cortical bidirectional systems, through specific and nonspecific sensory-motor and motor-sensory fields in cortex and subcortex. The transaction is completed in the response, i.e., in the act of perception, inner language or explicit expression. In the transaction, the cortex has not "abdicated," although it no longer holds exclusive rights over language learning. Its new role may be described as a merger, a coopera-

tive movement, in which its circuits participate with all sectors of the CNS. Contributing to the success of the transaction are homeostatic (controlled lability), altering or set-to-attend, feedback or fixation mechanisms.*

Although Berry continually cautioned her students to think in terms of a continuous, circular process and interaction of a whole series of neural events, she set the stage for viewing language processing as a complex series of stages where breakdowns could occur at one or multiple stages.

More recently, Wiig and Semel (1976) have also presented language disorders in children and adolescents as multistage processing problems where dysfunction may occur at numerous stages in the system. Figs. 2-2 and 2-3 present Wiig and Semel's illustrations of language comprehension and language production. They discuss in detail the processes outlined in these models and provide extensive assessment and remediation approaches aimed toward each of the processes.

Finally, Muma (1978) established a bridge between the "day of linguistic-psycholinguistic description" and the "search for processing explanations." He presented what he calls a "cognitive-linguistic-communicative systems and processes" orientation to child language disorders. Although Muma's approach is drawn largely from the literature on normal child development, he does incorporate explanatory processes for language disorders in children. His referent for processes, however, is behavioral and psychologic rather than physical and neurologic.

While Morley, Bangs, Berry, Wiig and Semel, and Muma stand out as prominent examples of speech-language pathologists who have provided multistaged processing explanations for child language disorders, nu-

---

*From Berry, M.F., *Language Disorders of Children.* New York: Appleton-Century-Crofts, 110 (1969).

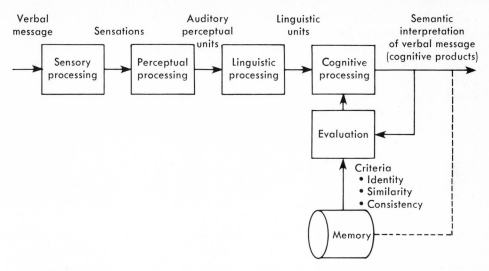

FIG. 2-2. Illustration of the relationships between sensory, perceptual, linguistic, and cognitive processing in language comprehension. (From Wiig, E.H., and Semel, E.M., *Language Disabilities in Children and Adolescents*. Columbus, Ohio: Charles E. Merrill Publishing Co. [1976].)

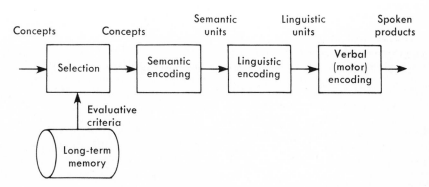

FIG. 2-3. Illustration of the relationships between cognitive, linguistic, and expressive aspects in language production. (From Wiig, E.H., and Semel, E.M., *Language Disabilities in Children and Adolescents*. Columbus, Ohio: Charles E. Merrill Publishing Co. [1976].)

merous professionals beyond the confines of child language disorders have offered processing explanations for speech, language, hearing, and communications. Psycholinguists (Clark and Clark, 1977), neurolinguists (Brown, 1977; Whitaker, 1970, 1971), and other speech-language pathologists (Mysak, 1966; Nation and Aram, 1977) have all provided perspectives toward language processing and dysfunction.

The search for processing explanations for child language disorders has been a continuous line of inquiry, and the quest goes on, armed with the knowledge and technologic capabilities available from each period of study.

SUMMARY: HISTORIC CONTRIBUTIONS TO THE PRESENT

This chapter has summarized a series of stages in the history of child language disorders. First, nascent roots were scattered but visible in neurology, other medical disciplines, and education of the deaf. These disciplines provided a source of knowledge and experience for the work of McGinnis, Myklebust, and Morley, whom we have credited with establishing the field of child language disorders. The work of these three pioneers (in particularly Myklebust), in stressing differential diagnosis of language disordered children in terms of primary etiology gave way to an era of etiologic typologies that largely resulted in the dead-end practice of pigeonholing children. Perhaps in part due to the nonproductivity of this earlier preoccupation with etiology, but certainly strongly influenced by the linguistic and psycholinguistic revolution underway, our field entered and continues in "the day of linguistic and psycholinguistic description." Paralleling these stages have been numerous attempts to provide processing explanations for child language disorders, although no particular period was dominated by such attempts.

Where have all these past practices and continuing trends led us today? In sum we see these past stages influencing our present and future study in the following ways. Our roots continue to span many disciplines as did the early influences that gave rise to this field. Understanding the complexity of child language disorders requires a multiperspective approach where ideas from diverse sources are brought together to better explain and remediate the many-faceted problems these children present. While child language disorders as a field has borrowed heavily from the social and behavioral sciences, much less effort has been given to applying information from the biologic and other physical sciences.

The founders, Myklebust, McGinnis, and Morley, established a tradition of detailing behavior as they saw it and juxtapositioning information from divergent disciplines, both traditions that are as valid today as they were in the 1940s and 1950s. The unfortunate practices evolving from differential diagnosis based on gross etiologic categories resulted in an abandonment of concern about etiology. Today we know little more about etiologies that cause children to develop disordered language than we did 50 years ago when the field was only emerging. Equally lamentable is the tendency for any flicker of concern for etiology to appear outside of rather than within our own discipline.

The developments in linguistic and psycholinguistic description during the past 15 years have brought a new level of sophistication to this field. Important contributions have accrued from the exacting attention to behavioral description of the various levels of language, the systematic assessment tools developed, and the theoretically consistent remediation approaches being developed.

Although periodic stabs at providing processing explanations have been offered in the past, none singly or collectively has exerted sufficient influence to provide a dominant thrust toward viewing child language disorders as processing disruptions. Further development of processing theories is a perspective toward child language disorders that we consider important and therefore develop in this book.

On balance, we see the current state of the art in child language disorders as providing well-developed theories or at least directions for understanding and describing language behavior. Our field, however, remains in the beginning stages of providing a comprehensive view of child language disorders that explains the processing of underlying disordered behavior and advances study of the etiologic factors responsible.

chapter 3

Many faces and facets of child language disorders

DIVERGENCE IN NEED OF CONVERGENCE

In the past two chapters the variability of children with language disorders has been introduced, and the divergent perspectives that have been applied to their study have been traced. The divergent perspectives have arisen from the professionals' studying the complexity, the many faces and facets of child language disorders. For the most part these divergent perspectives continue as contemporary lines of study. All have shaped and advanced our understanding and provide information needed for arriving at a comprehensive view of language disordered children.

To approach child language disorders from any orientation that considers these children as a homogeneous group is, in our way of thinking, an exercise in unreality. What can be said for one language disordered child may or may not hold true for another. What is needed is not simply a description of child language disorders but an appreciation for the complexity and variability inherent in this group of children.

We suggest that the study of child language disorders needs to hold on to this diversity. Yet

we need a guide for organizing, assimilating, and maintaining these divergent perspectives.

This chapter is intended to provide a framework toward child language disorders that maintains a multifaceted perspective toward the problem but provides an organizing principle around which child language disorders can be studied. This framework draws from and depends on historical and contemporary lines of study. From these divergent lines of study we aim to develop a convergence of information that allows for a more comprehensive view than is afforded by any single line of study. Currently this coalescence seems essential if we are to arrive at a view of child language disorders that represents many important types of information: the biologic mechanisms; the role and influence of factors extrinsic to the child; the relation between language and other aspects of child development; and centrally, the child's language performance.

The quest for describing, understanding, and treating child language disorders is ongoing. Therefore any approach to the study of this topic must be dynamic and have as its aim the provision of an orientation toward available information and uncharted territory. It must be an open-ended orientation that can transform its elements by adding new information, deleting information as its invalidity is demonstrated, and permutating elements as new combinations offer more consistent and powerful explanations. We intend to provide in this chapter an orientation that can guide the student of child language disorders in bringing together the divergent information he will confront. Our hope is that the orientation presented here will provide an anchor for the student's developing skill in understanding, diagnosing, and treating children with language disorders, a guide that will be useful not only today, but tomorrow, and years to come.

WORKING DEFINITION OF CHILD LANGUAGE DISORDERS
Terminologic confusion

Multiple terms and labels have been used to refer to and classify children with language disorders, many of which arose early in our history and have been maintained by tradition. In tracing our field's heritage in Chapter 2 we saw a concentration on etiologic typologies and differential diagnosis that led to one type of traditional terminology. Children were given an etiologic label under which their language problems were but one symptom. Therefore we have mentally retarded children whose language problems are prominent, children with "minimal cerebral dysfunction" whose language is one of a complex of problems, children whose major "psychoneurologic" learning disability is language, "Strauss syndrome" children, "autistic" children, and so forth, all of whom may be called something else but who also have a language disorder.

We saw that the study of child language disorders almost became synonymous with the study of childhood aphasia, incorporating such qualifying modifiers as developmental and congenital. This term continues to be used to denote a neurologic basis for language disorders. It also continues to present terminologic confusion. What Hardy said in 1965 seems true today.

It seems clear that any abstract term such as *aphasia* can mean to any of us whatever we wish it to mean. Most of us have some of the tendencies characterized by Humpty Dumpty. The meaning is a product of concept and usage, of training, of experience, and of intention. . . .

In recent years the literature has included subcategories like "basically a receptive problem with expressive aspects" or "mainly an expressive difficulty with receptive manifestations." Unfortunately this is comparable to what it must surely be like to try to play patty-cake with an octopus.*

This lack of clarity in use of terminology in child language disorders has impeded research and the development of effective remedial techniques. Which children are lumped together under the label "language disordered" may vary widely. Yet homogeneity of the group studied is often crucial in both research or in application of specific therapeutic approaches. All too frequently subject specifications are not included, a problem particularly notable in research and one explored in depth by Stephens (1979).

Apart from the terminologic confusion that stems from etiologic classification, we see confusion stemming from the use of the term language when referring to child language disorders. More often than not, modifiers accompany the term: language disordered, deficient, disabled, impaired, dysfunction, delay, retardation, and infantile language (speech).

Words such as delay, disorder, dysfunction, and infantile seem to imply an understanding of the nature of the language behavior pre-

---

*From Hardy, W.G., On language disorders in young children: A reorganization of thinking. *J. Speech Hearing Dis.,* **30,** 4-5 (1965).

sented, that is, delay suggests a slowed down rate but an expected pattern of development. Similarly, disorder or dysfunction seem to imply that language behavior is different in kind and not merely in degree. Although some discussion has been directed to the implications of the terminology used (Benton, 1964; Chappell, 1970; Hardy, 1965; West, 1962) and some fruitful research has been directed to the distinction between delayed versus deviant language (Leonard, 1972; Ludlow, 1980; Menyuk, 1964; Morehead and Ingram, 1973), these terms are frequently used with little regard for their implications for differentiating among the population of language disordered children.

Nondiscriminate and interchangeable use of these terms suggests that speech-language pathologists either cannot or do not make differentiations in terms of degree or kind of language presented by these children. This failure to use discriminating terminology may be related to the inertia of tradition, but more importantly may be attributed to an unclear knowledge base from which such distinctions are made.

This book intends to provide a framework through which distinctions in language disordered children and the terms reflecting these distinctions can be made. In Chapter 1 we introduced our working definition of child language disorders. The remainder of this chapter expands upon this definition, providing an overview of the authors' perspective.

A working definition

Our working definition as it appeared in Chapter 1 follows: *Child language disorders include children with disordered language behaviors related to language processing dysfunctions that appear as variable patterns of performance and are shaped by the developmental context in which they occur.*

This definition, which delimits our view of child language disorders, can be broken down into five principal working parts.

Working Part I: Children
Working Part II: with disordered language behaviors
Working Part III: related to language processing dysfunctions
Working Part IV: that appear as variable patterns of language performance
Working Part V: and are shaped by the developmental context in which they occur

Through amplification in the remainder of this section, these working parts will provide the vehicle for organizing the many faces and facets of the study of child language disorders; it is our attempt to bring convergence from divergence.

WORKING PART I: CHILDREN

Child language disorders is the study of children with disordered language. Although at first glance this statement seems obvious, on second thought the obvious becomes fuzzy. What defines childhood? Is it the legal 18- or 21-year designation? Or is there a developmental and biologic difference between childhood and adulthood that provides a logical basis for differentiating between child and adult language disorders?

Fortunately, a major difference exists between child and adult language disorders that may serve as a useful starting point in clarifying "children." The vast majority of children with language disorders are those whose disorder is developmental. The basis of these child language disorders is often viewed as "congenital," present presumably from birth and manifesting itself during the period of language development. Child language disorders are predominantly developmental in nature. This sharply and quite practically distinguishes most child language disorders from adult language disorders, which occur after language has been acquired. The distinguished feature here is that the child with a developmental language disorder does not acquire language normally.

☐ **At what age is primary language acquisition completed? Is there any controversy over this issue?** *(See Bloom and Lahey, 1978; Chomsky, 1969; Dale, 1976; Menyuk, 1977.)*

Although the distinction between developmental language disorders and acquired language disorders in adults is useful in clarifying the population of child language disorders, the boundaries become blurred by two major categories: (1) those children who acquired language disorders as preschoolers, as school-aged children, and as adolescents; and (2) those whose developmental language disorder continues into adulthood. Here the lines of demarcation become less clear; yet these fuzzy groups can be included within the scope of child language disorders.

The first major category, those with acquired language disorders, must be broken into two subgroups: (1) those who acquired the language disorder during the period of language acquisition and (2) those who acquired the language disorder after the primary period of language acquisition but before being old enough to be considered as adults. The first subgroup of children started on a presumed normal course of language development that was interrupted by some factor, be it an encephalitis virus, gunshot wound, or regression for unknown reasons. Thus the normal course of language development was not completed, and the child will conclude the period of language acquisition on a disordered course. In continued language learning the child straddles two processes: recovery of functions lost and learning of language never acquired.

The second subgroup of children presumably have completed the primary period of language development and then sustain damage that results in an acquired language disorder. In this way they often appear quite similar to adults with acquired language disorders. However, their age denotes that they are children and will be treated as such in therapy programs. Furthermore, the age limits of cerebral plasticity and reorganization are not fully understood. Some degree of language recovery based on cerebral plasticity may be expected, yet the age limits and completeness of recovery remain controversial points. It is, however, well established that age is important to language recovery in adult aphasia; the younger the individual the greater the chances for recovery.

The second major category, adults who continue to manifest the residuals of developmental language disorders, is difficult to include within the scope of child language disorders. In order to do so we have to close our eyes to chronologic age. We are not suggesting that they be viewed as children but that their language disorder is more closely akin to children with developmental language disorders than to adults with acquired language disorders. These adults have proceeded through language development in a non-normal manner and their language disorder as adults is characteristically different from acquired language disorders in adulthood. They are language disordered children grown up.

This category constitutes a rarely recognized or described group of individuals. A few are known to speech-language pathologists who have followed up clients over a 15- to 20-year span. From firsthand experience they know that some children never acquire normal language, despite intensive therapeutic efforts. Occasionally these adults turn up as "men of few words" who have developed the style of saying very little to prevent their inabilities from becoming obvious. At times these adults appear as the father or less frequently the mother of a language disordered child (Aram, 1979; Healy, 1980). When they describe their own history of language/learning problems, they are observed to use unelaborated syntax, have word finding problems, omit syllables, and may present a disordered sound system.

We also have been impressed by the number of young adults who seek speech-language therapy in conjunction with job training programs. Frequently these young adults have had years of therapy in the elementary grades, drifted in and out of therapy during junior and senior high school, and find when they seek jobs that their inability to express themselves intelligibly drives them back to seek therapy for their long-standing problem.

We do not feel we have resolved the issue of what children with language disorders are, but we can justify including the following four groups within the scope of this book:

1. Children with language disorders whose problem is manifest during the early stages of language development
2. Acquired language disorders in children during the period of language development
3. Acquired language disorders in children, after the primary period of language development but prior to entering adulthood as determined by chronologic age
4. Adults still manifesting the effects of developmental language disorders

WORKING PART II: WITH DISORDERED LANGUAGE BEHAVIORS

An indispensable aspect of the study of child language disorders is to make an observation of disordered language behavior. This task is easier said than done, since it assumes we have a completed normal data base from which to make these observations.

Referent for disordered language behavior

Although we can now more clearly specify many aspects of normal language behavior in children than earlier in our professional history, huge gaps continue to exist in this normative base. For example, syntactic stages of development have been studied in detail, and much descriptive information allows us to specify the normal order of development of verb phrases, yes-no questions, wh-questions, and so forth. However, much information crucial to our understanding of disordered language remains to be gathered. For instance, what range of language variance constitutes normal behavior? Frequently speech-language pathologists see 2-year-old children who have not yet begun to express meaningful speech, yet language comprehension and nonverbal communication appear to be normal. Is this "disordered language"? Clearly it is not usual or expected, but is it disordered? We all can point to neighbors' children, nieces and nephews, or clients who did not talk until after age 2, then proceeded to develop language normally and finally went on to acquire exceptional verbal and scholastic abilities. Are these 2-year-olds language disordered? We do expect that most 2-year-old children have considerable vocabularies and are using two- and three-word combinations. We cannot, however, say that all 2-year-old nonverbal children are language disordered. Some may be, but others may simply represent the lower end of a normal continuum of age of onset of language.

This example raises the delayed-deviant issue that was addressed earlier in this chapter. Should children who are delayed in the development of language but are developing according to expected patterns be considered language disordered? Or should the concept of disordered be reserved only for those children who are developing a deviant pattern of language?

With the diversity seen in child language disorders it is most likely that this population includes a range of distinctions: children who represent the lower end of the normal distribution, children who are clearly delayed but who are developing along an expected pattern, and children whose pattern of language behavior is clearly deviant for their age or stage of development.

These distinctions and probably others must serve now as referents for child language disorders since at the present time there is no set of standardized categories for language disorders in children, a point emphasized by Morehead (1975).

☐ **Literature has appeared that addresses the delay-deviant issue. What conclusions have been drawn thus far? What weaknesses are evident in the research that has been done?** *(See Leonard, 1972; Lee, 1966; Menyuk, 1964, 1978; Morehead and Ingram, 1973.)*

Another referent to be considered for determining disordered language behavior is related to expectations for language development in respect to a child's entire developmental context. This is a concern that will receive greater attention in Working Part V of our definition of child language disorders.

Since the relationship between language development and other dimensions of child development are not precise, we suggest using a floating referent for comparing a child's language behavior to other developmental areas such as mental, motor, cognitive, social, and so forth. The language behavior observed is then compared and evaluated in a broader developmental context.

In this way it will be kept in mind that the referent for disordered language is in terms of a particular child, not purely in reference to normative data for other children of the same age. Many children may fall below chronologic age expectations in language behavior and still not be considered language disordered if all other skills appear in keeping with language. For instance, mentally retarded children may or may not be language disordered, depending on the uniformity or scatter seen in various areas of development.

Our position is to view a retarded child's language as disordered if other cognitive areas are appreciably higher or more advanced than his language abilities, even if no area falls within normal limits. On the other hand, if all cognitive areas (including nonverbal or performance skills) are relatively comparable to the language deficits, that retarded child in our opinion would not present a language disorder. Here the determining criterion is the child's internal variations among skill areas, not externally validated norms against which he would be found to be retarded in every respect. There is no reason to assume that retardation and language disorders cannot occur simultaneously. On the contrary, the same etiologic agent that causes retardation may well cause a language disorder. Furthermore, the term mental retardation implies a cognitive disorder and language constitutes one important part of cognition.

☐ **What conclusions have been drawn about the language behavior of children classified as mentally retarded?** *(See Graham and Graham, 1971; Lackner, 1968; Naremore and Dever, 1975; Yoder and Miller, 1972.)*

Thus we essentially have two referents to use to observe disordered language behavior; first, an external referent based on normative information about language development, and second, a referent internal to the child and based on language behavior compared to other aspects of development. Given these referents, we can now turn to the levels of language behavior that can be disordered.

Levels of disordered language behavior

Although it resulted from a unified, indivisible process, language behavior has been subdivided for ease of description and study. Here we retain the levels of language behavior identified in our discussion of the day of linguistic and psycholinguistic description. The levels of language summarized in Chapter 2 include (1) the phonologic level, which concerns features of individual speech sounds and rules and processes involved in connecting these sounds in running speech; (2) the syntactic level, including word order, inflectional endings and functional words; (3) the semantic or meaningful level of language, including meaning of single words (the lexicon) and meaning derived from semantic relations; and (4) the pragmatic level, focusing upon the functions that language serves and the modifications induced by contextual considerations.

☐ **Not all writers cast language behavior into these parameters but use other typologies that fit their approach to language and language disorders. How do Bloom and Lahey (1978) and Muma (1978) approach categorization of language behavior?**

Although the phonologic, syntactic, semantic, and pragmatic levels of language may all constitute disordered behavior, variation is observed among language disordered children in terms of the relative deficit at each level. Some children's primary deficit may be pragmatic; they have difficulty adapting their language to the social context of the communication. Others' primary deficit might be phonologically revealed in poor performance on phoneme discrimination and phoneme selection and sequencing; whereas still others are primarily involved syntactically or semantically.

We refer the reader back to the summaries of these levels of language in Chapter 2 where references for further reading relevant to the normal acquisition of each have been included. Although each of these levels of language can be disordered in children, we will defer further consideration of the disorders seen until Chapter 6, when we will discuss disorders of language behavior in the context of processing disruptions.

WORKING PART III: RELATED TO LANGUAGE PROCESSING DYSFUNCTIONS

In Chapter 2 we addressed "the search for processing explanations" for child language disorders emphasizing two views: (1) auditory processing explanations as exemplified by Eisenson (1972) and (2) multistage processing explanations represented by Bangs (1968), Berry (1969), Morley (1957, 1965, 1972), and Wiig and Semel (1976).

Despite the multiplicity of influences that shape any aspect of behavior, ultimately behavior is a product of nervous system processes. Therefore central to our orientation to child language disorders is that language disorders in children are fundamentally related to dysfunctions of neurologic and psychologic processing. The disordered language behavior observed is the end product of more fundamental processing dysfunctions. Therefore no matter what other explanations may be offered, the speech-language pathologist must account for disordered language behavior in terms of differential functioning of processes internal to the child.

The use of models to portray the processes hypothesized to account for language has been present throughout the historical attempts toward processing explanations. Several of these models have been referred to in Chapter 2. Although the use of models allows us to organize information and schematically represent the interface between language and inferred underlying processes, models also have problems inherent in their use. First and probably foremost is that models represent abstractions of complex behavior in which detail is sacrificed and the abstractions formed are from the perspective of the model maker. Not only is "the map not the territory" but as with the two blind men examining an elephant, each may only be in contact with one part of the whole picture. Second, models are static and in themselves cannot capture the interaction among parts or the changes that evolve as new information is learned. Only the model user can impute a dynamic element into a model, which allows for interaction among parts to emerge and updating as the knowledge base changes. Third, many models exist, including those in speech-language pathology as well as other disciplines. What criteria direct the choice of one model over another? Earlier (Nation and Aram, 1977) we suggested a series of seven considerations for critical evaluation of a model's usefulness to the speech-language diagnostician. We suggest these considerations also hold for model selection in child language disorders and summarize them below:

1. For a model to be maximally useful it should focus on speech and language.
2. Since the auditory-oral modalities are basic in speech and language and the first to develop, these may justifiably serve as the primary modalities explicated in a model.
3. A diagnostically useful model should carefully describe and delineate observable speech and language behavior.
4. A model should allow for specification of the anatomy and "physiology" underlying language—the hypothesized internal language processes.
5. The diagnostic model should assist in developing the interface between the physical basis for language—anatomy and internal processing—and the observable speech and language behaviors.
6. The model should help the diagnostician understand causal factors and hypothesize cause-effect relationships.
7. A diagnostician's model should help him develop ways of measuring speech and language disorders.*

*From Nation, J.E., and Aram, D.M., *Diagnosis of Speech and Language Disorders*. St. Louis: The C.V. Mosby Co., 32-33 (1977).

With these considerations in mind, in 1977 we presented a Speech and Language Processing Model (SLPM) that offered a processing orientation (Fig. 3-1). This model was designed primarily for diagnostic purposes, illustrating how the diagnostician could relate observable behavior to underlying processing as well as how to analyze cause-effect relationships. The model was intended for use across the spectrum of speech and language disorders.

Here we will develop another model representing a processing orientation accounting for child language disorders. This model evolves out of the SLPM and is essentially an expansion of the Central Language Segment of the SLPM. The adaptations made derive from the focus here on child language disorders, on underlying language processes as opposed to physical processes, and on the need to incorporate advances made in relating language processes to language behavior.

The child language processing model (CLPM)

The Child Language Processing Model (CLPM) is a language processing/performance model that represents the language processes and behaviors the child is developing as he moves toward his adult language system. The CLPM has neurologic implications in that it could represent cerebral hemisphere processing; however, that is not its primary intent. A normal child would be expected to develop the sequential aspects of language processing in the left cerebral hemisphere, but a child with a language disorder may be presenting a different neurologic organization.

Thus, the CLPM focuses on the underlying language processes in relationship to the behaviors observed. This may be occurring in cerebral structures differently from what is expected. The model provides the speech-

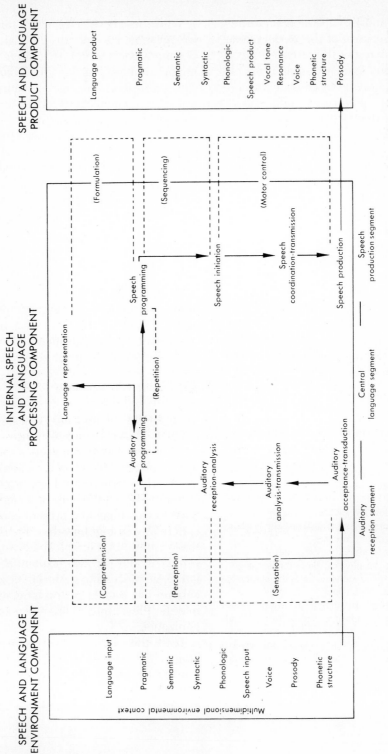

FIG. 3-1. Speech and language processing model. (From Nation, J.E., and Aram, D.M., *Diagnosis of Speech and Language Disorders.* St. Louis: The C.V. Mosby Co. [1977].)

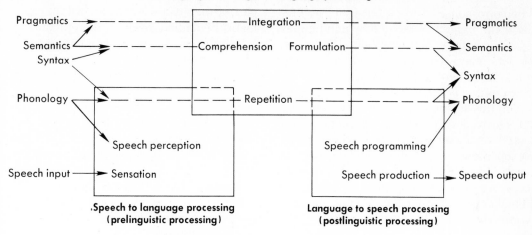

OBSERVABLE RESPONSE TO LANGUAGE   OBSERVABLE USE OF LANGUAGE (PRODUCT)

FIG. 3-2. Child language processing model.

language pathologist with a way of ordering and relating (1) language behavior, (2) language processes, and (3) underlying neurologic organization.

The schematic of the CLPM (Fig. 3-2) is composed of three units:

1. *One major processing unit* composed of three interrelated processing segments
   a. Speech to Language Processing Segment
   b. Language to Thought to Language Processing Segment
   c. Language to Speech Processing Segment

   Making up these processing segments are a series of processing stages
   a. Sensation
   b. Speech perception
   c. Language comprehension
   d. Language integration
   e. Language formulation
   f. Speech and language repetition
   g. Speech programming
   h. Speech production

2. *One observational unit* that focuses on the verbal and nonverbal responses that reveal the processing of language input
3. *One observational unit* that focuses on the verbal and nonverbal responses that reveal the processing of language output

Processing unit. The major processing unit made up of three segments is viewed as a series of continuous and overlapping transductions needed to receive, comprehend, integrate, repeat, formulate, and produce messages.

SPEECH TO LANGUAGE PROCESSING SEG-MENT. The Speech to Language Processing Segment involves prelinguistic processing of the language message before meaning is abstracted. At least two processing stages occur within this segment: (1) sensation and (2) speech perception.

Sensation here refers to the child's response to the intensity of the auditory stimulation at a range of frequencies. Sensation therefore is confined to behavioral reports of the intensity and frequency of sounds heard.

Reports of quality are not assumed by us under sensation. Any occurrence that reduces a child's response to the intensity of a stimulus or the frequency range to which he may respond interferes with sensation. Sensation disorders may arise from conductive, sensorineural, or central auditory pathology.

Speech perception as the second processing stage in this segment transduces the acoustic data received as intensity, frequency, and spectral characteristics into a speech code. Five operations are enumerated as part of speech perception and as basic to language processing since they appear to be implicated in breakdowns of language: (1) *auditory attention,* the ability to select and alert to one stimuli over another; (2) *auditory rate,* accommodating to a rapid temporal pattern of acoustic input; (3) *auditory discrimination,* sorting between speech and nonspeech signals; (4) *auditory memory,* retention of auditory information; and (5) *auditory sequencing,* holding auditory information in order of presentation. The Speech to Language Processing Segment overlaps with the next segment, the Language to Thought to Language Processing Segment. This processing overlap is necessary because of the interaction between language and speech perception in linguistic tasks. Chapter 5 examines each of these auditory operations and their disruptions in detail.

LANGUAGE TO THOUGHT TO LANGUAGE PROCESSING SEGMENT. The Language to Thought to Language Processing Segment interprets the speech code processed by the previous segment. This central language processing incorporates the structural and meaningful aspects of the message as related to the language users' past learning and experience. This segment incorporates four processing stages: (1) speech and language repetition, (2) language comprehension, (3) language integration, and (4) language formulation.

Speech and Language Repetition, placed as it is in Fig. 3-2, is the lowest and least complex of the processing stages within this segment. Repetition involves the reproduction of a heard speech and/or language stimulus. This repetition may be meaningful, in which case language comprehension, integration, and formulation are involved, or it may be nonmeaningful, in which case it is hypothesized that repetition occurs largely without reference to higher language processing stages, and that phonetic elements are merely reproduced. Repetition is a "borderline" processing stage, potentially operating as a prepostlinguistic operation, tying together speech perception and speech programming, or as a linguistic operation involving language comprehension, integration, and formulation.

Language comprehension implies that the listener has understood the words and grammar of what he has heard; that he has successfully analyzed the words and sentence structure that has made up the message. However, this processing stage does not imply that the listener has fully interpreted the message and will respond appropriately.

Language integration refers to the listener's ability to take what he has analyzed and relate that information to past experience, to information from other sensory modalities, and to other aspects of cognition. Language integration takes comprehension of the words and sentences one step farther. The listener now juxtaposes the words and sentences heard with what he knows (from experience and from his stage of cognitive development) and with what he simultaneously is seeing and feeling. He interprets the message.

For example, when a 3-year-old is asked to put the ball under the box he must understand the meaning of the words *ball* and *box* as well as the spatial relationship implied by *under.* These words need to be connected with the child's experiences from other sensory channels. Presumably the child also interprets this request in terms of past experiences with balls, boxes, and placing one object under another. The child must integrate all of these parts in his mind, possibly through visualizing these relationships, if he is to demonstrate his understanding through some motor response.

Language integration then implies that the words and sentences that have been comprehended are also interpreted in light of information from other sensory modalities, past experiences, and cognitive abilities. This processing stage is often implicated in the failure of children to perform higher level language tasks and is often seen in children with subtle language-learning deficits.

For example, one older adolescent, when asked to respond to the *Detroit Tests of Learning Aptitude* (Baker and Leland, 1967) test item, "If you stand exactly in the middle of the street, which side would be closer to you?", responded "Bagley Road." When the clinician tried a second time to explain what was being asked and encouraged him to consider any street at all, for example the ones outside the speech center, he responded, "I don't know the names of the streets around here." While this adolescent demonstrated that he knew the meaning of street, closer, and middle through picture identification and object manipulation tasks, he was unable to interpret how all these concepts fit together and could hypothetically be applied to an abstract problem. He was unable to abstract from the words and logically solve the task with which he was presented. The language integration he did demonstrate was in terms of a personal association to a street nearest his home.

In addition to providing an interpretive reference of past experience, other sensory data, and cognitive information, the language integration processing stage serves as the source of ideas to be communicated. As such, it serves as the first processing stage in output, providing the intentions and thoughts to be formulated into language.

Language formulation involves the selection and retrieval of words and the organization of these words into a logically acceptable and syntactically appropriate form. Language formulation translates the speaker's intentions and messages into language structure. Chapter 6 is devoted to further treatment of the Language to Thought to Language Segment.

THE LANGUAGE TO SPEECH PROCESSING SEGMENT. The final processing segment is primarily considered a postlinguistic sequence of processing stages. Here the language code is changed into a sequential set of motoric events. Two processing stages are included within this segment: (1) speech programming and (2) speech production.

Speech programming straddles the Language to Thought to Language and the Language to Speech Segments. Speech programming has been placed in this overlapping role in recognition that both language based and motorically based operations occur in this processing stage.

Speech programming provides a phonologic code for the syntactic and semantic message that has been formulated. In addition, it provides a transduction from this phonologic representation to the motor commands necessary for production. Speech programming therefore is an active selection, retrieval, and ordering of phonemes as well as an automatic, passive transduction of the phonemic sequences into motor commands for execution. Thus this processing stage provides the last stage of language processing and the first stage of speech output processing.

These two aspects of speech programming are interesting to view developmentally since the disorders resulting from disruption of the speech programming process in adults and children seem so dissimilar. Children acquire adult "speech programs" over time and appear to be acquiring speech programs through the continued interaction of what they know about the sound system of language and what they are learning about producing sounds.

Speech production, a postlinguistic processing stage, involves the entire set of neuromotor events required to produce the speaker's message. Here the speech response is initiated, coordinated, controlled, and actualized based on the planned sequence of serial events preprogrammed during the speech programming processing stage. These Speech to Language Processes form the topic of Chapter 7.

Observational units. The model presented here is intended to provide a representation of language processing, both when a child responds to the language of another speaker and when a child initiates language. Further, we suggest that the levels of language can be differentially attributed to the various processing stages outlined previously. While it must be reiterated that in reality language is an integrated, interactive system, different levels of language may be more closely attributed to certain processing stages than others. Therefore two observational units relate behavioral responses to these processing stages.

RESPONSES THAT REVEAL LANGUAGE INPUT PROCESSING. When listening to speech, the child primarily receives auditory information that represents language. Although he also is receiving other sensory input that will be of importance for message interpretation, it is the acoustic signal of speech that enters his ear for processing.

An observer can witness the child's responses to different levels of language that are related to the different stages of processing.

In Fig. 4-2 the language levels related to the processing stages are outlined to the left on the CLPM. We are suggesting that responses to phonologic information are primarily a result of speech perception. Syntax most centrally involves language comprehension; semantics relies on both language comprehension and integration; and pragmatic responses yield information about the language integration processing stage.

The child's responses may be verbal or nonverbal, allowing the observer to infer the intactness of various processing stages based on what he says or does. For example, if a child is prodded by his mother when she says, "What do you say when someone gives you candy?" and the child responds, "Thank you," the observer hears the child's verbal response and may infer that the child has related the current situation of receiving candy to similar past experiences. The observer infers from the child's "thank you" that *integration* of receiving candy with his mother's prodding language input has occurred. Such an observation thus tells the observer something about his *integration* but also about his responses to various levels of language input. For example, the child is shown four pictures, and one of them is of a ball. When the child is asked to touch the ball, the observer notes the child's pointing response to the processing stage of comprehension and learns that the child knows something about the semantics of the language input.

RESPONSES THAT REVEAL LANGUAGE OUTPUT PROCESSING. When a child produces speech, an observer can view that speech output in terms of the levels of language used. We are suggesting that phonologic output is primarily the result of speech programming, syntactic output derives from language formulation, and semantic output results from both language formulation and integration.

Pragmatic output is an expression of the processing stage of language integration. Here too the child's response may be either verbal or nonverbal. Verbal responses, along with contextual information, allow relatively direct observations of the four levels of language, which then can be tied to their respective stages in output processing. Nonverbal responses also permit observation of at least the higher levels of language output and stages of language processing. For example, a nonverbal child who excitedly makes his hand soar through the air like an airplane and pulls at his mother's arm demonstrates through his nonverbal behavior that he has formulated a response, even though that response has not been processed through speech programming or speech production. The child has pantomimed a pragmatic and semantic message although not verbally.

Providing a means whereby we can observe both the child's response to language as well as his use of language (language input versus language output) holds important implications for the study of child language disorders. It suggests, or at least leaves open, the possibility that a common unitary process does not necessarily underlie language comprehension and formulation. Thus a child's response to syntax may be quite different from his use of syntax. For example, Aram (1979) described a group of eight children with developmental verbal apraxia who had no difficulty with syntactic comprehension while all demonstrated marked disorders of syntactic formulation. Similarly a child's response to phonology may be different from his use of phonology, or semantic comprehension and formulation may not be parallel. The later is seen to occur in children who have anomic or word finding problems when they search for words for expression but who present no difficulty when more passive comprehension tasks are required. Therefore description of children's language must be done both in terms of their response to language as well as in terms of their use of language, because differences may exist.

WORKING PART IV: THAT APPEAR AS VARIABLE PATTERNS OF LANGUAGE PERFORMANCE

Language processing in language disordered children may be disrupted at multiple stages resulting in varying degrees of difficulty in responding to or using language. The patterns of language performance among them will differ. As every speech-language pathologist working with children can attest, the children they treat will range from those not being able to comprehend, repeat, or formulate language to those having relatively circumscribed disorders, possibly even limited to a single level of language behavior.

In our historical review we saw that those who viewed child language disorders from a processing perspective repeatedly reported contrasting language performance dependent on the point of breakdown in language processing and provided descriptions of these divergent patterns (McGinnis, 1963; Morley, 1957, 1967, 1972; Myklebust, 1954).

These writers provided rather detailed information about the aphasic child, describing patterns of differential behavior primarily through describing children as receptive or expressive aphasics. Myklebust (1954) added descriptions for the "mixed" and "central" aphasias. Morley (1957, 1967, 1972) provided more inclusive groups of language disordered children and described patterns of language performance in "apraxic, dyslalic, and dysarthric" children as well as the "receptive and executive" aphasias.

□ **Return to Chapter 2 to study these three authors, and using their books chart the patterns of language performance in the children they studied.**

After the early descriptions of McGinnis, Myklebust, and Morley, surprisingly little attention was given to identifying contrasting patterns of language performance based on a language processing–behavior analysis. More attention was focused on providing detailed linguistic descriptions of the levels of language behavior. Studies tended to treat language disordered children as a homogeneous group. Linguistic analysis often seemed to be a tool aimed at describing general properties of disordered language levels rather than capturing the differences between disordered children. While speech-language pathologists gained precision in their description of language disorders, differences among children were obscured. However, terminologic issues revolving around whether or not these children's language was delayed or disordered evidenced that differing patterns of language performance were being considered by investigators of child language disorders.

Aram (1972), recognizing that differences existed among language disordered children in their language performance, undertook a study to identify recurrent patterns of language performance and processing deficits in an etiologically heterogeneous group of children. Because the findings are central to this part of our working definition, the study will be treated in some detail here.

Forty-seven preschool children between the ages of 3 and 7 years old served as subjects for this study. All children were receiving therapy for language disorders, had normal hearing, and had not yet been in a formal school program. Fourteen language tasks were chosen to measure nine language dimensions: three processes (comprehension, formulation, and repetition) and three language levels (semantic, syntactic, and phonologic). The language tasks chosen are summarized in Table 3-1.

The measures chosen for semantic comprehension were restricted to lexical comprehension and included the Peabody Picture Vocabulary Test (PPVT) (Dunn, 1965) and the vocabulary portion of the Assessment of Children's Language Comprehension (Foster, Giddan and Stark, 1973). The two to four elements portion of the Assessment of Children's Language Comprehension and the receptive portion of the Northwestern Syntax Screening Test (Lee, 1969) served as measures of syntactic comprehension. Phonologic comprehension, in actuality a phonemic discrimination task, used two administrations of Templin's Picture Sound Discrimination Test (1957), the second presentation modifying the standard administration and the first naming the two pictures prior to asking the child to select the designated phonemic contrast.

An attempt was made to select formulation tasks that would closely parallel the comprehension tasks. Therefore an expressive adaptation of the PPVT was chosen, the Vocabulary Usage Test (Nation, 1972), and the vocabulary portion of the Assessment of Children's Language Comprehension was also modified requiring the children to name rather than identify by pointing to the items. Again only lexical formulation was tapped through these measures. Syntactic formulation tasks included again an expressive adaptation of the two to four elements of the Assessment of Children's Language Comprehension as well as the expressive portion of the Northwestern Syntax Screening Test (Lee, 1969). The phonologic formulation measure required children to name the pictures included in Templin's Picture Sound Discrimination Test. Repetition tasks were confined to repetition of the Northwestern Syntax Screening Test's expressive items and repetition of 19 phonemes, each followed by

TABLE 3-1. *Language tasks used as measures of language dimensions*

Comprehension	Formulation	Repetition
Semantic		
Peabody Picture Vocabulary Test	Vocabulary Usage Test	Peabody Picture Vocabulary Test: Adapted repetition
Assessment of Children's Language Comprehension: Vocabulary	Assessment of Children's Language Comprehension: Adapted vocabulary	
Syntactic		
Assessment of Children's Language Comprehension: Elements	Assessment of Children's Language Comprehension: Adapted elements	
Northwestern Syntax Screening Test: Receptive	Northwestern Syntax Screening Test: Expressive	Northwestern Syntax Screening Test: Adapted repetition
Phonologic		
Picture Sound Discrimination 1 Picture Sound Discrimination 2	Adapted phonologic formulation	Adapted phonologic repetition

ʌ/ (for example, /pʌ/). These six patterns, isolated through factorial analysis, were described as (1) nonspecific formulation-repetition deficit, (2) generalized low performance, (3) repetition strength, (4) comprehension deficit, (5) specific formulation-repetition deficit, and (6) phonologic deficit (Aram, 1972; Aram and Nation, 1975).

Nonspecific formulation-repetition deficit

Probably the most common pattern of language disorder seen is what we have called the Nonspecific Formulation-Repetition Deficit. Children who may be characterized by this pattern of language performance have their greatest difficulty in language formulation and repetition tasks but also show some limitations across all language tasks. These children may be considered to have a generalized language disorder. That is, there are no great strengths in any area but they are particularly weak in formulation and repetition. Thus these children had only mild deficits on the comprehension tasks but moderate to severe disorders on all formulation, and repetition tasks. This group appeared to have a breakdown in output processes superimposed upon a more generalized processing inefficiency. Our research (Aram and Nation, 1975) is not the only work that suggests that these children are the most numerous of language disordered children. The work of other writers (Wulbert, Inglis, Kriegsmann, and Mills, 1975) supports our findings.

Generalized low performance

Generalized low performance across all language tasks is a second, frequent pattern of language disorders presented by young children. Nonverbal skills of these children may range from well above normal to significantly retarded, with language performance at a uniformly lower level than nonverbal performance. We tend to see this pattern break into two subgroups. The first subgroup is made up of very young children. Our experience has suggested that often young children present generalized language deficits across all language processes. Not only can they not talk or formulate language; they also have difficulty repeating and do poorly on tests of language comprehension. Thus the first subgroup of children presenting generalized low performance on all language tasks is the young (3 years old or under) language disordered child.

The second subgroup of children presenting generalized low performance are children with more global retardation but whose language performance is lower than other aspects of development as measured by nonverbal intelligence tests. Significantly retarded children (that is, children functioning on the TMR level) often present difficulties with all aspects of language comprehension, formulation, and repetition that fall well below nonverbal skills.

Repetition strength

Other less common patterns of language performance are seen in smaller numbers of other children. Probably one of the most notable in terms of the attention paid by researchers and writers, although not a highly frequent pattern, is children presenting an unusually developed repetition strength. This remarkable ability to repeat stimuli at a more advanced level than apparent on either comprehension or formulation tasks has been described by numerous writers, including ourselves (Aram and Nation, 1975; Fay, 1966, 1967 a, b, 1973; Fay and Butler, 1968; and Fay and Coleman, 1977). For example, one child was not able to successfully complete any of the syntactic comprehension or formulation tasks. However, the child was able to repeat all 40 of the stimulus items on the expressive portion of the Northwestern Syntax Screening Test (Lee, 1969), although he was not able to relate these repetitions to the pictures they depicted.

Comprehension deficit

Another infrequent but intriguing group of children present comprehension deficits, but their formulation (when self-initiated) and their repetition skills appear amazingly intact. A number of hypotheses have been advanced to explain this apparent discrepancy between comprehension and formulation, running counter to the traditional language acquisition dictum that comprehension precedes production (Fraser, Bellugi, and Brown, 1963). Suggestions have been made that the higher performance on formulation and repetition tasks than on comprehension tasks may be explained by extralanguage factors. Aram and Nation (1975) offered the following interpretation:

First, the comprehension tasks required less active involvement of the children. Reduced motivation and attention, as well as intervening internal stimuli, may have interfered with performance on the comprehension tasks. The formulation and repetition tasks required a verbal response before proceeding to the next item and thus may have been more actively involving of some children. Another explanation for this language pattern may have to do with the nature of the tests themselves. Comprehension tests generally require higher level performance than do formulation tests for children of a given age, since children's comprehension of language is typically expected to be at a somewhat higher level than their formulation. However, it is possible that some children, . . . formulate language essentially simultaneously with their ability to comprehend language, so that comprehension and formulation are at a relatively equal level. It is therefore possible that these children's seemingly lower level of comprehension may only be a function of the expected normal discrepancy between comprehension and formulation tests.[*]

Besides the explanations we have offered for this unusual performance pattern, other writers addressing normal language acquisitions are questioning the traditional view of

---

[*]From Aram, D.M., and Nation, J.E., Patterns of language behavior in children with developmental language disorders. *Journal of Speech and Hearing Research* **18,** 240 (1975).

comprehension preceding production (Bloom, 1974; Chapman, 1974; Ingram, 1974).

Specific formulation-repetition deficit

A further, infrequently encountered pattern of language performance presented by language disordered children is that of a very specific problem with language formulation and repetition with relatively intact language comprehension. This has been referred to by the early writers in child language disorders as "expressive aphasia" (McGinnis, 1963; Morley, 1957, 1965, 1972; Myklebust, 1954). Just as the observant parent reports and the skeptical speech-language pathologist finds, these children really do understand "about everything" in contrast to their marked deficits in formulation and repetition. Although this specific formulation-repetition deficit is quite uncommon, probably representing no more than 5% to 10% of the entire population of language disordered children, such children have been described quite convincingly by Myklebust (1954) and Aram and Nasson (1979).

Phonologic deficit

The final pattern of disordered language presented by our group of language disordered children was a phonologic deficit that cut across comprehension, formulation, and repetition. While other levels of language were intact (little difficulty experienced with semantics or syntax), these children had difficulty on phonemic discrimination tasks as well as on phonologic use, either in spontaneous formulation or repetition tasks. Unlike the other patterns that generally demonstrated interference with a process affecting multiple levels of language, these children seemed to have a deficit confined to a specific level of language, probably related to a rather discrete processing stage.

In summary, our study demonstrated that the comprehension, formulation, and repetition language processes may vary independently or together. For example, although a child or group of children may be exceptionally good in comprehension, another child or group of children may have comprehension as their lowest area. Or repetition may be the outstanding ability in some disordered children, while for others this is one of the areas of low performance. Also, these language processing deficits will be seen differentially in the levels of language behavior affected.

In the last few years we have seen several additional attempts to identify subgroups of language disordered children in reference to their language performance. For example, Rapin and Allen (working paper) identified four groups of language disordered children using a mix of language and etiologic characteristics. These groups included (1) a group in which an expressive disorder appeared to predominate, which included three subgroups: (a) phonologic-syntactic syndrome with or without oromotor apraxia, (b) severe expressive syndrome with good comprehension, and (c) a syntactic-pragmatic syndrome; (2) a group they diagnosed as presenting verbal auditory agnosia that they characterized as an early stage linguistic processing deficit that interferes with phonetic decoding and thus precludes comprehension and verbal expression, although visually presented language is completely or partially preserved; (3) an autistic group, associated with profound deficits in affect and cognition, subdivided into one subgroup with mutism and a second subgroup with echolalia; and (4) a group with a semantic-pragmatic deficit without the severe affective deficits seen in autism but characterized by echolalia, deficits in semantic abilities, and inappropriate use of language in certain contexts.

A further attempt to identify subgroups of language performance in language disordered children was reported by Wolfus, Moscovitch and Kinsbourne (1980). Through a discriminant analysis, these investigators identified two groups: (1) an expressive group primarily characterized by deficits in the production of syntax and phonology and (2) an expressive-receptive group with deficits in phonologic discrimination, digit span, and semantic ability coupled with global syntactic deficits.

The growing number of studies demonstrate that children with language disorders present variable patterns of performance and must be viewed on this basis. Language performance must be considered an interrelationship between language processing and language behavior. The different frameworks and measurements in the above studies make it difficult to enumerate patterns common to all. We hope that patterns recurring across different populations and measures will become apparent through further research into this area.

WORKING PART V: AND ARE SHAPED BY THE DEVELOPMENTAL CONTEXT IN WHICH THEY OCCUR

Quite often the many developmental problems a given child may be experiencing are seen to stem from his language/communication disorder. Parents often lament: "If only my child talked better, everything would be all right." "Harold can't play with other kids because he can't talk." "We can't toilet train Todd because he doesn't understand what we tell him." "Troy can't go to kindergarten because the teacher can't understand him." Thus, talking is frequently viewed as the reason for the child's other problems as well as the key to their removal.

Although there may be instances where a language disorder appears to be isolated from the remainder of a child's development, the fact is that language does not develop and language disorders do not occur in isolation from other aspects of a child's development. Child language disorders must be viewed within a developmental context where language is seen as an early, fundamental relationship with other cognitive functions. Language disorders may reveal cognitive problems that are pointing the way to later potential learning problems.

In addition, child language disorders occur within a context of multiple extrinsic environmental circumstances and experiences that uniquely shape the course of development over time. Children also bring to language learning a set of individual intrinsic emotional and physical conditions that may aid or complicate learning language.

These three contextual aspects of child language disorders (cognitive development, extrinsic experiences, intrinsic conditions) must be viewed over time, within a longitudinal perspective. Often language disorders in children extend beyond language and beyond childhood.

Language development: a window to cognitive growth and failure

A major accomplishment of most children during their preschool years is developing an effective, highly elaborated language system. Although they also achieve other cognitive and motor skills during this period, development of language provides a fantastic avenue of interaction, understanding, and expression. Language learning is a pivotal accomplishment, both as a channel to demonstrate more general cognitive development and as a fundamental skill underlying much future learning, particularly during the school-aged years. Language development is a window to cognitive growth and failure, and the student of child language disorders must appreciate the relationship between language and cognition in order to appropriately identify and effectively remediate these disorders. Students of child language disorders need to develop a perspective toward the relationship between language and cognition. When language is disordered, what is the disorder—cognitive, language, or a combination?

Language and cognition. The relationship between language and cognition has been treated from numerous perspectives. Many writers, notably those of a Piagetian orientation, see language as an expression of more general cognitive development (Sinclair, 1969, 1971; Clark, 1973). Others have viewed language as uniquely distinct from other aspects of cognition (McNeill, 1970). Still others suggest that considerable overlap exists between language and other cognitive functions, but that cognitive development is not sufficient to explain language development (Bloom, 1974; Brown, 1973; Cromer, 1976; Slobin, 1978). This latter orientation has come to be known as the weak cognitive view of language. That is, although by and large cognitive development determines language, there are specific linguistic aspects to language development that are not reflected in more general cognitive development.

☐ **For a comprehensive review of the relationship between language and cognitive development, the student is referred to the references in this section and the chapters by Bowerman; Clark; Morehead and Morehead; Schlesinger; and Staats in Schiefelbusch and Lloyd (1974).**

Although we consider language to develop from more general cognitive roots, we do not see language as merely an expression of the symbolic function. Therefore we are aligned closely in viewpoint to Cromer's (1974 a and b; 1976) "weak form of the cognitive hypothesis" which he summarized as:

It [the weak form of the cognitive hypothesis] asserts essentially that although the study of cognitive structures and operations and the cognitions to which they give rise are of central importance in understanding the language acquisition process, these cognitive entities by themselves are not sufficient to *explain* that process. Our abilities 'make available,' so to speak, certain meanings to be encoded, but we must also possess certain specifically linguistic capabilities in order to express these meanings in language . . .

It may also be that the mechanisms and strategies of learning are different for language acquisition from those used for other types of cognitive attainments.[*]

Thus while children may have language delays and disorders as an expression of more general cognitive limitations, language can be impaired in relative isolation from other cognitive abilities. Cromer (1974, b) expresses this point:

While cognitive operations of particular types can be shown to be a necessary prerequisite for the acquisition of language in general or for the acquisition of particular grammatical features, there may be something more specifically linguistic which is also necessary for language acquisition to occur. In other words, the possession of a sensorimotor intelligence cannot in itself explain the *expression* of that intelligence in language. When examining some of the impaired processes found in different types of subnormality, it will be of interest to keep this in mind. Some groups may suffer from an impairment of one type of cognitive process or another while other groups of subnormals may lack language altogether because of more specific linguistic handicaps.[†]

☐ **Slobin (1978) has reported an interesting study that addresses the relationship between cognition and language in children whose native languages were Serbo-Croatian and Hungarian. What language-cognition position does his study support?**

---

[*]From Cromer, R.F., The cognitive hypothesis of language acquisition and its implications for child language deficiency. In D. Morehead and A. Morehead (Eds.), *Normal and Deficient Child Language*. Baltimore: University Park Press, 326 (1976).

[†]From Cromer, R.F., Receptive language in the mentally retarded: Processes and diagnostic distinctions. In R.L. Schiefelbusch and L.L. Lloyd (Eds.), *Language Perspectives-Acquisition, Retardation, and Intervention*. Baltimore: University Park Press, 248 (1974 b).

Yet, since language development is related to more general cognitive development, deficiencies in the latter will be reflected in the former, thereby stressing the importance of evaluating a child's language in reference to other measures of cognitive attainment. Through such a comparison, the aim would be to identify specific language disorders versus language disorders merely reflective of overall cognitive retardation.

Attention also has turned to evaluating the language disordered child's stage of cognitive development, often through various Piagetian tasks (Swope and Liebergott, 1977; Uzgiris and Hunt, 1975) in an attempt to identify and develop cognitive prerequisites for language.

Although the dependence of language on cognitive development is particularly notable in very young and/or low functioning children, this close relationship between language and cognition again becomes striking in language/learning impaired adolescents. In these adolescents the subtle language problems in tasks such as verbal analogies and understanding verbal absurdities often seem to reflect more general cognitive limitations such as more general deficits in logical relations and seriation in time and space (Wiig and Semel, 1976).

Language development: fundamental for later learning. In the previous section language was viewed as resting upon other more general lines of cognitive development. In this section the dependent relationship is reversed, viewing language as fundamental for academic learning. This fundamental position accorded to language in defining the learning disabled child is reflected in the definition used by the National Advisory Committee on Handicapped Children:

> Children with special learning disabilities exhibit a disorder in one or more of the basic psychological processes involved in understanding or in using spoken or written languages. These may be manifest in disorders of listening, thinking, talking, reading, writing, spelling or arithmetic. They include conditions which have been referred to as perceptual handicaps, brain injury, minimal brain dysfunction, dyslexia, developmental aphasia, etc. They do not include learning problems which are due primarily to visual, hearing, or motor handicaps, to mental retardation or to environmental disadvantage.[*]

As long as learning disabilities have been described, note has been made that many of the children having difficulty in school had histories of being late to talk or had difficulty with language as preschoolers (Chalfant and Scheffelin, 1969; Klassen, 1972; Kolers, 1972; Warrington and Kinsbourne, 1967). Although the implication that language difficulties "cause" other learning problems has been a controversial subject, this particular co-occurrence has been gaining increasing support in the literature.

Stark (1975) has suggested that reading failure is a language-based problem. Similarly, Vellutino (1977), through a critical review of various theories of dyslexia, has presented evidence in support for a verbal deficit hypothesis underlying dyslexia. Although not all reading specialists ascribe to this orientation, many do consider reading to be highly dependent upon the syntactic and semantic command that a child has of his language (Goodman, 1969; Goodman and Goodman, 1977; Kolers, 1972; Smith, 1971). Therefore it appears that one reason children have difficulty reading is because their command of language is insufficient. An important recent perspective on the relationship between lan

---

[*]From National Advisory Committee on Handicapped Children, January, 1968. First Annual Report, "Special Education for Handicapped Children." National Advisory Neurological Diseases and Stroke Council. *Human Communication and Its Disorders—An Overview.* A report prepared and published by the Subcommittee on Human Communication and Its Disorders. National Institute of Health, HEW Bethesda, Maryland, (1969).

guage and reading is that reading depends on a metalinguistic awareness of that which is read (an ability to reflect upon and analyze language as a symbolic system), rather than the more primary linguistic process of language comprehension and production. This view was initially advanced by Mattingly (1972) and more recently by others (Synder and Johnston, 1980).

In addition to the literature supporting the viewpoint that a language problem underlies reading problems, the language difficulties experienced by children identified as learning disabled have been described in some detail (Johnson and Myklebust, 1967; McGrady and Olson, 1970; Meier, 1971; Semel and Wiig, 1975; Warrington and Kinsbourne, 1967; Wiig and Semel, 1976).

□ **Kavanagh and Mattingly (1972), Vellutino (1978), and Wiig and Semel (1976) present extensive information about the relationship between language and learning disorders. How do these authors view the relationship between a child's ability to formulate and express language and his ability to read?**

A great deal of information is thus available demonstrating that cognition, language, and learning are fundamentally related to one another. However it is yet unclear how these relationships are expressed in language and learning disorders in children. More documentation is needed to determine how cognitive deficits become language deficits that may then become learning deficits and how any or all of these deficits might be overcome through remediation efforts. Yet in spite of the lack of definitive information, it is clear that "language is a window to cognitive growth and failure." Development is a reaching toward or an evolution toward maturity. What a child undergoes during cognitive development has some essential relationship to the onset and development of his language system and his later academic learning.

Extrinsic environmental interactions

Children with language disorders, like children without language disorders, must learn and use language within the framework of a multidimensional environment. The language disordered child is in continuous interaction with many significant environmental variables that provide his communication context and to which he must respond. Nation and Aram (1977) developed a schematic for viewing this multidimensional environment as it relates to speech and language disorders. Fig. 3-3 is a representation of that viewpoint, emphasizing environmental contexts and reflecting past, contemporary, or immediate factors. We present this diagram (Fig. 3-3) to assist in understanding the interaction of environmental circumstances to speech and language disorders.

Here we will focus on two important functions that people in the child's environment provide: (1) the speech and language stimulation, the raw input data from which children learn their language; and (2) the interpersonal context of communication.

Speech and language stimulation. That children learn the language spoken in their environment is an observation that far predates any scientific understanding of cause-effect relationships. Although it has been taken for granted that a German-born child will learn German, a French-born child will learn French, and a Polish-born child Polish, the process by which children extract the "primary linguistic data" from others in their environment has only received major study in the last 10 to 15 years.

Numerous studies have described how parents (particularly mothers) modify their speech, sensitively calibrating their language to provide models appropriately suited for the child's age and stage of language development (Broen, 1972; Cross, 1975; Moerk, 1974, 1975; Phillips, 1973; Snow, 1972). The

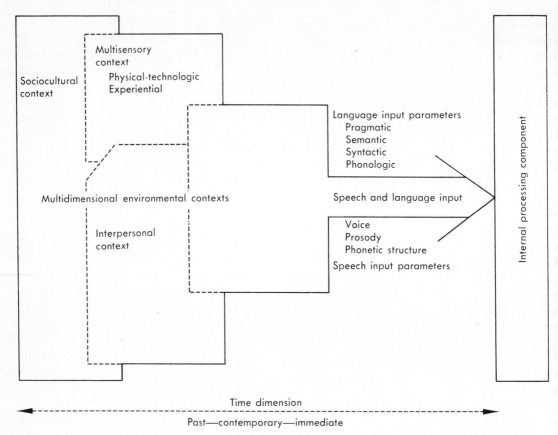

FIG. 3-3. Speech and language environment component of the SLPM. (From Nation, J.E., and Aram, D.M., *Diagnosis of Speech and Language Disorders.* St. Louis: The C.V. Mosby Co. [1977].)

characteristics of mothers' and recently fathers' speech to their young children is now a developed knowledge base in normal language development (Snow and Ferguson, 1977; Waterson and Snow, 1978).

Language disordered children also must extract information about the language they are to learn from important speakers in their midst. There have been suggestions that at least for some language disordered children the language environment is not as optimally suited for language learning as for the normally developing child (Inglis, Kriegsmann,

Mills, and Wulbert, 1975), but research in this area is only beginning to accrue, and it is premature to draw any generalizations about the adequacy of language input provided language disordered children.

Most researchers and clinicians would probably agree that much variation exists. Just as parents of normally developing children vary in the amount, quality, and appropriateness of the language stimulation they provide their child, so also must parents of language disordered children. Although some parents are unable to judge the level of comprehension of their child and modify their speech appropriately, many do an amazingly sensitive and effective job (Van Kleeck and Carpenter, 1980). Trying to calibrate one's language input in these circumstances is a less than exacting process for parent or professional; yet it comes as no surprise that the raw data base available to children with language disorders is an important variable for their development.

Interpersonal context. The second important function served by persons in the child's environment in reference to language learning is that these persons provide an interpersonal context for communication. The communicative interaction between caretaker and child before development of meaningful language is being described in detail by observers of infant and child development such as Bateson (1975), Bruner (1975), Condon and Sander (1974), Greenfield and Smith (1976), Halliday (1977a), Ninio and Bruner (1978), Ratner and Bruner (1978), and Stern, Jaffe, Beebe, and Bennett (1975).

These writers along with others have shown that even very early in life young infants' movements are synchronized with adult speech, thus laying the groundwork for interactional participation and language acquisition (Condon and Sander, 1974). Bruner (1975), Ninio and Bruner (1978), and Stern, Jaffee, Beebe, and Bennett (1975) have described the very early vocal dialogues established between mothers and their infants, referring to these early dialogues as the ontogenesis of communication patterns. Bateson (1975) and Bruner (1975) have studied the nonvocal as well as the vocal beginnings of communicative interaction.

Although studies of vocal behavior during infancy of language disordered children have not been described in detail, reports of high-risk babies and retrospective examination of the histories of many language disordered children suggest that even very early nonvocal communicative interaction (for example, shared attention or synchronized bodily rhythm and speech patterns) have been deviant. Many language disordered children have been described by their mothers as unusually quiet infants or as not responding to attempts at vocal interaction. Other children with language disorders, for example children diagnosed as autistic, are notably deviant even in communicative interaction before the age of 1. A few studies have demonstrated the communicative interaction between parents and older language disordered children to be different from that of normally developing children (Hetenyi, 1974; Marshall, Hegrenes, and Goldstein, 1973; Seitz and Marcus, 1976), but communicative interaction between language disordered children and their parents has not been extensively detailed.

Even though the speech and language abilities of the parents of language disordered children may be quite normal (that is, they can provide adequate amounts and types of stimulation and appropriate learning experiences), the fact that the child has a language disorder affects the interpersonal context of the communications that take place. The child with the disorder is a part of this interaction. His difficulties with language will affect the interaction and most likely the nature of the language input provided in subsequent communications. Parents of these children are at a disadvantage in knowing what form of communication will be best. The child may give back no response, even nonverbally, and the parent may at times be stuck upholding both ends of any communicative interaction. Communicating with a noncommunicating child becomes frustrating and at times intolerable for even the most stimulating, resourceful parent.

Because parents vary in the kind of communicative interaction they engage in with their child, the direction of any causal relationship for this interaction can flow from the child to the parent as well as from the parent to the child. Even if communicative differences exist between language disordered children and their parents when compared to normal children, one cannot simply deduce that the parent was responsible, or for that matter the language disordered child. Writers discussing normal language acquisition (Nelson, 1973) as well as those concerned with personality and temperament development (Thomas, Chess, and Birch, 1968) have stressed the importance of the match between parent and child in their style. For example, Nelson (1973) concluded that those children whose communicative style (expressive, referential) differed from that of their mothers were slower in acquiring their first 50 words than if both parent and child operated with the same style, either referential or expressive. Similarly Thomas, Chess, and Birch (1968) have reported that those children most at risk for development of personality problems were those whose temperaments were "out of sync" with their parents.'

Van Kleeck and Carpenter (1980) put to test the hypothesis that children's level of language comprehension was a major determinant of the modifications in language directed to language disordered children. These investigations compared the structural and pragmatic aspects of the language of adults speaking to children of two differing comprehension levels. The results of the study provided only partial support that children's level of language comprehension is the *crucial* factor accounting for the adjustments made in language directed to children. The investigators suggested that the variations in children's comprehension *strategies* rather than level of language structure provided a better explanation of the adjustments in the adults' language.

Thus language disordered children's communicative interaction may vary from that observed for normally developing children, both in terms of the absolute characteristics of that interaction as well as the match or mismatch in styles of the child and his caretakers.

Intrinsic lines of development

Thus far we have discussed how language development and disorders are shaped by interactions with cognitive development and extrinsic environmental contexts. Language development and disorders are also shaped by simultaneous interactions with other emotional and physical lines of development, here viewed as intrinsic to the child.

While a number of intrinsic lines of emotional and physical development might be considered and may well influence language development, the most frequently encountered problems are often in peripheral sensory development, motor development, development of behavioral control, development of the neurologic organization for language, and development of neurologic stability.

Limitations in peripheral sensory development. Many children with language disorders also have accompanying peripheral hearing losses, visual acuity problems, and reduced tactile-kinesthetic sensitivity. Although each of these sensory restrictions can in itself contribute to a language disorder, one or more of these sensory restrictions and a language disorder may co-occur. If present, the sensory restriction complicates and modifies the expression of the language disorder.

For example, the language deficits in children with peripheral visual problems are beginning to be documented (Fraiberg and Adelson, 1973; Fraiberg, 1975; and Kastein and Gillman, 1976). Not only does the condition of blindness appear to be a limiting factor upon language acquisition, but in addition whatever caused the blindness (e.g., rubella) may also cause further central nervous system damage providing an additional basis for a language disorder. Thus the language disorders of many blind children arise from both the blindness and subsequent restrictions in motility and development of perceptions and self-image, and also may be causally related to other language processing disruptions.

The pervasive effect of peripheral hearing losses on language development is an extensively documented relationship that comprises its own area of professional study, particularly language and speech development of the deaf (Ling, 1976; Ling and Ling, 1978; and Russell, Quigley, and Power, 1976).

Tactile-kinesthetic problems have been implicated in children described as apraxic, and indeed this population seems to vary on the basis of the presence or absence of such a concomitant problem (Jaffee, 1979). Understandably, receiving reduced information as to touch and position in space only complicates an already complicated disorder.

All other things being equal, peripheral sensory problems usually add to the severity of any language disorder, add to a more guarded prognosis, and add to the demands of diagnosis and therapy. How much of a child's problem can be attributed to peripheral versus central limitations is a recurring, perplexing problem that often cannot be answered with assuredness and that continues to surface throughout the child's developmental course.

Limitations in motor development. While subtle and minor motor problems may be more the rule than the exception with children with language disorders, some children present overt motor problems. These motor problems are the major defining condition of the handicap referred to as cerebral palsy, a motor problem originating during the developmental stages stemming from central nervous system involvement. Some of these children's motor problems may completely inter-fere with or prevent any oral expression. When the handicap is severe, such children may require nonverbal modes of communication ranging in sophistication from electronic systems to simple communication boards.

Limitations in behavioral control development. Some language disordered children present a range of problems both in responding to sensory input and in controlling the level of motor responsiveness. Although these children's sensory and motor systems may be intact, they often demonstrate attentional disturbances and deviant levels of motor activity.

Children whose language disorders arise from neurologic dysfunction frequently display these behavioral control problems (Kinsbourne and Caplan, 1979). Such children's attention may be brief and readily disrupted by extraneous stimuli. Others may overattend to a restrictive range of input, having difficulty shifting attention to new items. These children may seem to block out other things and persons and attend only to what they themselves have chosen or to objects or events of high-stimulus value. Deviant levels of motor behavior may range from hypoactive to hyperactive. Some children are quite lethargic in the way they greet the world, presenting limited activity and behavioral response to people in their environment. These children are often overly cautious and nonexploratory. At the other extreme are children who are in constant motion, darting from one thing to another, never engaging in any one activity more than a fleeting moment. Such children may be called "hyperactive" or perhaps more benignly, "overactive." When exaggerated activity level combines with a limited attention, a child may have difficulty sitting still or watching long enough to learn.

Other children present problems with affect, again probably best represented by a continuum of behavior from too little to too much. Some of these children, often coming from deprived environments, may sit passively and sullenly for long periods, never engaging in activities that surround them. Still others present what appears to be overaffection or perhaps more accurately nondiscriminating affection, kissing or hugging anyone in sight or wanting to be held excessively by anyone and everyone. Such children often do not show appropriate stranger anxiety and also seem not to have formed appropriate attachment to family members. The emotionally labile child presents still another set of challenges to the speech-language pathologist. Fleeting or prolonged tantrums may be triggered by seemingly insignificant factors. Or the child may alternate between hugging and biting, or kissing and kicking.

These deficits in behavioral controls often cloud and complicate a child's language disorder. Frequently management of these behaviors becomes an initial and an ongoing issue that the clinician must circumvent or work through in the course of diagnosis and treatment of the language disorder.

Development of neurologic organization for language processing. To be able to process language normally, children require a specialized organization of higher brain structures, notably the cerebral cortex. We are still in the beginning stages of understanding how language is processed in the brains of normal children developing language and how much and what kind of compensations occur if the neurologic processing is impaired. Based on our present level of understanding, however, several conclusions can be drawn from the literature.

CONCLUSION 1: *Innate or very early cerebral specialization for language processing exists.* Arguments have ranged from the concept of nonspecialization (equipotentiality) of the cerebral hemispheres for language at birth (Krashen, 1975; Lenneberg, 1967) to the idea of highly developed innate specialization (Kinsbourne, 1975; Kinsbourne and Hiscock, 1977). However, the evidence most strongly supports the position that the left cerebral hemisphere is destined for language processing and that this organization is present innately or very early in life. The theory of cerebral equipotentiality for language processing appears to be on less than sound experimental and clinical ground.

The preliminary evidence supporting this implication derives from the investigations of anatomic and functional cerebral asymmetry. The anatomic evidence is significant in pointing out that the anatomic differences in adults are also found in neonates, particularly the anatomic differences in the left temporal area, indicating that more space may be available in the left temporal areas for language processing (Galaburda, Sanides and Geschwind, 1978; Galaburda, LeMay, Kemper and Geschwind, 1978; Geschwind and Levitsky, 1968; LeMay and Geschwind, 1978).

The evidence from functional studies also supports the presence of very early left hemisphere specialization for language. Refer to Segalowitz and Gruber (1977) and Witelson (1977 b) for detailed discussion of this evidence. All in all, both anatomic and functional studies indicate that the adult neurologic model is a viable model for viewing the language processing of young children; that is, language processing is organized predominantly in the left cerebral hemisphere even in young children.

CONCLUSION 2: *Certain aspects of language processing are contributed to by both cerebral hemispheres.* When language processing is viewed from a cognitive base as opposed to only an auditory base, it appears that certain aspects of language may be contributed to by both the right and left cerebral hemispheres. That both hemispheres work together in processing linguistic data has been demonstrated by Molfese (1979). The pragmatic and semantic aspects appear to require less sequential and analytic processing and thus may be less left hemisphere-dependent than the phonologic and syntactic aspects (Moscovitch, 1977). This supposition is also supported by findings from children who have sustained right versus left cerebral hemisphere dysfunction (Dennis and Whitaker, 1976; Dennis, 1980; Rankin, Aram and Horwitz, 1980). This evidence indicates that the syntactic and possibly the phonologic aspects of language are more dependent upon left hemisphere intactness, whereas the semantic ability is not differentially affected by damage in either hemisphere (Dennis, 1980).

CONCLUSION 3: *Reorganization of specialization for language is a characteristic of the cerebral hemispheres when damage or dysfunction exists.* This conclusion stems from the large amount of literature available about language learning and language recovery in the presence of congenital and acquired cerebral disturbances (Dennis and Whitaker, 1975; Hecaen, 1976; Rasmussen and Milner, 1977). This evidence allows us to conclude that if the cerebral hemispheres are damaged, either right or left, the remaining cerebral structures allow for anatomic and functional reorganization; that is, plasticity of function is a characteristic of cerebral structures but within certain limits.

Because of the greater degree of language recovery in children than adults, it appears that the immature cerebral hemispheres have greater plasticity of function than the more mature cerebral hemispheres (Hecaen, 1976). Thus the age at which cerebral disturbance occurs will affect the ability of the remaining cerebral structures to take over the function assumed by the area damaged. Plasticity of function decreases with age; however, the age limits for recovery of function are unclear, ranging from birth to puberty. Since the evidence does not point to an absolute age range for recovery of function, it is likely that the ability of the cerebral hemispheres to reorganize following dysfunction is best viewed at this time as a continuum. Most likely a number of variables intervene in determining how much cerebral reorganization can take place, importantly the location and extensiveness of cerebral dysfunction.

It is unclear as to what cerebral structures are involved in takeover of functions (Kohn, 1980; Rasmussen and Milner, 1977). It appears that for a child any one of three possibilities may occur: (1) complete takeover of language processing by the opposite hemisphere, (2) residual structures of the damaged hemisphere assuming the entire responsibility for language processing, and (3) some bilateral hemispheric organization for language.

What the evidence does point to is that following damage there may be less complete and less efficient language processing as well as effects on other nonlanguage processes; the need to take over language processing by cerebral structures not initially destined for language processing will be done at the expense of other functions such as visuospatial processing. Thus the ultimate amount of language learning may be reduced in these children.

This evidence then indicates that both hemispheres have the capability to assume language processing functions, but they are not equal in their ability to do so. If damage occurs, congenitally or acquired, the amount of recovery depends on two factors: what cerebral structures are called upon to assume these language functions and how the assumption of these functions will affect other functions ordinarily assumed by those cerebral structures.

CONCLUSION 4: *The higher incidence of language disorders in boys than in girls may be accounted for on the basis of differences in neurologic organization between the sexes.*

There has been much documentation of differences between boys and girls in many phases of development (Buffery and Gray, 1972; Maccoby and Jacklin, 1974). The same holds true for differences in language learning and language disorders. The evidence available allows us to imply that boys may have different degrees of specialization at different ages and for different functions than do girls. It appears that boys have earlier and more confined specialization for language and other higher cortical functions. Thus it is suggested that boys have less "uncommitted" hemispheric processing space if early damage occurs, thus accounting for the greater incidence of language disorders in boys than in girls (Witelson, 1976).

CONCLUSION 5: *Language disorders in children with and without documented cerebral dysfunction can be viewed from a perspective of neurologic organization for language processing.* The information presented in the previous four conclusions leads logically to this fifth and final conclusion. All children, damaged or not, will be striving toward developing a communication system through language. To do this requires cerebral organization for language processing. If there is no cerebral dysfunction, one could expect in most instances of right-handed children that language processing is specialized in the left cerebral hemisphere with cooperation from the right cerebral hemisphere for certain aspects. If a child is damaged at birth or acquires cerebral dysfunction, a different neurolinguistic model for language will have to be entertained.

First of all, we cannot assume that if the left cerebral hemisphere is involved, the right cerebral hemisphere takes over the functions for language usually processed in the left; that is, we cannot assume total transfer of function. The damaged hemisphere may "persist" in its role in language processing or greater

bilateral functioning may occur. Second, we cannot assume that any reorganization for language processing will occur no matter what the age of the child is.

We do know, however, that language recovery does occur in children who acquire cerebral lesions. Our orientation must take this into account while at the same time remembering that the language recovery may be incomplete and at the expense of other functions. A number of considerations must be kept in mind: innateness of cerebral organization, plasticity of cerebral structures, the age at which the disruption occurs, and the degree and location of the cerebral dysfunction.

Therefore in the child who is damaged we cannot simply utilize a normal neurologic processing model, nor can we simply say that the right cerebral hemisphere is to blame. It is most likely that considerable neural reorganization has taken place. A processing model to account for the underlying neurologic organization for these children must await considerably more evidence than is now available.

When there is no documentation of neurologic dysfunction in children, it is more difficult to derive a neurologic processing orientation to their language disorders. Unlike adults or older children with acquired language disorders, the vast majority of children with language disorders reveal no clear-cut neurologic findings suggestive of a specific, localized lesion. Clinical findings other than the language disorder are often absent or subtle. Brain scans usually come back read as within normal limits, and electroencephalogram (brain wave) findings tend to be equivocal at best. However, we must start with the orientation that these children must utilize cerebral structures for processing language and that presumably they are moving toward the adult model.

The information that we have about language disorders in children with documented cerebral dysfunction can help us with our orientation to the child with no documented dysfunction. The presence of a neurologic basis for the language disorder is often inferred on the basis of the presented behavior rather than demonstrable by independent clinical or laboratory findings.

The evidence from anatomic and functional asymmetry could lead to the assumption that some of these language disordered children present less than adequate structures for specialization. There may be different degrees of cerebral specialization from birth that result in less than adequate language acquisition. Thus some of the delays and disorders seen may be related to this lack of cerebral specialization (Galaburda, LeMay, Kemper and Geschwind, 1978; Hier, LeMay, Rosenberger and Perlo, 1978; Witelson, 1977a). Apparently in these children the environmental stimulation has not circumvented problems that arose because of the lack of cerebral asymmetry.

Some of the language difficulties may stem from specialization occurring in the "wrong" hemispheres (Witelson, 1977a). Some of the information from studies with dyslexic children implicate this as a possibility. If for some reason language becomes specialized in the right hemisphere, the child will encounter difficulties with language processing, especially for syntax, as well as with other aspects of learning and development. Processing mix-ups, confusions, and competition may exist leading to language delays and disorders. This disrupted processing could result in language disorders affecting various aspects of language. The nature of the language disorder could well provide us with information about the underlying processing disruptions.

Our orientation, of course, must also include those children in whom there is no underlying neurologic basis for the presented language disorder. In these instances we must introduce other bases for the disorder; however, at the same time we must be willing to accept that any deficit that exists, intrinsic or extrinsic to the child, has a potential effect on his language processing mechanisms.

Limitations in development of neurologic stability. In addition to considerations of neurologic organization for language, some children with language disorders present a fluctuating or degenerative neurologic condition. An example of such a fluctuating neurologic state encountered is that of children with seizures. A speech-language pathologist could be the first to note petit mal seizures in which there may be a transient loss of consciousness; the child's attention becomes fixed and a blank stare is seen. These fadeout periods may intermittently and unsuspectingly come and go. Other children's uncontrolled seizures may manifest themselves as grand mal seizures or in other clearly observable forms. In such cases these uncontrolled seizures may stem from nonidentification of the seizure activity or failure to arrive at effective drug control of the seizure disorder. In such cases the uncontrolled seizures interfere with attempts to learn new behaviors and may destroy established learning.

Summary

Working Part V of our definition of child language disorders has emphasized how the language of the child is shaped by development that includes (1) cognitive development; (2) extrinsic environmental interactions; and (3) intrinsic sensory, motor, behavioral, and neurologic lines of development. Although each of these has been treated somewhat distinctly in our discussion, it is clear that all these aspects of development are interactive. Seldom do we see a child with a language disorder who has no difficulties in other aspects of development. Difficulties in one aspect of development will likely have consequences for other simultaneously developing aspects. Understanding how these interactive lines of development influence one another and coexist presents a theoretic, diagnostic, and treatment challenge for the speech-language pathologist.

☐ **Berry (1969) was an early major advocate of viewing the extrinsic and intrinsic lines of development in relationship to language. Study her "The Profile of David: Language Disorder Associated with Genetically Determined Deficits of the Nervous System" as it relates to Working Part V of our definition of child language disorders.**

A LONGITUDINAL PERSPECTIVE OF THE LANGUAGE DISORDERED CHILD

One of the pleasures and glories of working with children is that change is a "cardinal rule" of childhood. Change, as an inevitable aspect of childhood, contributes to the many faces and facets of child language disorders. How a language disorder looks today may not be how it will look in 2, 6, or 12 years. At different stages in the child's life, his language disorder affects him differently. The 2-year-old does not confront classroom learning, but the 6-year-old is faced with a real, often troublesome academic demand—reading, writing, mathematics, and spelling. Also, the influence a language disorder exerts on other domains, such as social relationships, takes quite different forms at different ages. Similarly, vocational concerns present a new demand in the late teen years that previously did not have to be met.

One of the shortcomings in the profession of speech-language pathology has been a failure to collect and report longitudinal data. Little literature has addressed the long-term outlook for language disordered children. Yet most clinicians in practice for extended periods of time have their private store of anecdotes about successes and failures; the children who went on to graduate with their class in school and were esteemed by their classmates, but also the ones who dropped out of school, became isolated misfits, or disappeared into the community with no record of their ability to adjust. Beyond the personal successes and failures accumulated by clinicians, little documentation is available for speech-language pathologists seeking a long-term understanding of the effects of child language disorders.

A longitudinal perspective of child language disorders is needed if we are to guide our language disordered children and their parents beyond the preschool years. This section will present the information available focusing on (1) what is known about the changes in their language over time and (2) the problems they often encounter in school, employment, and social adjustment. The studies presented below generally addressed both of these issues to some extent. We will separate the content into the two categories above.

Changes in language over time

Weiner (1972, 1974) provided both a well-documented case study of a single child followed over a 12-year period and a follow-up study of seven children over 2 years. Weiner's case study (1974) details the variety of long-standing problems of Art, a child followed from age 4 to 16. At age 4 Art was seen because of his severe language difficulties, and at age 16 even though he had "grasped the essential nature of the language he is using" he still demonstrated many difficulties, among them inadequate use of determiners, plural inflections, copula, tense, and other syntactic forms.

In his 1972 study Weiner reported on seven language disordered children (dysphasics) as compared to a normal control group over a 2-

year span. Many tests were given concentrating on auditory-vocal and oral-motor functioning. A test of language comprehension was also included. The first and second year comparisons between the dysphasics and the normals were similar; the dysphasic children performed inferiorly compared with the normal children on almost all tests requiring auditory and oral-motor functioning. Of striking importance were the two-year comparisons on the dysphasic children; their deficits remained essentially unchanged and persistent.

Similarly, Menyuk (1964) noted that the language disabilities of the children in her study remained relatively static across the age groups studied. She reported that her infantile speech group seemed to be using the most generalized rules or first approximations to rules to formulate their sentences. Furthermore, as they grew older they seemed unable to move beyond these elementary and generalized rules.

Wolpaw, Nation, and Aram (1977) reported five-year follow-up data on 30 of 47 children whose pattern of language performance had been described by Aram and Nation (1975). These 30 children were given the same test battery as administered during their preschool years. Two thirds of these children continued to demonstrate some form of language problem. Although all but one of the children's test scores had improved, some changes from initial patterns of performance were noted. Essentially two groups were identified: (1) those termed static and (2) those termed shifters.

The children who fell into the static group, whether they had high or low scores originally, tended to retain the pattern of language performance seen initially. The children identified as shifters fell into two subgroups. First, there were those children whose shift was reflected as a leveling off of language performance. Some of their early language deficits

were brought more into line with their early language strengths. These children tended to equalize their overall language performance, although they did not achieve normal language abilities. The second group of shifters were those who dramatically changed in some aspect of their early language performance, although the aspect varied from child to child.

Two other retrospective studies whose focus was more toward academic problems experienced by language disordered children also add information. Hall and Tomblin (1978) investigated the communication status of 36 adults who had been seen as children. They retrospectively grouped them as language impaired (19) and articulation impaired (18). Their findings revealed that the 18 adults considered as language impaired were reported to persist in presenting articulation and language problems as adults more frequently than the 18 identified as articulation impaired. Aram and Nation (1980) followed up 63 children who in their preschool years were diagnosed as language disordered. All 63 children were now attending school. The results of this study indicated that up to 49% of these children were continuing to experience language problems depending on what level of language was being considered.

Finally, De Ajuriaguerra and his co-workers provided longitudinal data about 17 language disordered children followed over a two-year period. These findings have been presented in a chapter entitled "The Development and Prognosis of Dysphasia in Children" (1976).

Language disorders and their subsequent educational, social, and vocational implications

Many preschoolers with language disorders will go into the school years and present learning disorders in addition to or in place of their earlier language problems. Although this continuum of language-learning disorders is frequently observed and occasionally reported, documentation and systematic study of this relationship has been sparse. Aside from Weiner's (1974) very detailed longitudinal study of Art, clearly demonstrating ongoing language-learning and social problems, few such studies have appeared in the literature.

Of the 30 language disordered children studied by Wolpaw, Nation, and Aram (1977) only 10 were functioning acceptably in normal classrooms. The remaining 20 were presenting academic difficulties along with their language difficulties. In addition, from parental and teacher reports it was suggested that these children were also experiencing social and behavioral problems.

Based on the Aram and Nation (1975) and Wolpaw, Nation, and Aram (1977) studies, Aram (1977) reported that preschool measures of nonverbal intelligence, as measured by the Arthur Adaptation of the Leiter International Intelligence Scale (1949), coupled with the level of performance on any of a variety of comprehension tests (Assessment of Children's Language Comprehension, Foster, Giddan and Stark, 1973; Peabody Picture Vocabulary Test, Dunn, 1965; Northwestern Syntax Screening Test, Lee, 1969), were strongly related to subsequent educational placement in regular, LD, or EMR classrooms. That is, if a child scored at a high level on language comprehension tasks and had a relatively high Leiter score as a preschooler, the probability was high that in elementary school he would be in a regular classroom. However, if a child performed at a moderate or low level on comprehension tasks and did not have an exceptionally high Leiter score, he would probably be educated in an LD or EMR classroom, depending on how low both comprehension and nonverbal intelligence were.

In the Hall and Tomblin (1978) study of 36

adults the 18 identified as language impaired also had more subsequent academic difficulties (particularly in reading) than did the 18 identified as articulation impaired, and differed in the types of postsecondary education attempted. It is important to note that the 18 adults identified retrospectively as language impaired may have presented only mild language disorders as children.

☐ **The Hall and Tomblin (1978) study is interesting to evaluate from a research design point of view. How did they determine the initial diagnosis of these 36 adults?**

Approximately 40% of the 63 language disordered children followed up by Aram and Nation (1980) presented reading, mathematics, and/or spelling problems. Preschool levels of language comprehension, formulation, semantics, syntax, phonology, and speech production were all found to be moderately correlated with the subsequent level of class placement in the elementary grades. Duration of preschool therapy, however, was not related to follow-up language measures or to level of class placement.

The studies presented clearly indicate that much needs to be learned about the longitudinal perspective of child language disorders. From what has been presented we conclude that children with preschool language disorders are at risk for subsequent academic, social, and vocational achievement. We can also conclude that these language disorders are not easily resolved even with therapy, since many of the reports indicate continued problems with language and communication. Many questions arise from this information, for example:

1. What is the relationship between the type and severity of the language disorder to subsequent learning difficulties?
2. How effective is language treatment for preschool language disorders?

3. Can language treatment circumvent subsequent learning, social, and vocational problems?

These are only a few of the important unanswered questions that remain. They suggest research directions that would provide basic information about the course of child language disorders over time. We hope such information will be forthcoming in the near future.

GARY: A LANGUAGE DISORDERED CHILD GROWN UP

We will close this chapter with a narrative about an adult who was a language disordered child. Gary's case study is a sobering one; his problems help those who undertake study and work with the language disordered child to more fully appreciate that language is central to much of what is human and to much of what is rewarded in our society. This narrative reveals the interactions of the working parts of the definition of child language disorders presented in this chapter.

Now 25 years old, Gary has seen his share of speech and language clinicians. The whole process began at age 1 when his mother first questioned his ability to hear. An answer to that question was debated for some years. At age 2½ he was first tested by an audiologist who obtained responses to free field testing suggesting a moderately severe hearing loss. Although not fitted with a hearing aid, Gary spent the next several years in a preschool class for hearing impaired children. During his time in that program he was reported to be understanding some words and a few simple commands, and he started to use several single words. However, the master teacher noted that he did not learn as readily as most other hearing impaired children. In addition, she noted that he was unable to tolerate any kind of interruption in his activity, had an unusual fascination with lights, and drooled excessively.

In order to better understand why Gary was not using more language or learning more quickly, he was referred for the first of a series of neurologic examinations. The neurologist suggested that the fact that Gary's mother had taken iodine for asthma during her pregnancy with Gary and that he was born with a congenital goiter may lie behind Gary's developmental problems. An electroencephalogram also obtained at this time evidenced cortical and subcortical encephalopathy in the right temporal areas.

At age 7, Gary was referred to a day treatment program for atypical retarded children, because his behavioral problems were of increasing concern. Here he began joining words together but continued to make very slow progress in other language areas, and continued to be described as a diagnostically perplexing child. The consulting psychologist who studied Gary at the center for mental retardation through the elementary grades was later to remark, "I never was comfortable with the diagnosis of emotional problems and mental retardation."

Over the years Gary was to have numerous hearing tests with contradictory findings. If he did or did not have a hearing loss was an unsettled question that kept him from having a hearing aid. Finally one resolute audiologist insisted, and at 11 years old he received his first hearing aid, a monaural aid for the left ear. About this time he was transferred to the public school system, where for a few years he attended classes for slow learners but ultimately graduated from high school with a low B average.

Throughout his years in public school, Gary was in speech therapy, usually with one or two others. Although apparently therapy focused on his seemingly minor articulation distortions, notably sibilants and /r/ distortions, the therapists' notes suggested that his language structure was poor, that he had a poorly developed vocabulary, and that he often did not seem to understand what was said to him.

Multiple psychologic examinations throughout his school years continued to reveal a marked discrepancy between his nonverbal and verbal skills. For example, the last Wechsler Adult Intelligence Scale (Wechsler, 1955) administered to him at school at age 17 yielded a verbal IQ of 90, a performance IQ of 124, and a full scale IQ of 108. Despite his very good nonverbal ability, Gary persisted in being a loner and being considered "strange" by his peers, teachers, and other adults who knew him. The examining psychologists remarked that Gary's most pronounced weaknesses included deficiencies in use of common sense, judgment, and reasoning as well as a poor ability to understand words and draw from a fund of information. Despite his high nonverbal IQ, in grade 11, Gary's reading, spelling, and arithmetic were no higher than a sixth grade level. Not only did Gary finish high school with these learning deficits, but he was also a social isolate. He regarded retarded children as "dumb" but was not accepted by his normally developing peers.

After completing high school, Gary went from one job training program to another, gaining temporary but unsuccessful employment in a variety of semiskilled jobs. At age 20, he performed at a 12-year level on all subtests of the Peabody Individual Achievement Test (Dunn and Markwadt, 1970) (reading recognition, mathematics, and spelling), except for general information. He had now become "an intensive, almost compulsively nonstop talker, about mostly trivial and previously reported information, yet he had nothing to say in group discussions." Again the

psychologist noted that in regard to social and personal perceptions and behaviors he appeared more like a 10-year-old than the 20-year-old that he was.

Despite numerous though sporadic stabs at speech and language therapy since his preschool years, today, at age 25, Gary continues to present significant language difficulties. A year ago, largely in hopes of aiding his poor social adjustment, Gary's mother again turned to a speech-language pathologist for help.

When examined, Gary's language skills were found to cluster between the 6- and 10-year level, seriously deficient when contrasted to his above average nonverbal ability. His speech was described as low pitched, mildly nasal, and monotone. Sibilant sounds were frequently distorted or omitted. His comprehension of syntax suffered primarily from his not differentiating between inflectional markers such as "the boy writes/the boys write." Similarly he failed to use many inflectional markers in his expressive syntax; for example, he often did not mark subject-verb agreement. Probably the area in which he was found to be having the most significant difficulty was in vocabulary, verbal integration, and abstraction. He had notable difficulty with verbal opposites and was completely unable to abstract likenesses and differences between words. For example, when asked what the important similarity between egg and apple were, he responded, "they're hard." He answered questions requiring concrete information quite adequately (month, season, year, time, etc.) but seemed to lose the point when asked for any relationship. For example, when asked if he were to work every day, could he do more work in a month or a week, his answer was a week.

Because of these very noticeable language deficiencies, Gary was enrolled in speech and language therapy with a private clinician and was seen for a comprehensive audiologic re-evaluation.

The audiologist recommended that he continue to wear the binaural amplification as he had been doing since he was 17 years old. With such amplification his hearing was within normal limits, and he had excellent speech discrimination. Unaided he presented a moderate to severe bilateral sensorineural hearing loss for pure tones, but he reached considerably better speech reception thresholds, suggesting at worst a moderate unaided level of hearing.

Speech and language therapy during the past year has focused on his very notable semantic and pragmatic deficits. Therapy has been oriented toward daily life issues, addressing current and very real problems in Gary's life. For example, early in therapy, the State of Ohio driver manual served as content for vocabulary training since Gary had never been able to pass the written examination required for a driver's license. Although he could "read" the entire manual, it soon became apparent that he did not know what many crucial words meant, such as "pedestrian," "intersection," and "caution." However, as a prelude to approaching the task of vocabulary development, the speech pathologist had to painstakingly confront the concept that words have meaning. Gary responded blankly when asked what a word "meant," or he provided an associative response. For example, when asked what "pedestrian" meant, he would respond, "Pedestrian crossing." One useful approach in therapy has been to encourage him to draw a picture of whatever the word represents and then to describe what he has drawn. Social connotations of words have also been emphasized. Although having women friends has been a focal concern of Gary's, he does not understand what he has been told when for example one young woman stated that she wanted to be "just friends" or when another said she was "busy."

Besides tackling the major semantic deficits that Gary presents, therapy also addressed the pragmatic aspects of his communication. Described by his speech-language clinician as "totally insensitive to other persons and the impact of his behavior upon them," Gary does not grasp the subtleties of communication in a social setting nor does he modify his language or other behavior according to the social demands of a setting. Recently having been admonished for barging into the clinician's office upon arrival with no regard for who else might be in the office at the time, Gary was told by the clinician to knock before coming in. He now knocks and then barges in, sitting down with little heed of who may be there or what else may be going on.

Frequently Gary is at a loss for how to respond in social situations. Although he frequents discos, he doesn't know what to say to the people he meets, and when he does talk, he comes across as literal and strange. Because of the significant interpersonal problems he experiences, the speech pathologist has recently requested that a psychotherapist act as a consultant to her in working with his many interpersonal problems.

Although Gary has managed to hold a job as an electrical transformer repairman, he finds the job "boring" and would like to secure more challenging employment. Such a possibility is improbable at least for the present, since he is a trying employee for even the most accepting foreman. For example, having been told at least a dozen times not to do some metal grinding near a particular machine so that the metal shaving would not get into the machine, the usually mild mannered boss yelled, "If you do that one more time, I'll fire you." Stunned and at a loss for what to say, Gary cried. In such situations it is difficult to know if Gary was listening, how much he did or did not understand, or if he understood but simply didn't modify his behavior. In any event, given sufficient warning he did not appropriately modify his behavior in response to the language he heard. The speech pathologist notes that she is puzzled and frustrated by Gary's failure to listen even when he clearly hears and understands what is said to him. He frequently yawns and seems to tune out others when they talk.

Twenty-four years after his mother raised questions, Gary continues to present a host of language, learning, social, and vocational problems. Although he is gainfully employed, talks in sentences, has completed high school, and occasionally dates, he has not grown out of or been remediated out of the language and learning problems he presented as a young child. Although he has made immeasurable progress, using all aspects of development as a floating referent, he has never been able to close the gap between himself and his peers. Gary continues to be a language disordered child grown up. As he grew up, he took on a wider spectrum of experiences. The focus on his initial language problems shifted to learning problems, and finally to major vocational and social problems. Other language disordered children may have different long-term courses, but for Gary and many others, the language disorder continues to have impact in adulthood.

chapter 4

Causation and child language disorders

The first three chapters of this book discussed a number of perspectives on child language disorders leading to a working definition. The vital issue of causation has not been addressed directly although it becomes clear that much of the information in these chapters has a bearing on cause-effect relationships in child language disorders. In this chapter we will focus on causation, directly ending with an interactive-developmental orientation to causation.

We will be drawing principally from two sources. First, we will be applying the information presented in the first three chapters to the issue of causes of child language disorders. Here we will not be presenting new information, but rather integrating the earlier information around cause-effect relationships. Second, we have devoted entire chapters in our earlier book *Diagnosis of Speech and Language Disorders* (Nation and Aram, 1977) to the study of causation and cause-effect relationships in speech-language pathology. We will be basing much of this chapter on that earlier work, because we have found such an orientation to be as useful to the study of child language disorders as it is to other areas of speech-language disorders.

THE CONTEXT OF CAUSATION

Causation as an issue in speech-language pathology has yet to be resolved to the satisfaction of the professionals involved. Some speech-language pathologists have suggested that concern with causation is irrelevant to the study of speech and language disorders, while others have maintained that causal relationships are an integral part of understanding and treating individuals with speech and language disorders.

Prevailing practices in child language disorders

In child language disorders the prevailing practices applied to causation are similar in many respects to those found in the more general field of speech-language pathology. Here we will draw attention to these practices and provide both criticism and support of them. We will also make reference to previous chapters, where some of this material has been discussed.

□ **We (Nation and Aram, 1977) have discussed the state of the art of causation in speech-language pathology, reviewing a number of practices that have developed in our profession over the years. We have concluded** that a set of "dead-end" practices have been used including cataloging of etiologies, etiologic classification systems, and dichotomizing functional-organic etiologies. Why have these practices led to a limited understanding of causation?

Etiologic typologies. As discussed in Chapter 2, our field passed through an "era of etiologic typologies and differential diagnosis." Child language disorders were classified, diagnosed, and treated primarily from a static etiologic orientation. The focus of this practice was more toward mutually exclusive etiologies than toward the language disorder, and it led to a simplistic view of causation, searching for *the* cause of *the* language disorder—a view that led some to conclude that causation was irrelevant to the study of child language disorders.

Yet we cannot ignore that this practice holds real meaning to the profession of speech-language pathology. Etiologic classifications do exist. For example, journals have been created around them *(Mental Retardation, American Annals of the Deaf, Journal of Autism and Childhood Schizophrenia)*; work settings are frequently described and funded accordingly (mental retardation unit, programs for the hearing impaired); training of professionals occurs along etiologic lines (teachers of the hearing impaired, mental retardation specialists); and many diagnostic and treatment protocols derive from etiologic classification.

Speech-language pathologists often operate in terms of a ready-made etiologic classification of child language disorders: the mentally retarded, the autistic, the emotionally disturbed, the hearing impaired, and the culturally deprived. Because of the assumptions implied about the homogeneity of the children so classified, these etiologic classifications have limited usefulness for diagnosing, assessing,

and treating child language disorders. In Chapter 3, we pointed out in our working definition that multiple patterns of language disorders exist and may be related to variable points of processing breakdowns. The failure to relate language behaviors to etiology underscores the limitations in an etiologic approach to causation and child language disorders.

Yet because these terms are still used, the speech-language pathologist should learn to function with them. This may require a reinterpretation of the etiologic terms from a more dynamic causal orientation rather than relying on a static set of assumptions.

Contagious cataloging. Another dead-end practice has been listing and cataloging etiologies. This practice has already resulted in a long list, a list that may be endless, of etiologies to be considered for language disorders. We believe that this practice often stems from the underlying assumption that a language disorder can be understood simply by knowing the etiology rather than knowing how the etiology disrupted the speech and language processing system.

A prevailing practice now appears to be "contagious cataloging," where children are grouped on the basis of a known or presumed etiology. The children are thus thought to be similar, and then their language behavior is studied. Thus in some of the literature we see language disorders described for various etiologically categorized groups, for example: the Laurence-Moon-Biedl syndrome (Garstecki, Borton, Stark, and Kennedy, 1972); premature children (deHirsch, Jansky, and Langford, 1964; Ehrlich, Shapiro, and Huttner, 1973); DeLange syndrome (Moore, 1970); myelomeningocele and hydrocephalic children (Schwartz, 1974); and so on.

Major criticisms of contagious cataloging are first, the assumption made about the homogeneity of the population and second, the lack of attention that might be paid to other important variables such as concomitant causal factors, age, intellectual status, and social circumstances.

Yet again, this approach has merit since it focuses attention on various causes of child language disorders, a focus that can move our profession toward a fuller understanding of the diversity of causes that may result in child language disorders. It brings to light the range and variety of factors that can have an effect on the development and use of language. What is needed is a dynamic interpretation of how these diverse etiologic factors may have interfered with language development by disrupting underlying language processing. Such interpretation must replace a static interpretation that simply associates etiology and the described language disorders. A list of symptoms associated with a list of etiologies provides little understanding—only lists.

Causation does not matter. Those who ascribe to the view that causation does not matter are those who focus almost exclusively on the behavior of language disordered children (Bloom and Lahey, 1978; Trantham and Pederson, 1976). The extralanguage information reported by these investigators is usually confined to detailed demographic data, for example age, sex, socioeconomic status, and race. This approach is closely aligned with the "day of linguistic and psycholinguistic description" that was presented in Chapter 2.

Interestingly, in studies presentd by adherents of this approach we often see in the subjects studied the exclusion of language disordered children who have been defined as mentally retarded, emotionally disturbed, hearing impaired, neurologically impaired, and so forth (Leonard, 1972; Morehead and Ingram, 1973). In ruling out such language

disordered children, adherents to the "causation does not matter" view are narrowly classifying child language disorders, representing only one subset of the larger population. This approach promotes determining language disorders primarily based on such characteristics as mean length of utterance and syntactic and semantic characteristics. The assumption made from this data is that the children are all alike in the way that they process language for communication. The overwhelming merit of this information, however, is that it has provided invaluable descriptive detail of language behavior.

Processing starts. In Chapter 2 we discussed what we believe to be a re-emergence, though not a dominant approach, of studying child language disorders and their causes from a processing orientation. The focus of much of this work was on aphasic and other brain-injured children exhibiting difficulties in language and other learning tasks. From this work, both uni- and multi-stage processing hypotheses were derived.

In Chapter 3 we provided a Child Language Processing Model and discussed the intrinsic and extrinsic developmental contexts in which these processes emerge. We suggest that this model provides a means for developing an interactive-developmental perspective toward causal factors, a subject to which this chapter is devoted.

PERSPECTIVES ON CAUSATION
Causation does matter

Even though causation as an issue in speech-language pathology has not been resolved, and although some professionals do not believe it is crucial for understanding child language disorders, we take the position that causation does matter.

If the basis for the child's problem is not

understood, inappropriate, long-term remedial approaches may persist.

> Bill remembers his life as a continuous series of temper tantrums: 11 years of physical therapy, steel leg braces and corrective surgery during which he never learned to walk; 11 years of speech therapy during which he never learned to talk; 11 years of occupational therapy during which he never learned to use his hands. . . . The headstick was the first thing he had ever succeeded at. It was, he says, "like coming out of solitary confinement."*

Several major principles in the study of causality in child development and child language disorders keep us wary of main effects interpretations, (that *a* cause creates *an* effect on language). First, it is generally clear that one cause can be responsible for different primary effects; second, that one cause can be responsible for multiple effects; third, that a variety of causal factors can create the same primary effect; and fourth, that whatever the primary historic cause, it may not be the best explanation of the current status of the child's development.

The fact that causation is complex and often unclear is not justification for discarding it as an important issue in child language disorders. An orientation that helps us to study and interpret these complexities is needed. To this end we will develop an orientation that picks up on the view introduced in the first chapter of this book: that language disorders in children are the result of a series of complex cause-effect interactions over time.

We will present this orientation by first developing three perspectives on causation: (1) a processing perspective, (2) an interactive perspective, and (3) a developmental perspective. We will then draw these perspectives together into an interactive developmental orientation to causation.

---

*From "The Expanding World of Bill Rush," LIFE © 1980 Time Inc. Reprinted with permission.

Processing perspective

Our processing perspective stems directly from our working definition for child language disorders as presented in Chapter 3. The perspective must incorporate language disordered children as those "with disordered language behaviors *related to language processing dysfunctions* that appear as variable patterns of language performance and are shaped by the developmental context in which they occur." This major point of our working definition of child language disorders is that language disorders are a reflection of disrupted underlying processes.

Nation and Aram (1977) developed a major processing perspective on cause-effect relationships. It is notable, however, that many writers and investigators taking a causal orientation have come from outside the profession of speech-language pathology. For example, Rapin and Wilson (1978) express a similar view when they state:

> . . . failure to develop language is always, except in rare instances of extreme environmental deprivation, the consequence of neurological dysfunction affecting pathways which transmit information from the ear to the brain, within the brain itself, or from the brain to the muscles of articulation.*

This perspective, therefore, requires that we view the variety of causal factors that can have an impact on language in terms of their effect on underlying language processing. Our working definition implies that the disordered language performance is a result of these disrupted processes. Also, this perspective must provide a way to view the variety of causal factors for use in our interpretation of

---

*From Rapin, I., and Wilson, B.C., Children with developmental language disability: Neurological aspects and assessment. In M. Wyke (Ed.), *Developmental Dysphasia.* New York: Academic Press, Inc., 13 (1978). Copyright by Academic Press Inc. (London) Ltd.

ausation. This will be done by discussing what both the child and the environment bring to language development and disorders.

The child. The child brings to language learning a set of intrinsic biologic and psychologic mechanisms necessary for language processing. Children will differ in terms of the intactness of these substrates for language. What the child brings to this task has been discussed in previous chapters and will only be outlined here for causal focus.

1. The child brings an intrinsic processing system. The Child Language Processing Model was developed in Chapter 3, focusing on underlying language processes related to language performance and behavior.
2. The child brings intrinsic cognitive mechanisms that shape language learning and use. A discussion of cognition and the relationship between language, learning, and cognition was developed in Chapter 3.
3. The child also brings a set of other intrinsic physical and psychologic mechanisms. Again, these were discussed in Chapter 3 and were presented as intrinsic lines of development including peripheral sensory development, motor development, development of behavioral control, development of neurologic organization for language processing, and development of neurologic stability. All these also shape the child's language development.

The status of these intrinsic biologic, psychologic, cognitive, and physical mechanisms determines what a child can and will learn. There are a variety of causal factors and means that can affect these intrinsic mechanisms, resulting in disruptions of the language processing system. These causal factors can be present at birth, as when any of the intrinsic mechanisms are damaged, or acquired at some time during childhood. Some are direct; for example, neurologic disease or trauma that directly disrupts central nervous system mechanisms. Others are more indirect; for example, an endocrine disorder that makes the child listless and therefore less responsive to the language learning process.

Some of these causal factors are more obvious in their effect on language processing than others. For example, the child with a bilateral cochlear degenerative process will be different in his language and his ability to learn language than a child with no problems of the peripheral auditory pathways. Similarly, a child born into a family where his father, paternal uncle, grandfather, and brother all were delayed in language acquisition and presented language learning difficulties may well come genetically wired for a language learning problem whereas a second child may have no known genetic basis for his problem.

An organization of the vast array of potential causal factors is needed. A portion of Nation and Aram's (1977) scanning device for searching out and cataloging causal factors that affect intrinsic mechanisms is outlined below*:

I. Scanning device for potential intrinsic causal factors
   A. Given biologic makeup
   B. Structural defects and growths
   C. Nutrition
   D. Diseases, infections and allergies
   E. Physical traumas and accidents
   F. Drugs and irradiation
   G. Psychologic-emotional mechanisms

The causal factor categories in the scanning device must be considered in light of their effect on language processes. The basic

---

* From Nation, J.E., and Aram, D.M., *Diagnosis of Speech and Language Disorders*. St. Louis: The C.V. Mosby Co., 124 (1977).

relationship to be expressed is the following: cause → affected intrinsic mechanism → disrupted language process → language behavior.

☐ **The student should develop a list of intrinsic causal factors that have been cited as important to child language disorders. Following the development of the list, categorize each into the scanning device and then consider the cause-effect relationship expressed above for each of the causal factors. Nation and Aram (1977) would be a useful first resource.**

The environment. Children, both intrinsically intact and not intact, are born into and live in an environment that may change drastically over the course of language development. This environment with all its people, things, and events must be viewed in terms of what it offers or does not offer to the child learning language. One would hope that the environment of language disordered children is not unlike that of most normal children. However, it is unlikely that any child with a language disorder would be reacted to in the same way as a normally developing child.

In Chapter 3, we discussed extrinsic environmental interactions and developed the theme that direct speech and language stimulation and the interpersonal context of communication serve in an instrumental way for the child to learn and process language. This section should be reviewed as it relates to extrinsic environmental causal factors.

Consistent with our working definition of child language disorders, extrinsic environmental factors must be considered in causal relationships to the language processing system. The implication expressed here is that language processing and resulting language behavior can only reflect the quantity and quality of the information put into the child. For example, Schiff and Ventry (1976) have documented the communication problems of hearing children of deaf parents. Further re-

search needs to address the relationship between environmental variables and disordered language.

Therefore organizing the many environmental variables of importance to language learning and use is complex and difficult. Earlier we (Nation and Aram, 1977) set about this task by first developing an environmental component to our speech and language processing model. The illustration of that component appeared as Fig. 3-3. We based this component on the primacy of speech and language input data as the crucial environmental determinant for learning speech and language. This variable also has the most direct relationship to underlying language processing.

From this component we derived a scanning device for searching out and categorizing environmental causal factors applicable to children with language disorders. This device has been adapted and is outlined below*

II. Scanning device for potential extrinsic environmental causal factors
  A. Speech and language input
    1. Quality
    2. Quantity
    3. Nonverbal communicative interaction
  B. Interpersonal factors
    1. Parents and parenting
    2. Sibling relations
    3. Other significant relationships
  C. Multisensory factors
    1. Physical-technologic
      a. Physical environment
      b. Technologic possessions and use
    2. Experiential
      a. Significant and abrupt changes
      b. Sensorimotor stimulation and exploration
  D. Sociocultural factors
    1. Income, economic status
    2. Education-occupation of parents and others
    3. Racial, ethnic practices

---

*Modified from Nation, J.E., and Aram, D.M., *Diagnosis of Speech and Language Disorders*. St. Louis: The C.V. Mosby Co., 124 (1977).

Considering the causal factor categories in the extrinsic scanning device requires that they be analyzed in relationship to underlying language processes. The basic relationship implied is: extrinsic environmental factor → disrupted language process → language behavior.

□ Again it is recommended that the student develop a list of extrinsic causal factors cited and discussed in the literature from which the causal relationship expressed above can be analyzed. For starters we suggest the language of deaf parents, bilingualism, television, and maternal deprivation.

In summary, the processing perspective requires the speech-language pathologist to view what the child brings (his intrinsic mechanism) and what the environment provides (his extrinsic conditions) in causal relationship to language processes as a means of interpreting disordered language performance and behavior. Each specific intrinsic and extrinsic factor suspected of being causally related to the language disorder must be interpreted on the basis of its impact on language processing.

Interactive perspective

The interactive perspective on causation in child language disorders stems from the principle that language behavior does not always reveal which cause came first, or what might be thought of as the primary cause. Language disorders rarely can be explained on the basis of a single variable or determinant.

The majority of children with language disorders come with a complex of multiple, potentially contributing influences upon their language development. No single clear cause can be identified; rather, several possible causes may be suggested in varying degrees of probability. Differences in the child's biologic and psychologic mechanisms, differences in speech, language, and other be-haviors, and differences in environmental circumstances all interact in dynamic, complex combinations resulting in a diversity of language disorders. The reciprocal actions and influences among these factors that make up the interactions must be explored to understand the language disorder.

Developmental perspective

Our developmental perspective draws upon the information presented in Chapter 3, the working part of the definition of child language disorders that states that child language disorders are "shaped by the developmental context in which they occur."

Children, by definition, mature in a developmental context. Both the child and the environment are subject to the effects of time and timing, the modifications, and the adaptations (both positive and negative) that take place. Time passes and changes occur. Development modifies, restructures, and alters the way in which any child will continue to process and use language. Many of these adaptations are creative attempts to maintain homeostasis, allowing the child and his family to shape their lives and responses to the language disorder and its causal basis in a positive direction.

□ The developmental perspective relates to the entire issue of child care practices in relation to developmental disorders. How does Sameroff (1975) treat this issue in his discussion of a continuum of caretaking causality?

Even when a specific causal factor was known to have an immediate effect on language processing, that effect will be modified over time. Other adaptations will enter into development and influence both the original cause and the original effect. In a sense, the cause and the effect will develop and modify both in relationship to one another. For example, a child's language disorder may be related to his seizure disorder, which may over time become controlled through medication, or conversely may become more frequent and less well controlled.

The changes that occur during development that provide the context that shapes and modifies how a child processes language is the perspective that provides us with a longitudinal view of child language disorders. Past events as well as current events can be analyzed and interpreted in relation to one another. What is going on with the child at the time he is seen can be analyzed in relation to events that took place in the past. The reader should return to Chapter 3 where this material is discussed in greater detail. Here we will focus on a causal issue that has been addressed at some length in the literature: time of occurrence of causation.

Time of occurrence of causation. In approaching time of occurrence of causation in child language disorders, tradition leads us to two major subdivisions of causation: (1) congenital and (2) acquired. However, as we addressed in our working definition, classification of child language disorders according to these two divisions becomes blurred. The reader should refer to that discussion in Chapter 3 as a basis for the following.

CONGENITAL CAUSATION. Congenital causes are generally considered to be present at birth, although they may not be identified until some growth and development has taken place. For example, if mental and physical problems are suspect at birth, they may not be revealed until certain cognitive and motor stages of development are expected. Or, in the case of neurolinguistic processing problems, may not be revealed until some measure of language comprehension and formulation can be taken. The congenital conditions may be genetically determined or may stem from prenatal or perinatal factors that disturbed what otherwise would have been a genetically normal child. The assumption made about the group of congenital causes is that the child does not bring to language learning and use an intact set of biologic and psychological mechanisms needed for normal development of language. According to the concepts presented in Chapter 3, children sustaining language disorders from congenital causes would be grouped as the following: (1) children with developmental language disorders whose causal basis was present at birth or (2) adults with persistent language disorders if the disorder is not resolved during childhood.

ACQUIRED CAUSATION. Acquired causal factors are those not considered to be present at birth but instead affect a normal child's biologic and psychologic mechanism after a period of more normal mental, physical, or language development has taken place. These factors disrupt language processing and interfere with language learning and use or create a regression in language development. The acquired group of causal factors occur after a substantial period of normal development, and they disrupt or diminish previously acquired language behavior. The assumption made about acquired causation is that the child initially had intact biologic and psychologic mechanisms, but some causal factor affected these mechanisms and interfered with language development.

To date, the majority of information addressing acquired forms of language disorder has appeared in the medical literature, and it is indeed surprising that the topic has received so little attention in speech-language pathology journals and texts. Only within the past few years have articles begun to appear that describe in detail the language loss sustained by children with acquired circumstances which disrupt language. While the potential number of acquired causes are many, the literature available has addressed the following primarily: (1) acquired central nervous system lesions, from trauma, infarcts and so forth (Alajouanine, 1965; Guttman, 1942; Hecaen, 1976; Lenneberg, 1967); (2) idiopathic EEG abnormalities associated with language loss (Cooper and Ferry, 1978; Gascon, Victor, Lombroso, and Goodglass, 1973; Landau and Kleffner, 1957; Shoumaker, Bennett, Bray, and Curless, 1974; Worster-Drought, 1971); and (3) regressive diseases and disorders, such as Heller's syndrome, or metabolic disturbances that manifest themselves only after a period of normal development (Aram, 1978; Courtney, 1978).

According to the concepts presented in Chapter 3, children sustaining language disorders from acquired causes affecting biologic and psychologic mechanisms could be categorized into any of the four groups described.

Although congenital versus acquired causation represents two clearly identifiable groups of causal factors, it is suggested here that these factors not be treated as discrete categories. Instead, they should be treated as opposite end points on a continuum. Although there are some important and very real differences between the language disorders associated with congenital and acquired causation (particularly in regard to the difference between interfering with language development and disrupting already acquired language and processing) an acquired causal factor also interferes with the ongoing development of language. For example, contracting meningitis at 3 years old may be categorized as an acquired causal factor; certainly the factor was not present congenitally or during development prior to 3 years old. Yet this acquired factor will go on to interfere with continued language learning that is still in a very active phase. Similarly, maternal death when a child is 2 years old may be viewed as a significant acquired factor that has a regressive influence on already acquired behavior but that also will have continued effect on future development. Thus, although there are theo-

retic and practical reasons for distinguishing between congenital versus acquired causal factors, it must be kept in mind that this distinction represents a continuum and not discrete dichotomy.

THE INTERACTIVE DEVELOPMENTAL ORIENTATION TO CAUSATION

From the preceding perspectives, it is clear that any view of causation that expresses a one-to-one relationship (one cause equals one effect) will not result in the best interpretation of a child's current language status. Whenever a child with a language disorder is seen, that child's language performance is a contemporary reflection of a series of events that have taken place over time. Thus a main effect analysis does not have the explanatory power of an interactive analysis.

Here we will bring the perspectives together into an interactive-developmental orientation to causation. This perspective focuses on the continous interactions between the child, his environment, and language behavior over time. These interactions are viewed as a succession of occurrences. Each new event adds to the nature and scope of the complex, continuous interactions. The orientation is designed to take into account the child's biologic and psychologic mechanisms, processing systems, environmental circumstances, language behaviors, adaptations over time, and the time of occurrence of causal factors. Consideration focuses on a child with a language processing disruption stemming from some intrinsic or extrinsic cause who presents faulty comprehension and formulation of language at one or more linguistic levels. This language disorder affects the environment and in turn is affected by the environment. Thus interactive-developmental cause-effect relationships occur. The speech-language pathologist can use this scheme to analyze and interpret the current developmental status of the child with emphasis on how any set of interactions have affected language processing resulting in disordered language behavior.

In Chapter 1 we illustrated this developmental interactive orientation through a simple figure (Fig. 1-1). These concepts will be amplified by adapting two figures from Nation and Aram (1977) that serve the two following purposes: (1) demonstrate plotting of causal factors according to the scanning devices and (2) develop a basic set of cause-effect interactions to guide our analysis and interpretation.

Plotting interactive factors

Fig. 4-1 plots a set of positive and negative factors over time that could be hypothesized for a child with a language disorder. The intent of plotting allows the speech-language pathologist to view any number of historical and contemporary factors that might be influential in understanding and interpreting the basis of the child's current language status. This plotting of factors only emphasizes the variables of importance apart from their effect on language processing or behavior.

Basic set of cause-effect interactions

In Chapter 1 we stated that complex interactions occurred between the following three points: (1) the multidimensional environment; (2) the language disordered child, including both biologic and psychologic mechanisms; and (3) the child's resultant speech, language, and other behavior. Chapter 3 expanded the aspects of the language disordered child's intrinsic language processing into what we termed the Child Language Processing Model. We now want to spell out more specifically the cause-effect interactions that may hold between the language processing of the child, his environment, and his language behavior. We have delineated the following four primary interactions:

1. Environment → Processing → Behavior
2. Processing → Behavior
3. Processing → Environment → Processing → Behavior
4. Behavior → Environment → Processing → Behavior

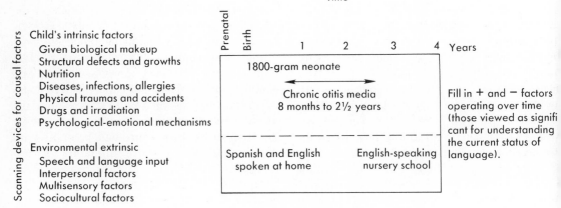

FIG. 4-1. Plotting interactive causal factors for a hypothetical 4-year-old child with a language disorder. (Modified from Nation, J.E., and Aram, D.M., *Diagnosis of Speech and Language Disorders*. St. Louis: The C.V. Mosby Co. [1977].)

In the following discussion we will describe each of these basic cause-effect interactions, further exemplifying our orientation to causation as an interactive-developmental orientation. These basic interactions may combine to produce a series of complex interactions accounting for involved interactions presented by some language disordered children.

Interaction 1: Environment → Processing → Behavior. Interaction 1 states that some environmental factor affects processing, which in turn results in poorer behavior. Although for language disordered children we usually think of these interactions in terms of negative effects that therefore lead to processing breakdowns and decreased language abilities, these interactions do not have to be in the negative direction. The fact that a particular child is doing as well as he is may be the result of a very "good" mother who intuitively has figured out how best to provide language input for her child. Although it is important to analyze both the positive and negative interactions that may occur, the majority of the examples presented here will stress negative influences, since we are attempting to identify factors that contribute to language breakdowns and disordered language.

As discussed in Chapter 3, the environment provides the data base from which children learn about their world and in particular their language. The environment and most importantly the people in that environment, especially parents, determine the amount, quality, and kind of learning experiences made available for a child. This interaction suggests that when environmental input is not optimal, language processing will be decreased, since the child does not have enough of whatever he needs to develop or use language effectively. This "whatever he needs" may involve the absolute language input made available as has been suggested by Schiff (1979) and Schiff and Ventry (1976),

who have studied the influence of deviant maternal language of deaf parents on the language development of their normally hearing children. The limitations provided by the environment may also be more related to limited diversity and experiences that language encodes, and thus the child may have less to process and less to talk about.

When environmental circumstances are extreme, as in the case of Arnold summarized in Chapter 1, these environmental restrictions may lead to actual biologic changes resulting from the environment (Fromkin, Krashen, Curtiss, Rigler and Rigler, 1974). For example, a mentally retarded mother may provide a poor diet for her 3-year-old son, which causes less than optimal mental and physical development and thus results in a language delay. A disturbed parent may repeatedly abuse her child by beatings that may lead to neurologic sequelae if sufficiently violent, which again in turn will affect language learning and use. A neglectful parent may ignore a child's ingestion of paint until accumulated lead has already affected the central nervous system, limiting further language and learning.

Karen, a 4-year-old, exemplifies Interaction 1. From all accounts, Karen seems to be a bright, responsive child; yet her general behavior and language immediately mark her as an unusual child. Although her hearing is normal, Karen habitually places her face as close as she can get to her listener and speaks in a loud, probably 70 decibel-level voice. The context of her language is hard to follow, consisting primarily of continual associations, often connected to occurrences during the first 3 years of her life. As the county welfare worker stated: "Karen has seen everything: sex, drugs, hunger, death—you name it." Although there is not evidence of intentional physical abuse, Karen experienced criminal neglect during the first 3 years, spending one night here, perhaps another week there, often left alone or in the care of children only somewhat older than herself. When removed from the natural mother at age 3, Karen was malnourished, filthy, and had received no medical attention since birth. She had few behavioral controls, talked incessantly but unintelligibly, flitting from one association to another, and did not respond appropriately when spoken to. After finally "becoming lucky" and having lived with a marvelous foster mother for a year, Karen now has put on weight, has learned to count to 20, knows the alphabet, is beginning to learn acceptable behavior, and displays in many ways her quickness in learning, but she continues to present a very striking language and social problem. Casting Karen into Interaction 1, we might summarize her situation in the following way: a disorganized, severely neglectful environmental situation, providing limited language and social learning opportunities and little data to be processed; poor nutrition that may have affected neurologic development; and no medical attention, the effect of which can only be speculative since we know nothing of the illnesses she may have had during this time. All of these have lead to a semantically disorganized, pragmatically unusual, and phonologically and syntactically deficient language behavior.

□ **The student is now referred back to Chapter 1 and the case study of Arnold. Cast Arnold's case history information into Interaction 1, specifying the environmental factors, probable processing effect, and resultant speech and language disorder. The student is referred to Fig. 4-1 for help in plotting causal factors as they occurred over time. What other hypothetic situations or real children with whom you have had experience would fit the interactions characterized in Interaction 1?**

**Interaction 2: Processing breakdown →
Behavioral disorder.** Interaction 2 states that some occurrence that directly causes a processing breakdown produces a behavioral dis-

order. This interaction is probably the most straightforward and common causal relationship that accounts for language disorders in children. Innumerable "organic" bases can be cited that create language disorders. For example, any form of conductive or sensorineural hearing problems that result in a chronic loss of hearing may cause a reduction in language abilities. Similarly, any abnormality of the central nervous system that reduces language processing will result in a language disorder, be they sensory limitations, motor limitations, or higher cortical function limitations. Thus a child with a brain stem tumor may have both reduced auditory processing as well as poor motor production, both of which may well affect the observed language behavior. Furthermore, any condition that leads to a more generalized impaired level of cognitive ability, such as Down's syndrome, often neurofibromatosis, or the Hunter-Hurler syndrome, will likewise result in disordered cognitive abilities, including language.

Stanley, Ruth, and Bill, all of whom were introduced in Chapter 1, can be seen to present cause-effect interactions where a processing breakdown was the primary causal factor leading to disordered language. It may be recalled that Stanley is an 8-year-old significantly retarded child who presents a very severely restricted expressive language consisting of 25 single words. Pregnancy with Stanley was complicated by severe toxemia and delivery was accomplished only after prolonged, arduous labor. The umbilical cord was tightly wrapped around his neck, and it was probable that he suffered anoxia during this process. Apgar scores* were 3 (at 1 minute

---

*An Apgar score is an evaluation of a newborn's condition with a maximum of two points assigned to each of five categories, including skin color, heart rate, respiratory effort, muscle tone, and reflex irritability. A score of 10 is perfect, with most normal newborns receiving scores of 7 or greater.

ute) and 5 (at 5 minutes), evidencing the rocky start with which he entered the world. These prenatal and perinatal events resulted in an impaired central nervous system that was revealed primarily as retardation and an even more pronounced expressive language disorder. In short, a central nervous system processing breakdown resulted in a range of behavioral disorders that included language.

☐ **Ruth and Alan are children presented in Chapter 1, each of whom had specific neurologic problems that resulted in reduced language ability. Ruth's problems were largely acquired, whereas Alan's were present at birth. Contrast the cause-effect relationships presented by these two children using Fig. 4-1 to plot primary causal factors as a function of time of occurrence. Drawing from the literature or real children with whom you have had experience, suggest other cause-effect relationships that may be cast into Interaction 2: Processing Breakdown → Behavioral Disorder.**

Interaction 3: Processing breakdown → Environment → Processing → Behavior. Up to this point the causal relationships specified have been relatively straightforward. However, often with child language disorders interactions do not proceed in one direction, as in Interaction 3. This cause-effect interaction states that some intrinsic mechanism that affects processing is impaired; this processing impairment affects the environment in such a way as to further reduce effective processing, ultimately resulting in disordered behavior. In Interaction 2, we examined how any intrinsic processing breakdown could directly result in disordered behavior. Here the interaction is not so direct. A processing breakdown (which in and of itself may also result in disordered behavior) feeds back to the environment in such a way as to further change processing, thus compounding already existing processing problems, all of which add up to disordered behavior.

Examples will help clarify this set of interactions. Eli, a 4-year-old, is a severely involved quadriplegic cerebral palsied child who ap-

pears to have aspects of normal ability particularly in areas of language comprehension, but who has very poor voluntary control of his motor system. Eli's 18-year-old mother is having difficulty enough coping with the facts of being a mother and a single parent, much less accepting and appropriately managing such a motorically impaired child. Deeply depressed and conflicted by her situation, the mother finds meeting Eli's most basic needs an almost impossible task. Thus he spends long hours in his crib with the television his most constant companion. The little interaction he has with his mother is perfunctory. She has not been able to sort out his abilities to understand and his needs for mothering from his very impaired motor ability. Thus what began as a motorically limited child evolved into an experientially and emotionally deprived child. The mother's reactions to Eli's processing deficits compounded the processing limitations, resulting in even more pervasive language deficits.

Such an interaction is not uncommon in the case of significantly impaired children where the environmental, often parental, reaction to an impaired child exacerbates an already existing problem. However, a feedback interaction from the processing of the child to the environment also can be observed in more subtle situations. Bill, introduced in Chapter 1, represents such a child. Bill entered this world with some mild processing limitations secondary to nutritional and possibly toxic effects of his mother's drinking. What was probably more important in contributing to Bill's language disorder was his mother's guilty reaction to what she perceived as a "damaged child" of her own making. With each new article she read documenting the effects of alcohol on unborn children, Bill became increasingly impaired in her perception. Although sober since his birth, she hesitantly evaluated his every ability, depriving both Bill and herself from spontaneous enjoyment and interaction with one another. Furthermore, she expected Bill to be retarded and therefore responded to him as if he were retarded and not capable of learning. Before a skillful therapist intervened, Bill was on the way to becoming the retarded child that his mother feared.

☐ **How might parents respond to an ostensibly normal child in such a way that further language processing might be impaired? Consider victims of child abuse, stepchildren, children with craniofacial abnormalities. What other examples come to mind?**

Interaction 4: Behavior → Environment → Processing → Behavior. Interaction 4 is similar to Interaction 3; however, in Interaction 3 it is the biologic or intrinsic child who influences the environment, further adding to processing deficiencies. In Interaction 4, it is some specified aspect of the child's behavior that sets off an environmental reaction which then in turn limits processing and adds to the behavioral deficit. The important distinction between Interactions 3 and 4 is that for Interaction 4 there is nothing intrinsically wrong with the child; the problem is that the parents or environmental circumstances do not respond appropriately to the child's behavior.

Two examples directed toward language behavior may further clarify this interaction. Two-year-old Todd's mother is a striving middle class mother, extremely concerned about Todd's failure to use connected speech. "How can we have a slow child, and if he is slow or can't talk, how can he go to Harvard Law School," is implicit in her questions and anxiety level. Todd's spontaneous attempts at communication are interrupted with constant admonishments to "Say hello to the doctor," "Did you say thank you?" "Tell the doctor your name," "Speak up so the doctor can hear you." And to the doctor, Todd's mother suggests, "I think Todd's stubborn, he just won't do what I tell him." Not only will Todd not talk when and as he is instructed, he also won't have his bowel movements where and when he is supposed to. Some time during his short 2 years, Todd seems to have learned that whatever he does is not quite right. He also has figured out that you can lead a horse to water but you can't make him drink, that if he does not act on cue, he becomes more powerful than if he attempts to comply with his mother's performance standards. In short, Todd's speech has become a concern for his mother, who has turned communication into a push-pull battleground. Todd has learned that withholding is as effective a strategy as he can come up with. While we rarely consider withholding language to be a primary factor in child language disorders, withholding more often may signal an area of difficulty for the child. In some infrequent situations, however, such a cause-effect relationship may account for the behavior presented.

More commonly encountered with children with disordered language are situations where the child's expressive language is taken as an indication of his level of comprehension and/or cognitive abilities. Although very little research has been directed toward describing the language environment of language disordered children (as noted in Chapter 3), such children must provide confusing signals for all but the most insightful parents. Should the child be spoken to at his level of language expression? Or language comprehension? How does a parent know how best to talk with a child who does not talk back? What keeps the parent motivated to keep talking when verbal communication is largely a one-way street? The language disordered child, particularly one with a significant discrepancy between his level of language comprehension and expression, may well be "spoken down to," thus being provided with less to process than what he is capable of. This in turn further adds to his already deficient expression.

□ Cramblit and Siegel (1977) have described the verbal environment of a language impaired child. How did this child's same-aged cousin, mother, father, and babysitter talk with the child? Was the verbal environment felt to have a facilitory or deleterious effect on the child's speech?

□ As a clinical exercise, briefly describe the language of the mother of a language-disordered child to her child. Is this mother directing her language to the child's level of comprehension? Expression? Or neither? Do you think her language helps or hinders her child's language development? Why or why not?

Multiple interactions over time

Above we have presented a series of four interactions that we consider to represent the basic cause-effect interactions accounting for child language disorders. We have presented these largely as discrete interactions, but we want to underscore the fact that for any one child several of these interactions may occur. Furthermore, the primary interactions occurring may change over time. At one point, for example, a mother may be primarily responding to the fact of having an impaired, possibly physically or mentally retarded child; later she may have successfully resolved her feelings of rejection and depression. At that point, the primary interaction operant may be Interaction 2, where the impaired processing results in impaired behavior, uncompounded by or even possibly facilitated by environmental contribution. Because multiple interactions may occur and these may change throughout the child's development, we have found it important to maintain a dynamic view of causation that allows for differing cause-effect relationships to surface as the environment, the child, and the child's behavior change.

What the orientation can do

Knowledge and insight about cause-effect relationships is vital to understanding how and why a child communicates as he does. The interactive developmental orientation presented here was designed to:

1. Be consistent with the language processing view taken in this book
2. Be dynamic and open-ended rather than static, increasing our understanding of causation rather than limiting it
3. Assist the speech-language pathologist in making the best estimates of the relationships among a variety of causal influences that can affect language development and use over time
4. Provide better insight and decisions about diagnosis and assessment of child language disorders
5. Lead to the most appropriate management and treatment objectives for each child with a language disorder

□ The student is encouraged to go back to Chapter 1 and trace the multiple cause-effect relationships that are stated or implied in the following case studies: Danelle, Bill, and Stanley. Hypothesize changed cause-effect interactions over time for at least one of these children.

□ Sameroff (1975) has written persuasively on causality in child development. How does he interpret cause-effect relationships in terms of biologic and environmental interactions? Compare his transactional model of causality with our interactive developmental model.

chapter 5

Speech to language processing disruptions

As part of our working definition of child language disorders we developed the Child Language Processing Model (CLPM, Fig. 3-2). This model incorporated a major processing unit with three processing segments as a way to view how children receive, comprehend, integrate, repeat, formulate, and produce messages. Our working definition emphasized that disordered language behavior in children is a reflection of disrupted language processes within these three segments. The processing segments can help us determine if the language disorder is related to the prelinguistic processing stages within the Speech to Language Segment, linguistic processing stages within the Language to Thought to Language Segment, or postlinguistic processing stages within the Language to Speech Segment.

Even when a process is not disrupted directly, whatever causal factors prevent a child from learning and using language appropriately will be reflected in his processing abilities. In Chapter 4 we developed scanning mechanisms to help understand and interpret the causal basis for the language processing disruptions.

In the next three chapters we will discuss the processing segments of the CLPM, focusing on how disruptions of language processing stages affect language learning and use in children. Chapter 5 will cover the Speech to Language Segment, Chapter 6 the Language to Thought to Language Segment, and Chapter 7 the Language to Speech Segment. Information about the processing stages within each segment will be amplified, incorporating theoretic information, research, and professional controversies about the relationship of language processes to language disorders in children.

A word of caution must be inserted for the reader in interpreting the information presented in Chapters 5, 6, and 7. Even though we are organizing our presentation of language disorders around processing disruptions within the three processing segments, we do not mean to imply that these are necessarily discrete relationships. Our intent is to provide a processing perspective to child language disorders and therefore we reiterate: language disordered children have many faces and facets. Each child must be assessed and treated individually in terms of his particular processing disruption and his unique interactive-developmental context.

DOMAIN OF SPEECH TO LANGUAGE PROCESSING DISRUPTIONS

Speech is an auditory event. It must enter and be transformed by the auditory modality before arriving at central language mechanisms for interpretation. The anatomy of the speech to language processing segment includes the bilateral auditory system, from the external ears to the primary auditory cortices. The anatomy of this complex, multiply crossed system is still incompletely understood. Chapter 9 in Daniloff, Schuckers, and Feth (1980) and Yost and Nielsen (1977) can be used as primary sources for review.

This Speech to Language Segment of the CLPM concentrates on two major processing stages: (1) sensation and (2) perception. Auditory operations within each of these two stages will be delineated. The purpose of this segment is to change the acoustic information in the incoming speech stimulus into a linguistic code by means of a series of auditory operations.

The processing stages within this segment are primarily prelinguistic analyses of the speech stimulus. These prelinguistic analyses act on the auditory characteristics of the stimuli, allowing the listener to derive sensory and perceptual information. Thus, this segment does not allow the listener to derive meaning from the message, but rather readies the auditory data for interpretation in the next segment.

A number of auditory operations have been identified as a part of this segment. The literature and the tasks used to measure these operations provide important background to this segment of the CLPM. Chapter 5 in Borden and Harris (1980) along with Daniloff et al. (1980) and Yost and Nielsen (1977) can serve as primary review resources. The function of this chapter therefore is to focus on the prelinguistic processes taking place within the

Speech to Language Segment and the disruptions that prevent the child from readying auditory information for further language processing by the next segment, the Language to Thought to Language Segment.

Although it would be infinitely simpler to demarcate this processing segment from the one that follows (Language to Thought to Language) by limiting it to prelinguistic processes, such a clear-cut division cannot be imposed strictly. The processing of phonologic information provides one example for this. Although phonology is considered part of the linguistic system, we are treating processing of incoming phonologic information within the Speech to Language Segment for several reasons. First, phonetic and phonologic processing are inextricably bound, and the overlap between prelinguistic and linguistic processing stages is most apparent when studying the parameters of the speech sound system. It therefore becomes cumbersome and artificial to separate phonetic and phonologic processing. Second, our clinical experience has led us to conclude that processing of phonologic data may be more closely akin to the "lower" processing stage of perception on the incoming side than to the "higher," more central language processes. Placing phonologic processing at the border between speech and language analyses is consistent with much of the theoretic and clinical data.

Theories of speech perception provide another reason these two processing segments cannot be strictly separated. These theories indicate that perceptual processing is aided by and done within a context of language. The results of prelinguistic processing of speech may not be simply fed forward; language processing (knowledge of syntax, semantics, and pragmatics) also appears to be fed back to aid perception. For example, a child's discrimination of *coat* versus *goat* may be aided by knowing what these words mean. Therefore, although the primary nature of Speech to Language Processing is preliminary to language processing, these prelinguistic processes are not divorced from language; rather, they are inextricably interdependent.

SENSATION PROCESSING STAGE
CLPM definition

Sensation, although activating all levels of the auditory system, is best viewed as primarily a peripheral rather than a central process. In its psychophysical sense it is a measure of absolute threshold. Sensation is considered a low level, behavioral response to the presence or absence of sound, an on/off reception of a stimulus. Any occurrence that interferes with a child's sensitivity to the intensity, range of frequencies, or total energy vibrations of the auditory stimulus will create a processing disruption of sensation.

Conductive and sensorineural disruptions

The study of conductive and sensorineural hearing losses form the basis of information for disruptions of the sensation processing stage. These peripheral hearing losses reduce the child's hearing abilities and thereby reduce the amount of auditory and language information available for further processing. These losses, depending on their types, severity, age of onset, and so forth, create a range of language and speech problems and require special skills in assessment, treatment, and education.

The study of deafness and hearing impairment, particularly from sensorineural hearing losses, and their relationship to language development and usage falls primarily within the professional area of audiology and education of the deaf. It is necessary, however, that speech-language pathologists keep in mind that language differences and disorders related to conductive and sensorineural hearing

losses are a part of their professional undertaking as well, and that these children comprise one subgroup of language disordered children. Our intent here is not to exclude them but to keep that information in professional perspective. It is assumed that the student will undertake study in audiology, aural rehabilitation, and speech and language of the hearing impaired. Berg (1976), Berg and Fletcher (1970), Ling (1976), Ling and Ling (1978), and Katz (1978) can be reviewed as primary resources for this information.

Before leaving the subject of conductive and sensorineural disruptions, we want to elaborate on an area of growing concern for the speech-language pathologist: the study of middle ear disease and conductive hearing loss and their effect on language development in young children. This study forms a large body of information in audiology and otolaryngology. Even though the effects of these ear problems on subsequent language and learning have been suggested, the primary effort has been principally directed to medical management, including drug treatment and surgical insertion of ventilating tubes.

One population of children of particular concern are those born with cleft lip and palate and other craniofacial anomalies. These children are known to have recurring, chronic bouts of middle ear disease with subsequent reduction of hearing (Paradise, Bluestone, and Felder, 1969). As the language differences became recognized, hypotheses relating the conductive hearing losses to the language differences were explored (Nation, 1970). For a major review of the subject of middle ear disease, hearing loss, and speech, language, and communication problems of the child with cleft lip and palate, refer to Graham (1978).

There is a growing recognition that middle ear disease and conductive hearing loss may be responsible for certain developmental delays seen in language. Rarely have such children been treated as hearing impaired, although hearing loss may have been present on a chronic or fluctuating basis over some time. Frequently these children appear for speech and language services with a history of ear infections but no current hearing loss. Middle ear disease and conductive hearing losses generally had not been considered high-risk indicators for language delays; however, recognition as such has recently been suggested by Brookhouser, Hixson, and Matkin (1979).

Most of the research thus far has been retrospective, taking a population of language delayed or disordered children and reviewing the medical histories for middle ear problems, or identifying a group of children who had early histories of middle ear disease and testing them on certain language measures. Ventry (1980) has provided a critical review of much of the recent literature. A workshop sponsored by the National Institute of Neurological and Communicative Disorders and Stroke on this subject was held in 1978 and its proceedings published in 1979 (Hanson and Ulvestad). In the summary of these proceedings, Ruben and Hanson (1979) state the following:

> While the literature is not definitely clear, the participants in this workshop, on the basis of literature reviewed, the presentations and discussion, reached the conclusion that temporary fluctuating mild hearing loss in the developing child, most usually associated with recurrent otitis media, may well have a significant effect on the child's development. The primary effect is probably on early acquisition of language skills. Indirect effects on cognition, social adjustment, school performance and academic achievement which are suggested by some studies could be related to delay in the normal maturation of language skills.*

Research is continuing to examine this relationship. A study by Johnson, Newman, and Glennan-Brethauer (1979) studied the relationship between otitis media, deficits in central auditory processing, and language deficits. They reported on four children with significant histories of otitis media. Although they found diverse profiles in the language behavior and central auditory test responses, all four children exhibited some positive central auditory findings and attentional deficits. They concluded:

> It is not our intention to suggest that all children with recurrent otitis media will have specific central auditory or linguistic deficits. However, these initial observations do imply that early identification and medical management of otitis media is important. In cases where conductive hearing loss has been established careful monitoring should be completed by the audiologist. These children should also be seen for speech and language screening so that appropriate intervention can be implemented.*

□ **What are some of the important issues raised by the workshop on otitis media and child development? What further research questions might be asked and how might the design of the studies meet the research design criticisms raised by the workshop participants (Hanson and Ulvestad, 1979)? Consult Ventry (1980) for his perspective.**

PERCEPTION PROCESSING STAGE
CLPM definition

Perception is the second processing stage within the Speech to Language Segment of the CLPM. As stated in Chapter 3, this processing stage is responsible for transducing the physical characteristics of speech stimuli into a speech code. Operationally, perception has included a number of hypothesized audi-

---

*From Ruben, R.J., and Hanson, D.G., Summary of discussion and recommendations made during the workshop on otitis media and development. *The Annals of Otology, Rhinology and Laryngology*, Supplement 60, Vol. 88, No. 5, Part 2, p. 111 (1979).

*From Johnson, A.F., Newman, C.W., and Glennan-Brethauer, N., Central auditory and language disorders associated with conductive hearing loss. Paper presented at the Annual Convention of the American Speech-Language Hearing Association, Atlanta, 6 (1979).

tory processes or operations. In the CLPM we have delineated these operations as prelinguistic; that is, analyses are performed on the auditory stimuli prior to derivation of meaning. Or, as Sanders defines it, "Auditory perception of speech is a process of interpreting the instructions imprinted on the acoustic wave by the speaker over a time span."[*]

Auditory processing and speech perception are areas of study basic to understanding disruptions of the perceptual processing stage of the CLPM. We recognize that hearing loss affects language by disrupting sensation. The assumption about auditory processing is similar. Disruption of auditory perceptual processes can interfere with the child's ability to comprehend, integrate, and formulate language. However, these relationships are not yet understood, the data is equivocal, and much work is being undertaken to clarify the many issues that exist.

Speech perception

Command of the subject matter of speech perception in normal children, particularly developmental aspects of speech perception, is important for the reader as a background for study of the language disordered child. The following will summarize some of the current theories of speech perception and speech perception research in infants and young children, and will point the direction for further reading in these areas.

Theories of speech perception. Speech perception has been actively investigated for some time, and numerous theories have been developed. Controversy has centered around a number of issues, including how active the listener is in forming his perception of speech, what role motor systems play in perception, whether perception is carried out in a serial

or simultaneous manner, and if perception represents a bottom-up versus top-down analysis.

The box on pp. 89 and 90 from Sanders (1977) presents a summary of some of the major theories of speech perception divided into active and passive theories. Other reviews of speech perception theories are available, including Pisoni (1975), Lieberman (1972), Massaro (1975), Darwin (1976), and Davis (1978). Here we will not discuss these theories of speech perception but will abstract some tentative and not universally held conclusions that have relevance for child language disorders.

First, it is probable that speech perception encompasses both active and passive processes. Specialized neurologic mechanisms within the auditory system may allow for the decoding of auditory information resulting in phonetic and ultimately phonemic identification. However, the presence of passive processes such as Abbs and Sussman's (1971) hypothesized feature detectors do not exclude the role of more active, listener-based perceptual strategies. Even if the listener possesses an auditory system uniquely designed to transform auditory information to linguistic information, what he knows about language may well provide a knowledge base that allows him to structure what he hears. A part of a listener's perception may well be shaped by what he knows about the formal rules of his language (as in an analysis-by-synthesis model of speech perception, Stevens, 1972; Stevens and Halle, 1967), or what he knows about producing speech (as in a motor theory of speech perception, Liberman, et al, 1967 a, b).

In either the active or passive approach to speech perception, it is likely that perception of incoming speech is modified by the listener's knowledge of speech and language. The ability to use language and to produce speech

---

[*]From Sanders, D.A., *Auditory Perception of Speech.* Englewood Cliffs, N.J.: Prentice-Hall, Inc., 98 (1977).

Abstract of major exponents of passive and active theories of speech perception[*]

PASSIVE THEORISTS (non-mediated, direct decoding)

Selfridge

"Pandemonium Model." Complex signal interrogated by "demons" (computational, cognitive, decision) to determine the presence or absence of the features they represent. System is tuneable by weighting relationship patterns between computational and cognitive levels.

Uttley

Neurological model based on mathematical classification of the CNS. Binary analysis leading to identification of a unique pattern of firings. Four requirements must be met:

(1) Input channels identifiable as active/inactive
(2) Multiple combination of inputs
(3) Indicator unit for each combination denoting *active* status of each component thus defining the pattern
(4) Storage capacity

Fant

Source (voice)/Filter (articulators and resonators) Model which uses distinctive-feature theory. Source characteristics:

(a) silence
(b) voice
(c) voice and noise
(d) noise.

Acoustic features mapped onto neurological features of auditory system. This results in internal auditory pattern representations. Acknowledges parallel encoding at phonemic level and need for syllabic processing.

Hughes and Hemdal

Computer-based Model. Acoustic signal analyzed in binary form according to distinctive features for categories of sound. Each decision determines the routing of subsequent interrogation. It does this by computing the probabilities of occurrence from the data already available. System is self-adjusting (tuneable) to allow for inter-speaker variation (normalization).

Abbs and Sussman

Neurological model. Feature detection based on auditory decoding. Features represented as specialized neural configurations. Parallel processing of information of transitional cues. Efferent control permits neural tuning through selective lateral inhibition. Rapid sorting of speech sounds into categories according to distinctive features.

[*]From Sanders, D.A., *Auditory Perception of Speech: An Introduction to Principles and Problems.* Englewood Cliffs, N.J.: Prentice-Hall, Inc., 100-101 (1977). *Continued.*

Abstract of major exponents of passive and active theories of speech perception—cont'd

---

ACTIVE THEORISTS (mediated, indirect coding)

Liberman et al. (Haskins Lab Group)

Postulate a motor theory based on the mediative role of the neuromotor rules of speech production. Propose that the model operates from phonemic to semantic levels of linguistic processing. Speech is perceived by reference to manner and place of production of the speech wave. Speech production and perception seen as unique process involving

    (a) a special function

    (b) a distinctive form

    (c) use of a special key to encode/decode

    (d) a special perceptual mode. Sees speech as hierarchically structured at all levels. Parallel encoding and decoding. Relates parallel encoding to co-articulatory function and syntax. Segmental analysis is recognized. Speech is perceived by running the production process backward.

Stevens and Halle

Analysis-by-synthesis model based upon hypothesis testing. This involves perceiving speech by comparing incoming signal (acoustically and linguistically) to internally generated patterns. These internal representations are generated according to rules selected on probabilities based on earlier data. Concur with Liberman that generative rules are highly similar to those used in production. Abstract representation of speech event fundamental to production and perception. Identification of appropriate generative rules permits invariance to be maintained through computing of error correction (normalization).

---

affects speech perception. For example, a listener may recognize a speech segment to be /flaɪ/ rather than /əlaɪ/ even if he does not hear the /f/ə/ distinction, since he knows /flaɪ/ is permissible in English phonology, whereas /əlaɪ/ is not. Or he may make reference to articulatory movements, realizing that he does not produce /ə + l/ combinations although an /f + l/ combination is acceptable. Or, if the sound sequences heard are coupled with what is seen, it would direct his perception to "fly" rather than "thly." It could be hypothesized that language disordered children are deficient in their biologic prewiring, not allowing them to passively decode the auditory signal into a speech form, or that their difficulties with language development prevent them from active speech perception.

Second, it appears that speech is not simply analyzed in a temporal, sequential order, but that multiple parameters of the stimulus may be decoded simultaneously. Thus, the speech stimuli is not simply decoded phoneme by phoneme; rather, phonetic analysis may be simultaneously analyzed along with semantic, syntactic, and possibly pragmatic information to form perceptual hypotheses about what has just been heard. Speech perception may involve informational analysis at each level simultaneously.

Third, it may be that various strategies of speech perception change during development. For example, the degree to which an individual relies upon passive versus active strategies or motor reference versus semantic reference may vary depending on the stage of development of the infant, child, or adult. It could be speculated that, for example, an 8-month-old relies on passive strategies since he has not yet learned language, whereas an 8-year-old with language uses more active strategies.

Fourth and finally, all language disordered children may not be equally dependent on the same perceptual strategy for understanding speech. Thus, it is conceivable although not objectively demonstrated that language disordered children with very little language comprehension may be operating primarily on the basis of passive prewiring. Or alternatively, children with good comprehension but limited articulated speech, as in severe developmental dysarthrias or apraxias, may have to rely on perceptual strategies that do not make reference to motor production, since motor ability is impaired in these children. Although such differences in speech perception strategies need to be demonstrated through further research with language disordered children, the possible occurrence of alternative strategies for speech perception in children with developmental language disorders raises an intriguing research question.

Developmental aspects of speech perception. An active area of research has been the study of infant speech perception. Here the intent has been to chart what parameters of acoustic and speech stimuli infants and young children perceive and the developmental progression of their perception. Again, we will summarize some of the major findings and point the reader toward resources where he might fill out his background.

First of all, we know from both behavioral paradigms such as high amplitude sucking in which the infant's change in sucking is re-

lated to the stimulus presentation (Eimas, Siqueland, Jusczyk, and Vigorito, 1971), as well as from the use of auditory evoked potentials, which are the measurement of changes in electrical activity in the brain following stimulation (Molfese, 1977), that neonates can discriminate at least some phonetic distinctions such as voicing (Eimas et al., 1971). Furthermore, it has been shown that very shortly after birth, if not immediately, placement of articulation distinctions also are made, notably placement of stop consonants (Moffitt, 1971; Eimas, 1974a) and fricatives (Eilers and Minifie, 1975). It has also been demonstrated that infants, like adults, discriminate vowels in a continuous manner, whereas stop consonants are discriminated in a categoric manner (Trehub, 1973; Swoboda, Morse and Leavitt, 1976).

Much of this work demonstrating the very early capability of infants to make phonetic distinctions has been used as support for the presence of biologically determined, innate phonetic feature analyzers (Cutting and Eimas, 1975; Cole, 1977). Although it has been demonstrated that lower animal forms including the chinchilla and Rhesus monkey can make some of these distinctions such as voicing and place of articulation (Waters and Wilson, 1976; Morse and Snowdon, 1975; Kuhl and Miller, 1975), other distinctions have not been demonstrated except in humans.

While the work in infant speech perception has lent support for the presence of feature detectors (hypothesized intrinsic sorting devices for phonemes), the influence of the language environment on speech perception has also been demonstrated, lending some support for the theories suggesting that knowledge of language influences perception. For example, Streeter (1976) demonstrated that 2-month old Kikuyu infants were capable of making distinctions between prevoicing, voicing, and voiceless consonants, a voicing distinction present in Kikuyu but not English.

Other researchers, among them Eisenberg (1970, 1976) and Morse (1974), have examined and summarized other aspects of infants' and young children's responses to speech and other auditory parameters, such as frequency, intensity, and duration of the stimuli.

☐ **Refer to the following sources for further information relative to speech perception in infants and young children: Morse (1974, 1977), Eimas (1974b, 1975), Eisenberg (1976), and Cole (1977). What does Weener's (1974) article contribute to our understanding of the development of auditory perception?**

A search for auditory processes

A major thrust of the writings relevant to the perceptual processing stage and child language disorders has been to search for and define a series of auditory processes. Following is a listing of auditory processes as viewed by several major professionals working in this area:

Sanders (1977)
Aspects of auditory processing

1. Awareness of acoustic stimuli
2. Localization
3. Attention
4. Differentiation between speech and nonspeech
5. Auditory discrimination
   a. suprasegmental discrimination
   b. segmental discrimination
6. Auditory memory
7. Sequencing
8. Auditory synthesis

Weener (1974)
Basic components and measurement procedures of auditory processing

1. Echoic memory
   a. Duration
2. Discriminative filter
   a. Selective attention
   b. Phoneme and word discrimination
3. Structural analyzer
   a. Utilization of linguistic structure

Chalfant and Scheffelin (1969)
Auditory processing tasks

1. Attention to auditory stimuli
2. Sound versus no sound
3. Sound localization
4. Discriminating sounds varying on one acoustic dimension
5. Discriminating sound sequences varying on several acoustic dimensions
6. Auditory figure-ground selection
7. Associating sounds with sound sources

Eisenson (1972)
Perceptual functions underlying language acquisition

1. Selectivity
2. Discrimination
3. Categorization
4. Perceptual defense
5. Proximal and distance reception
6. Sequencing

Wiig and Semel (1976)
Auditory-perceptual processing

1. Attention
2. Localization
3. Figure-ground
4. Discrimination of nonverbal stimuli
5. Discrimination of verbal stimuli
6. Sequencing
7. Synthesis: resistance to distortion
8. Segmentation and syllabication

Butler (1975)
Subcomponents of auditory perception

1. Auditory vigilance
2. Figure-ground
3. Auditory analysis
4. Auditory discrimination
5. Auditory sequencing
6. Sequencing unrelated speech sounds
7. Intonation patterns
8. Auditory closure
9. Auditory synthesis
10. Auditory memory (for nonsense multisyllable words)
11. Auditory association

Bangs (1968)
Avenues of learning

1. Sensation
2. Perception
3. Memory-retrieval
4. Attention
5. Integration

When outlining a series of auditory processes, most writers caution that the series they enumerate must be treated as highly interdependent, overlapping processes rather than discrete, steplike occurrences. For example, Sanders (1977) cautions use of his list with the following reservation:

> Thus, while our consideration of speech perception is strongly supportive of a holistic treatment of incoming speech data, it would be unrealistic to claim that there do not exist identifiable components in this process. The problem is that *at this time we do not know the specific nature of each function, nor do we understand how each interacts with other functions*. An attempt to describe the components makes apparent the fact that each is so intimately involved with all other aspects of processing that it is impossible to define any as truly autonomous.*

As can readily be seen from these lists, a wide variety of auditory processes have been hypothesized reinforcing the reservations expressed by Sanders (1977). It must be kept in mind that the auditory processes viewed by each of the authors stem from their theoretic view of auditory processing as well as its relationship to language learning and use.

Many of the processes have been derived from tasks used to measure some parameter of auditory stimuli—nonlinguistic, prelinguistic, and linguistic. Thus when research is conducted in auditory processing, it is frequently defined in terms of the auditory tasks used rather than assuming a true auditory process is being measured. Therefore the search for a series of or stages of auditory processes must be interpreted as such, rather than as demonstrable, proven, and discrete auditory processes that explain language development, usage, and disorders.

□ Referring to the preceding list of auditory processes, explore the following:
1. Each author has referred to auditory processing in a somewhat different manner, defining the processes as aspects, components, tasks, and so forth. What subtleties in orientation may be implied by these differences?
2. How do the authors of these lists define each of the processes specified: by theory, tasks, or measures?
3. Examining the list, what similarities and differences do you see that are evident? Is it possible to arrive at a composite list that incorporates all these processes? Would the composite list be more or less inclusive?

Disruptions of auditory operations

If the relationship of auditory perceptual disruptions to language disorders in children is to be studied, the components of this perceptual processing stage must be examined, as Sanders did in 1977. Even though the research is unclear at this time, a list of auditory processes, here termed auditory operations, is presented below as a means to discuss auditory processing disruptions and their relationship to child language disorders.

We have proposed five auditory operations, recognizing that these are not mutually exclusive nor are they necessarily considered to be hierarchical stages of perceptual processing. The five auditory operations follow:
1. Auditory attention
2. Auditory rate
3. Auditory discrimination
4. Auditory memory
5. Auditory sequencing

These auditory operations are represented in Fig. 5-1 as a circle to prevent viewing them as hierarchical stages. Quite likely they are simultaneous operations, interrelated in a complex and continuous manner. Therefore we do not want to imply that attention, for example, must precede the other operations. Therefore in our discussion of these auditory operations we will be assuming a relationship between the operations and child language disorders.

We offer pragmatic rather than purely theoretic justification for our selection and concentration of these five operations. First, these

---

*From Sanders, D.A., *Auditory perception of speech: An introduction to principles and problems*. Englewood Cliffs, N.J.: Prentice-Hall, Inc., 201 (1977).

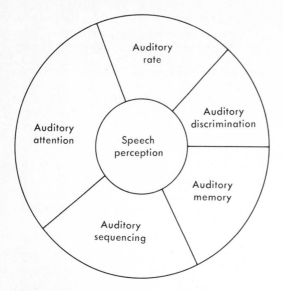

FIG. 5-1. Five basic auditory operations that are interdependent for prelinguistic perceptual processing of speech (auditory) input information.

operations represent aspects of clinically observable perceptual problems. There appear to be children whose chief perceptual problem is attending to what is said. When they are attending, the message seems to get through, but there is a problem in gaining and maintaining attention. Similarly, there are children whose chief perceptual problem is adapting to the rate at which speech stimuli are presented. Still others seem to have difficulty forming perceptual categories or having difficulty discriminating among them. Some children seem not to be able to retain speech stimuli long enough to abstract information from it. These children present the memory problems that are often implicated in language disordered children. Finally, there are those in our clinics who seem to retain auditory information but get the order jumbled. Since there are clinically based justifications for our choices of auditory operations, it is believed that many speech-language pathol-

ogists will recognize children who have problems with these specified auditory operations. We do not know whether these operations will be borne out by future research; however, at this time they allow for clinically useful subdivisions of auditory perception.

Apart from clinical utility, our choices of auditory operations were guided by the theoretic and research literature. These five auditory operations encompass a body of information important to understanding the relationship between auditory processing and child language disorders. In the next section we will review this literature for each of the auditory operations.

It must be stated at the outset that the available literature does not address a wide range of child language disorders and in some instances focuses primarily on children defined as learning disordered, minimally brain injured, or having minimal cerebral dysfunction. At times it is not known whether these clinical groups have language disorders along with the learning disorders. Other literature focuses heavily on children classified as aphasic. Thus we draw upon a range of literature that often says little about the nature of the language disorder and seldom compares language disordered children, with and without demonstrable brain dysfunction, to normal children. We are a long way from knowing how important each of these operations is for normal and disordered language. With this in mind we will give a summary of pertinent literature for each of these auditory operations.

Auditory attention. Attention as an auditory phenomenon usually incorporates such concepts as selective attention, the ability to ignore irrelevant auditory stimuli and to separate auditory figure-ground relationships. When listening to speech the listener presumably separates the important auditory speech signal from any ambient, interfering background stimuli.

Although many writers note the frequent occurrence of attentional deficits in language disordered children, surprisingly little research has been directed toward its study. Several commercial tests are designed to test auditory attention and have been used with language disordered children, leaving us with a situation where most of what we know about language disordered children's attentional problems derives from their performance on these tests. Thus auditory attention becomes operationally defined as what the attention tests measure. Little research data is available aside from performance on these standardized tests.

For example, Costello (1977), in discussing the development of the Flowers-Costello Test of Central Auditory Abilities (Flowers, Costello, Small, 1970), noted that many children with language and reading problems exhibit difficulty with selective or attentional listening. She commented that these children may function acceptably in ideal listening conditions, but they manifest difficulty in conditions of acoustic distortion, visual distraction, and other kinds of confusion. Terming this a difficulty in selective or attentional listening, she and Flowers developed a test battery that would allow them to compare a child's response under ideal listening conditions to his performance in conditions requiring increased levels of attentional listening (including frequency distortion using low-pass filtered speech) and competing messages.

After the Flowers-Costello Test of Central Auditory Abilities was developed, it was presented to various groups of speech and/or language disordered children (Flowers and Costello, 1963; Thies and Thies, 1972) who were found to perform more poorly on these tests. It was then concluded that these language/speech disordered children presented difficulties with auditory attention.

One study that may be as much a study of

auditory discrimination as one of auditory attention was done by Brotsky (1970). A test of auditory figure-ground perception was developed and was used to compare 26 aphasic children with 26 normal children in their ability to discriminate spondee words (two-syllable words having equal stress on each syllable, such as *baseball*). These words were presented with varying background noises (running water, traffic, a playground, and a carnival) at 60:45 dB HL signal to noise ratio. Although the groups were significantly different from each other, the complexity of the type of background noise did not affect discrimination performance significantly. Wiig and Semel (1976) and Berry (1969) speak of difficulties with auditory attention in language disordered children, but do not reference research findings. A review of the *Journal of Speech and Hearing Disorders* and *Speech and Hearing Research* uncovered no articles addressing auditory attention and language disordered children other than those who were of school age and were classified as learning disabled. Wiig and Semel (1976) also discuss research with learning disabled children (Lasky and Tobin, 1973; Ricks, 1974).

Exemplary of these studies is that of Lasky and Tobin (1973) who compared the ability of 11 normal first graders and 11 first graders who were suspected of being learning disabled. These investigators found that the suspected learning disabled children's performance was adversely affected by competing linguistic stimuli, but that white noise (nonlinguistic competing stimuli) did not affect their performance. Studies such as that of Lasky and Tobin demonstrate that learning disabled children may be negatively affected by tasks that compete for their attention, thus demonstrating auditory attention deficits. The nature of the attentional deficit in such conditions, however, remains unspecified. Is the learning disabled child having difficulty blocking out the competing stimuli and therefore responding to it, exhibiting a deficit in shifting attention? Or does he have difficulty focusing on either message, a failure to attend rather than a failure to shift attention? Questions such as these remain unanswered for language disordered children, although they may fail these auditory attention tasks when competing stimuli are introduced. Yet why they fail and what the basis of the attentional deficit is remains unknown. Auditory attention deficits, a clinical phenomenon in child language disorders recognized by most speech-language pathologists, remains largely an unexplored area of study.

Auditory rate. Clinicians working with both adults and children with language disorders have long noted that rate of presentation of auditory information seemed to be a variable relating to their client's ability to understand what was said to them. McGinnis (1963), for example, suggested that clinicians use slowed speech when talking with aphasic children.

Studies with normal children have shown that young children perform better on comprehension tasks when they are presented at slower rates (Berry and Erickson, 1973; Bonvillian, Raeburn and Horan, 1979). Furthermore, Tallal (1976) has demonstrated that only the oldest children in her study of normals, the 8½-year-olds, responded as well as adults to auditory patterns presented in rapid succession (8 to 305 millisecond intervals), but that normal 6½-year-old children could respond correctly to the same patterns if presented more slowly. Thus it appears that our ability to respond to auditory information at increased rates shows a developmental trend.

Unlike the situation in attention, auditory rate and its relationship to comprehension in both normal and disordered populations has been researched considerably. The study of auditory rate and its influence on language has revolved primarily around artificially altering the rate of presentation of the stimuli, including lengthening and shortening various parameters of both speech and nonspeech auditory stimuli.

Two very active groups of investigators have dominated much of the experimental work pertaining to rate alterations and their effect on language comprehension. One group has concentrated on time compressed speech, and the second has systematically lengthened and shortened both speech and nonspeech stimuli.

COMPRESSED SPEECH. The early work with time-compressed speech was largely devoted to two undertakings. The first was directed toward the development of time-compressed procedures, discussed at length in Beasley and Maki (1976) and Beasley and Freeman (1977). While initially fast-slow playback techniques and chop-splice procedures were used to develop compressed speech stimuli, the development of the electromechanical time compressor expander (Fairbanks, Everitt and Jaeger, 1954; Lee, 1972) allowed for a mechanized means of shortening or lengthening the auditory stimulus. This equipment reduced the disadvantages of frequency distortions (as in fast-slow playback methods) and the time-consuming tape preparation in the chop-splice methods. Probably the most widely used time-compressed tasks include use of the Word by Picture Identification Index (WIPI, Ross and Lerman, 1971) and the PB-K 50 word lists (Haskins, 1949), at 0%, 30%, and 60% compression of normal duration.

These procedures were used with normal groups of children in order to establish normative data (Beasley, Forman, and Rintelmann, 1973; Beasley, Maki and Orchik, 1976; Beasley, Schwimmer and Rintelmann, 1972). For example, Beasley, Maki, and Orchik (1976) presented these two speech discrimination measures, the WIPI and the PBK-50, at 0%, 30%, and 60% compression to 60 normal children between the ages of 3½ to 8½ years. They reported that the average intelligibility scores increased as a function of increasing age and sensation level and decreased with increasing amounts of time compression. These procedures were also applied to various clinical groups, including persons with sensorineural hearing losses (Kurdziel, Rintelmann, and Beasley, 1975; Maki, Beasley, and Shoup, 1976), aging persons (Konkle, Freeman and Riggs, 1977), persons with known hemispheric lesions (Kurdziel, Noffsinger, and Olsen, 1976; Snow, Rintelmann, and Miller, 1977), children with acquired aphasia (Oelschlaeger and Orchik, 1977), children with reading problems (Freeman and Beasley, 1978), and children with auditory perceptual problems (Manning, Johnston, and Beasley, 1977).

It has been suggested that time-compressed procedures provide a useful diagnostic tool for determination of site of lesion in children with acquired aphasia. Results for an 11-year-old with an acquired left hemisphere lesion indicated significantly poorer speech discrimination at 60% compression in the ear contralateral to the left hemisphere (Oelschlaeger and Orchik, 1977).

In using time-compressed speech with children with auditory perceptual disorders (defined as normal performance on visual tasks but at least one year below chronologic age norms on two of the auditory subtests of the ITPA [Kirk, McCarthy, and Kirk, 1968] or the Full-Range Action-Agent Test [Gesell, 1940]), Manning, Johnston, and Beasley (1977) reported that their 20 auditorily impaired 6½- to 8½-year-old children showed no change in performance from 0% to 30% compression, but performed significantly poorer at 60% compression. The author's conclusion, that 60% compression interferes with comprehen-

sion due to difficulties in processing incoming auditory information at increased rates of presentation, appears to be consistent with other research in rate alteration. Their suggestion, however, that 30% compression aids the performance of language disordered children is provocative and much criticized (Tallal, 1979).

Tallal, for example, has criticized this interpretation of the findings on grounds that if the children with auditory processing difficulties showed no change at 0% to 30% compression, this does not evidence that compression aids processing. Tallal also has criticized the findings on methodologic grounds in that insufficient data were reported regarding selecting and matching criteria of the "normal" children to whom these children were compared. Furthermore, Tallal points out that although the authors report that the disordered group's performance was poorer than the control group's at 1% to 60% compression, both groups demonstrated considerable variability. The authors do not report whether the differences were in fact statistically meaningful ones or merely the result of random variation.

Although the interpretation of the failure to show deterioration in performance at 30% compression is open to question (Manning et al., 1977) the possibility should not be dismissed altogether. As we have noted repeatedly, different language disordered children present different processing abilities and disabilities. Although increased rate of presentation may well cause disruptions in accommodating to auditory rate, there is no reason for assuming that the relationship between level of processing difficulty and rate is linear. It is possible that children's performance may suddenly "decompress," or rapidly fall apart, when a critical rate-compression is passed. Furthermore, a child may present both a difficulty accommodating to rate and a short-term memory deficit. In such a situation, it may be that relatively small increments may aid comprehension while greater increments cause a rapid deterioration in ability. Although the evidence does not yet allow for such claims, Manning et al. (1977) have advanced a hypothesis worthy of further consideration.

OTHER AUDITORY RATE ALTERATIONS. The second group of investigators who have been particularly active in examining the effects of auditory rate on language performance in children are Tallal and her co-workers. They have studied the relationship of auditory rate and developmental dysphasia in a highly controlled, systematic, incremental manner.

Throughout their experimentation these investigators employed two nonverbal operant conditioning methods as response modes. The first method, the *repetition method,* required the child to associate the panel presses with the auditory stimuli to be discriminated. They were then required to repeat what they heard. This was done by successively indicating the panel presses that corresponded to the stimuli. Thus the children were required to respond with a successive motor response. The second method of response was termed the *same-different technique.* It simply required that the children press one panel if the two stimuli presented were the same and the other panel if the stimuli were different, thus not requiring a sequential motor response.

These investigators have systematically studied dysphasic children's ability to handle alterations in the rate of auditory nonverbal stimuli, visual nonverbal stimuli, and alteration of various parameters of verbal auditory stimuli. In early reports Tallal and Piercy (1973 a, b) demonstrated that dysphasic children had difficulty discriminating nonverbal auditory stimuli when the duration of the stimulus elements themselves was decreased as well as when the interstimulus interval or time between stimuli (ISI) was decreased.

These authors hypothesized that aphasic children were unable to perceive auditory stimuli at a normal rate and suggested that this difficulty in auditory processing lay behind their language impairment. In discussing their findings, these researchers note that the adverse effect of the short interstimulus interval on the dysphasic children's performance was not absolute, since it could be compensated for by increasing the duration of the stimuli. Rather, it seemed to be the total duration of the two stimuli and the intervening interval that were critical for the performance of these language impaired children. Furthermore, Tallal and Piercy (1973b) found the effect of duration of auditory stimulus was specific to the auditory modality, since their children performed comparably to the normal control group on a rapid visual sequence task.

Tallal and Piercy (1975) have extended this early work with nonverbal auditory and visual stimuli to incorporate verbal stimuli. Using synthesized vowels (/ɛɪ/ and /æɪ/) and CV combinations (/ba/ and /da/), they demonstrated that dysphasic children are impaired in their ability to discriminate the format transitions in CV combinations. This difficulty was not because of an inherent problem in perceiving and discriminating transitions, but because of the very brief duration of this crucially important parameter of consonantal discrimination. When the format transitions of the synthesized consonant vowel stimuli were extended from 40 to 80 milliseconds, the dysphasics performed comparably to the normal controls. This demonstrated that the dysphasics could discriminate between speech sounds mediated by transitions, provided they were sufficiently long in duration.

More recently, Tallal and her co-investigators have demonstrated that these difficulties perceiving and discriminating the rate of auditory information extend to meaningful words (Tallal and Stark, 1979), and likewise that these perceptual difficulties are reflected in the children's speech production (Tallal, Stark, and Curtiss, 1976; Tallal and Piercy, 1978). Tallal et al. (1976, 1978) reported that the seven perceptually impaired dysphasic children studied were significantly worse than the seven perceptually unimpaired dysphasics and normal control groups in three areas: their production of isolated steady state vowels, stop consonants in both CV and CVC nonsense syllables, and stop consonants in clusters. They furthermore suggested that the dysphasic children's pattern of production corresponded to their perceptual impairment; that is, the production of isolated vowels and nasals was significantly less impaired than that of stop consonants, especially in clusters. Tallal and Piercy made the following conclusion:

> Those speech sounds incorporating rapid spectral changes critical for their perception are most difficult for dysphasic children to perceive and are also most often inaccurately produced. These results add further support to the hypothesis that developmental dysphasia can be accounted for, at least in part, by a failure to develop an auditory perceptual process necessary for the perception of speech.*

Tallal and her co-workers therefore have rather convincingly demonstrated that the absolute rate of auditory information affects at least some language disordered children's ability to discriminate between stimuli. Furthermore these investigators have shown that this difficulty with auditory rate is evidenced on both a nonverbal and verbal level and does not seem to arise from a difficulty with formant transitions if these transitions are extended in duration.

Auditory discrimination. Auditory discrimination has been one of the most studied audi-

tory perceptual operations in relationship to speech and language disorders and probably presents some of the most confusing literature. Much of this confusion stems from the variety of tasks for measuring auditory discrimination—tasks varying from discriminating between two pure tones to tasks requiring listeners to indicate whether two sentences were the same or different. Thus discrimination tasks range from nonlinguistic to linguistic to metalinguistic.

Here the auditory discrimination operation is considered prelinguistic, making discriminations among speech sounds without demanding that the listener derive meaning from what is to be discriminated. This operation includes phonetic, phonemic, and phonologic discrimination and programming.

Since the very early days of our profession, speech pathologists have assumed a relationship between a child's speech sound errors and his ability to discriminate between speech sounds. Many of the classic texts directed toward articulation therapy have advocated speech sound discrimination training, often referred to as ear training, before embarking on correction of the sound error (Berry and Eisenson, 1956; Van Riper, 1954). Through the years the relationship between discrimination of nonspeech and speech sounds to phonologic and phonetic errors has continued to be a highly controversial issue.

Weiner (1967) has provided an extensive review of much of this earlier literature relating auditory discrimination to articulation. He offers the following conclusions based on his analysis of the literature:

1. Auditory discrimination shows a developmental progression that peaks during the eighth year.
2. Children's performance ratings on nonsense syllable and word comparison discrimination tests are higher for children with higher socioeconomic status.

---

*From Tallal, P., and Piercy, M., Defects of auditory perception. In M.A. Wyke (Ed.), *Developmental Dysphasia*. New York: Academic Press, 75 (1978). Copyright by Academic Press Inc. (London) Ltd.

3. The relationship between auditory discrimination and intelligence seems to vary with the type of test.
4. In primary age groups of children younger than 8 or 9 years old, the relationship between auditory discrimination and articulation holds.
5. Studies with children who misarticulate multiple sounds (four or more) usually indicate a positive relationship between auditory discrimination and articulation, but this relationship usually does not hold when two or fewer sounds are in error.

Furthermore, the developmental phonology literature suggests that auditory discrimination of phonologic contrasts generally precedes production of those same contrasts (Edwards, 1974; Eilers and Oller, 1976; Menyuk and Anderson, 1969), and that during normal phonologic development, "perceptual difficulties probably play a substantial role in some childhood speech errors, but little, if any role in others" (Eilers and Oller, 1976). Thus although the relationship is far from understood and the controversy continues, we might tentatively conclude that at least some young children with multiple sound errors may present difficulty with auditory discrimination tasks.

As with attention, data regarding the relationship between auditory discrimination and language disorders in children have arisen from tasks designed to measure what each investigator defined as discrimination. The profession is overflowing with discrimination tests, but there is a notable lack of clear research demonstrating that discrimination difficulties are associated with, or more crucially, causally related to language disorders. Locke (1980a,b), while maintaining that analysis of a child's perceptual responses (in particular discrimination) provides one of the few good ways of inferring what a child knows about the phonologic structure of language, has questioned the validity of conventional discrimination tests. He argues that the commercially available tests do not identify clinically relevant perceptual disorders. To be clinically useful, he states, a phonologic discrimination test must be based on the production errors that the child himself makes in reference to the intended phoneme. In addition to presenting an approach to discrimination testing based on the child's errors, Locke also provides a critical assessment of current practices as well as the relationship between discrimination and production errors in children.

Several models of speech and language processing have assumed that auditory discrimination must be intact for the normal development and processing of language (Hardy, 1965; Morley, 1972; and others). In such models, hierarchical auditory stages are proposed. Information must first traverse a discrimination process before feeding information forward for language processing. Thus errors in auditory discrimination would be passed on to language processes and be reflected in language usage. Yet, as discussed earlier, theories of speech perception are not in agreement in terms of the recognition granted passive versus active speech perception mechanisms. The direction of information flow, from primarily a bottom-up dependency to a top-down interaction, is also a point of debate. The bottom-up models tend to stress the importance of prelinguistic auditory processing as a prelude and necessary prerequisite to linguistic processing, whereas the top-down models see linguistic knowledge as shaping perception.

We have already seen how prelinguistic auditory variables can influence the ability of normal and language disordered children to discriminate linguistic information as demonstrated in the research on auditory rate. We also have suggested that auditory attention problems can interfere with discrimination of linguistic information, although here the experimental support is weaker. Later we will document the findings that auditory memory can also interfere or limit discrimination ability. Thus there exists evidence that prelinguistic auditory operations that are viewed as acoustic (that is, not limited to linguistic information but extending to both linguistic and nonlinguistic auditory information) may well interfere with discrimination of linguistic stimuli.

Whether or not discrimination of speech stimuli exists in the absence of these acoustically based, prelinguistic processes is yet another question, and one for which the final answer is not yet found. Tallal and Piercy (1973 a,b; 1978) in their series of articles suggest that it does not, although Manning, Johnston, and Beasley (1977) found that even with no compression of stimuli, their language-disordered children performed inferiorly to normal children on discrimination of speech. Clearly, this question must be investigated further. In any event, substantial evidence suggests that acoustically based, prelinguistic processes may negatively influence speech discrimination.

Just as speech discrimination may be disrupted by bottom-up auditory operations, so also may top-down linguistic knowledge influence discrimination. In a classic study of discrimination ability, McReynolds (1966) reported that dysphasic children between 6 and 8 years old performed as well as normal children on discrimination tasks of isolated speech sounds but were significantly inferior when these same sounds were embedded in a phonetic context. Furthermore, Schwartz and Goldman (1974) demonstrated that normal children's discrimination of speech sounds is influenced by the linguistic context in which the discrimination is required. Chil-dren in nursery school, kindergarten, and first grade all made consistently more errors when the speech sounds were in contexts that supplied limited grammatic and phonetic cues. Similarly, Atchison and Canter (1979) reported that one subgroup of their learning disabled first graders performed significantly differently, depending on the degree of phonetic difference, the position of the contrast, and the degree of lexical familiarity of the linguistic stimuli to be discriminated. Studies such as these contend that language knowledge can influence discrimination ability. They also offer support for Rees' (1973) argument that auditory processing tests reveal the obvious— that the children have language-learning problems.

That children with language disorders present discrimination difficulties has been a long-standing assumption based on the clinical impressions of the writers who have addressed child language disorders (Eisenson, 1972; Johnson and Myklebust, 1967; Strauss and Lehtinen, 1947; Wiig and Semel, 1976). However, there are many difficulties encountered in studying auditory discrimination in language disordered children and in teasing apart the research findings. These difficulties are exemplified in a study reported by Wilson, Doehring, and Hirsch (1960). These investigators compared 14 receptive aphasic children to a group of nonaphasic hearing impaired children on their ability to discriminate a long tone, a short tone, a long noise, and a short noise from one another and to associate each tone with one of four randomly chosen letters. Results of this study were instructive in several respects. First, the aphasic children did not perform as a uniform group in that 5 of the 14 never reached criterion, and the three best aphasics equaled the performance of the three best hearing impaired children. Thus it was concluded that the aphasics were not homogeneous in their ability on this task.

Second, when the investigators modified the task by requiring the children to verbally respond "long tone," "short tone," and so forth upon hearing the stimuli, the aphasic children did so with no difficulty. Thus Wilson, Doehring, and Hirsch (1960) concluded that the initial inability resulted not from a discrimination deficit but from the complexity of the associative process required to match the tone with a letter.

At this point we must remain skeptical about any conclusions regarding the relationship of auditory discrimination to language disorders in children. The evidence suggests that auditory discrimination may be influenced by acoustic (nonlinguistic) parameters of the auditory stimuli as well as by the state of linguistic knowledge of the child. Whether a distinct auditory discrimination operation exists for speech sounds apart from other auditory parameters remains to be determined.

Auditory memory. A further auditory operation with much clinical support but confusing and controversial research findings concerns auditory memory and its relationship to developmental language disorders. Virtually all of the classic writers in child language disorders suggest that memory dysfunctions contribute to disordered language in children. McGinnis (1963) reported that children with motor aphasia were impaired in their memory for sequence of sounds and that poor memory for language lay behind the sensory aphasic's disorder. Eisenson (1968) maintains that the storage system for speech sounds is defective in aphasic children, and Bangs (1968) details memory retrieval as an "avenue of learning" that may be disrupted in language and learning disordered children. Numerous contemporary investigators have also implicated memory functions as causal bases for disordered language (Menyuk, 1964, 1978; Tallal, 1976, 1978). As with the other auditory operations, the investigations of auditory memory abilities of language disordered children have yielded equivocal results and interpretations. Several of the resulting issues are examined below.

WHAT IS AUDITORY MEMORY? A major difficulty in studying the relationship of auditory memory to language and language disorders centers around the definition of memory, since that definition reflects theoretic constructs about memory. There is no clear answer to this difficulty; however, most writers differentiate between long-term and short-term memory (Massaro, 1975). Again, as in the study of other auditory operations, we are frequently left with a series of tasks that have been used to measure what has been defined. In auditory memory these are often tasks that look at some dimension of recognition, retention, or retrieval of information as these dimensions relate to short-term and long-term memory. Questions arise about the ability to separate auditory memory from other auditory operations and whether there is one or many auditory memories.

Auditory memory tasks are intimately bound to auditory sequencing tasks, since memory measures usually include stimuli of varying length and complexity. When more than one auditory element is presented in memory tasks, it becomes clear that retaining the order of these elements is important to the interpretation of memory. However, in many of the studies of auditory memory the sequential order of the material was not carefully controlled, making it difficult to know if the problem was one of auditory memory or one of auditory sequencing.

Studies of auditory sequencing operations in language disordered children are numerous, and virtually all require both memory and sequencing abilities. That both auditory operations are required is noted at times, and sometimes the memory demands only confound the sequencing findings and vice versa. Because the investigators usually cite sequencing as the primary focus of their study, we will defer consideration of these memory sequencing studies until we discuss auditory sequencing.

Assumptions have been made that some type of absolute short-term memory exists separate from the auditory stimuli employed in the auditory memory tasks. McNeill (1966) suggested that separate production and comprehension memory spans may exist on the phonologic and grammatic levels, and it has been quite conclusively demonstrated with both adults and children that memory for sentences depends highly on semantic and syntactic features inherent in the sentences. Although the concept of multilayered, interdependent memory spans for language may exist and there is considerable experimental data with normal subjects supporting such a concept, this concept has not filtered down to practice with language disordered children. Instead, we still see general use of digit span, for example, to measure short-term memory deficits that are believed to be related to the language disorder, even though there is limited evidence to suggest such as relationship.

MEMORY AND LANGUAGE DISORDERS. Although deficits in auditory memory are frequently cited as causing child language disorders, we know of no clear evidence demonstrating such a cause-effect relationship. The co-occurrence of two problems does not mean one causes the other, merely that the two co-occur. Although one possible relationship between auditory memory and language disorders is that the former causes the latter, until this is demonstrated more clearly, other possible relationships must be seriously considered.

Olson (1973) has suggested that auditory memory differences between younger and older children could be attributed to the younger child's inability to organize, plan, monitor, and integrate information, therefore not remembering as effectively as older children or adults. He suggests that the classical findings on increased memory span as children get older merely reflect the development of the child's ability to handle verbal information rather than changes in memory. Olson hypothesized that a child's ability to retain increasing information demonstrates growth in internal organization and representation of that information rather than an increase in memory span per se. Olson's hypothesis, then, would suggest that language disordered children's language problems may even "cause" the memory deficits, or more probably that these children's difficulty in organizing, planning, monitoring, and integrating information is reflected in both language and short-term memory tasks.

In addition to hypothesizing that language disordered children present short-term memory deficits, Menyuk (1964, 1969) also has detained the interdependence of interaction between language and memory functions. In a series of elegant experiments, Menyuk and Looney (1972a,b) have shown how both the length and the linguistic structure of the stimulus sentence interact.

Menyuk and Looney (1972a,b) examined the ability of normal and language disordered children to repeat sentences of various types (active-declarative, imperative, negative, and question), varying the length of the sentences from three to five words. Unlike Menyuk's 1964 findings that the language disordered children's accuracy in sentence repetition correlated significantly with sentence length, which was not limited to five words, the 1972 work with Looney in which sentence length was limited demonstrated that their performance was more significantly affected by structure than by length. Therefore when length is controlled, Menyuk (1978) maintains that memory for sentences is determined by linguistic factors. She states:

> In summary, the above experiments seem to show that there is a hierarchical organization in the processing of information reflected in the immediate recall of sentences. Language disordered children preserve best the intention of the sentence (to command, declare, negate and question) and the main relations in the sentence (actor-action and frequently object). They also preserve the syntactic rule of *word order* to express this relation. They do not, however, preserve the transformational modifications used to express the intention and relations in the sentence, and the specific phonological segments of the speech signal.[*]

Because it seems clear that auditory memory is not a unitary operation, that many factors influence it, and that it is only beginning to be understood in relationship to child language disorders, we cannot ascribe to the claims that auditory memory deficits "cause" child language disorders.

However, selectively administered and carefully interpreted memory tasks can be useful in understanding some aspects of child language disorders. For example, some children consistently give back only the last part of a given auditory stimulus, providing data relevant to what and how much these children are retaining from whatever is said to them. Similarly, other children may present an exaggerated auditory memory span in contrast to some of their other linguistic abilities, but such a skill may be found to be a rote auditory-motor skill with little intervening comprehension or integration of information.

Hermelin and Frith (1971) compared intellectually normal and subnormal children of the same mental age to a group of autistic children in their ability to repeat from memory several meaningful or syntactically ordered tasks, versus random word strings. These experimenters found that even very young and very retarded children were able to process material by making use of structure and organization. Autistic children, however, seemed less efficient in their ability to make use of meaning or structure to aid short-term memory tasks. When presented with word strings, some sentences and others nonsentences (wall long cake send), normal children recalled sentences better than nonsentences independent of their position in the word list, whereas autistic children recalled the last words better than the first regardless of position or meaning. This finding suggested that the autistic children used their exaggerated memory like an echo rather than for reorganizing auditory information. Furthermore, when given lists of adjectives and nouns such as "cup, white, glass, pink, plate, blue," the normal and subnormal children recalled messages by clustering together words of the same category, whereas the autistic children tended to repeat exact word order.

Studies in which auditory memory tasks are used such as those of Hermelin and Frith (1971), although not yielding causal conclusions, can be used to gain insight into how language disordered children process or fail to process information in auditory memory. Continued research along these lines will be needed before we can conclude what relationships exist between auditory memory and child language disorders.

Auditory sequencing. A disorder in the perception of temporal sequence has long been suggested as a causal basis for developmental language disorders (Monsees, 1961). Following Efron's (1963) landmark study demonstrating that adult aphasics with left temporal lobe damage were significantly impaired in their ability to indicate which of two tones occurred first, numerous investigators have turned to studying auditory sequencing

---

[*]From Menyuk, P., Linguistic problems in children with developmental dysphasia. In M.A. Wyke (Ed.), *Developmental Dysplasia*. New York: Academic Press, Inc., 148 (1978). Copyright by Academic Press Inc. (London) Ltd.

abilities in language impaired children (Aten and Davis, 1968; Lowe and Campbell, 1965; Olson, 1961; and Stark, 1967).

Overall, the studies provide considerable evidence supporting an auditory sequencing deficit in some groups of language impaired children. However, frequently these studies confound a number of variables, making analysis and interpretation of the findings difficult.

As with the other prelinguistic auditory operations, any study of auditory sequencing cannot be isolated from the other auditory operations, most notably memory. For a child to sequence, he has to be able to hold in memory what he is required to sequence. Very little of the reported research differentiates between memory and sequence deficits; that is, rarely are the data presented in such a way that it is known if the child mixed up the sequence or if he reported fewer of the auditory stimuli presented, although in the correct order (e.g., Stark, 1967). Frequently input versus output sequencing requirements are not separated, and although a child may fail a task, it is not clear whether or not the failure arose from auditory sequencing, from executing output motor sequencing, or from both (Olson, 1961; Stark, 1967; Aten and Davis, 1968).

Furthermore, often the tasks require associate learning; that is, the child must associate a given tone, phoneme, or other auditory stimulus with a secondary representation such as blocks of varying length or color (Aten and Davis, 1968; Lowe and Campbell, 1965). In most investigations the children are required to demonstrate having made this association to some specified criteria. Yet clinical experience with language disordered children suggests that when tasks become difficult, they often lose their novelty or become tedious, and under such circumstances, language disordered children do not maintain performance as well as normal children. Thus failure on such tasks could be explained by failure to maintain associated learning requirements or attentional and motivational factors rather than a failure in auditory sequencing.

The Aten and Davis (1968) study is exemplary of much of the work that has been undertaken in auditory sequencing. These investigators compared 21 children with minimal cerebral dysfunction and learning difficulty to a group of normal children on three nonverbal and seven verbal sequential tasks. The three nonverbal sequential tasks were (1) rhythmic pure tone sequence (decoding), (2) absolute judgment of tonal duration sequence, and (3) rhythmic pure tone sequence (encoding). The seven verbal sequential tasks were defined as (1) nonsense syllables (repeated), (2) digits (repeated forward and backward), (3) noun sequencing (ordering pictures based on words presented), (4) multisyllabic word reproduction, (5) scrambled sentences (reordered into appropriate sentences), (6) paragraph recall, and (7) oral sequencing of syllables.

The results of this study demonstrated that the children with minimal cerebral dysfunction were significantly deficient in performance on all three nonverbal tasks and on the verbal tasks of backward digit span, noun sequencing, multisyllabic word reproduction, scrambled sentences, and oral syllable sequencing. A general conclusion drawn by us and one that seems quite reasonable from the data is that children diagnosed as having minimal cerebral dysfunction may have temporal ordering difficulties for both nonverbal and verbal auditory tasks. Although the children with minimal cerebral dysfunction clearly demonstrated significant difficulty with the required auditory sequencing tasks, performing significantly lower on 8 of the 10 tasks, the findings might be attributed to factors other then temporal ordering difficulties.

It is important to question whether these findings arose as a result of the different language abilities of the two groups involved. That is, the experimental and control groups were matched by IQ, socioeconomic status, and equal sex distribution, however not by any measure of language performance such as mean length of utterance or reported language tests. In fact, there was virtually no information about these children's language ability reported, even though deficits in auditory sequencing are called on to explain their problems in language learning.

Several other explanations might also be offered to explain the findings of the Aten and Davis (1968) study. First, the three nonverbal sequencing tasks required use of associative learning, either associating single or double tone bursts with blocks bearing single or double dots or with one or two verbally produced beeps, or associating tones of varying duration with blocks of varying length. Even though the children demonstrated this associative learning to a criterion of five correct responses for each task, it is possible that their reduced scores reflected reduced learning ability on an associative task rather than a sequencing disability. It must be kept in mind that these were learning disabled children.

Second, many of the tasks required the children to do some abstract organizing of information to be able to perform successfully, and in several cases this required knowledge of language structure. For example, the scrambled sentences required that the children make correct sentences from the scrambled sentences presented, a task that seemingly would make as much of a demand on metalinguistic knowledge of sentence structure as on sequencing ability. Similarly, saying digits backward required some ability to code and transform the presented digits, an ability that seems to go far beyond auditory sequencing as such.

Third, it is possible that oral or motor programming and sequencing problems might explain breakdowns on some tasks such as reproduction of multisyllabic words and oral sequencing of syllables. Still other interpretations could be offered from this data if one views the tasks that differed in relation to the tasks that did not. It is interesting, for example, that the scores of children with minimal cerebral dysfunction were worse on nonverbal auditory sequencing tasks. Could this be evidence of a cerebral laterality problem or an inability to process acoustic rather than linguistic data? The verbal tasks where there were no differences were digits forward, nonsense syllables, and paragraph recall. How can these nondifferences be accounted for in relation to those instances where differences occurred?

It is doubtful that a temporal ordering factor could explain the findings. No differences were found between the groups on repetition of nonsense syllables or forward digit span, two measures of auditory sequencing where linguistic factors presumably come less into play. If some general auditory sequencing factor were responsible for the differences, it could be questioned why it was not revealed on these two rather "pure" measures of linguistic ordering.

Thus, although Aten and Davis (1968) demonstrated differences in performance between normal and minimal cerebral dysfunction children, these differences may be explained on grounds other than auditory sequencing. It seems that any global interpretation may be misleading at this time. We suggest that until more data are available and a more systematic approach to the relationship of auditory sequencing to language processing and disorders is found, a more conservative stance regarding cause-effect relationships should be maintained.

As Cromer (1978) has so aptly stated in

his thorough discussion of sequencing and dysphasia:

It should also be noted however, that when experimentation has shown the deaf to be poorer than normal children in sequencing, no one supposes their inability to sequence to be a *cause* of the deafness! The experiments with dysphasic children are of an identical logical status, but this does not appear to prevent some theorists from adopting the position that a sequencing disability is the cause of the dysphasia. In fact the direction of causation may be reversed; it may be that lack of experience with the auditory information of language, in these children, may result in their seldom relying on temporal order to encode or understand the world.*

AUDITORY PROCESSING DYSFUNCTIONS DO/DO NOT EQUAL LANGUAGE DISORDERS

As realized from the preceding discussion, much information is available on auditory processing. Numerous professionals are searching for an auditory perceptual basis for language and learning disorders. Unfortunately, much of the work done in this area has not been clearly defined, and questionable conclusions are being drawn. Professional camps and controversies have centered around those advocating auditory processing breakdowns as the primary if not the only basis for child language disorders, versus those maintaining that auditory processing separated from linguistic processing is irrelevant and an invalid approach to children's language disorders.

Controversies

In Chapter 2 we discussed some of the attempts that have been made to search for a processing explanation for child language disorders. One of the views presented was that of promoting auditory processing disruptions

---

* From Cromer, R.F., The basis of childhood dysphasia: A linguistic approach. In M.A. Wyke (Ed.), *Developmental Dysphasia*. New York: Academic Press, 104-105 (1978). Copyright by Academic Press Inc. (London) Ltd.

as a primary if not sole basis for certain language disorders seen in children, particularly those diagnosed as aphasic. McGinnis (1963), Myklebust (1954), Hardy (1965), and Eisenson (1968, 1972) were instrumental in developing this viewpoint. As well, Benton (1964), in his early description of developmental aphasia, concluded that the evidence suggested that higher level auditory perceptual deficits are the basis for receptive and expressive aphasia.

As emphasized in Chapter 2, Eisenson (1968, 1972) represents one of the most extreme views, believing that developmental aphasia and auditory perceptual problems go hand in hand except in rare instances. This theme is developed extensively in his 1972 book, *Aphasia in Children*.

☐ **Of the auditory operations we have discussed in the preceding sections, which does Eisenson (1972) feel are implicated in childhood aphasia? Does he implicate others we did not enumerate?**

Rees (1973), however, questions the validity of attributing language disorders in children to failures in auditory processing. She maintains that the evidence is weak. Calling upon aguments from the literature in speech perception, she notes that normal children and listeners perceive speech in reference to what they know about language and how speech is produced. Thus she concludes that the inabilities of language disordered children on various auditory processing tasks reveal that these children's language deficit prevents them from effectively performing on the presented tasks. She sees the problem as a top-down (language influencing the auditory processing ability) rather than bottom-up (auditory processing creating the language disability) problem. Similarly, Sanders (1977) suggested that what have been called auditory perceptual problems are intimately related to language coding problems, and that study of such problems and their remediation must be done in the context of linguistic based information.

Tallal and Piercy (1978), in a thoughtful consideration of the relationship between language disorders (childhood aphasia) and auditory perceptual defects, analyzed four relationships: (1) the auditory defect may be a necessary cause of the developmental dysphasia, (2) the auditory defect might be a sufficient but not necessary cause of developmental dysphasia, (3) defective auditory perception might be secondary to a primary linguistic defect, and (4) the auditory defect might be a concomitant of the linguistic defect but not causally related to it. After evaluating these possible relationships, they concluded:

> . . . that *some* cases of developmental dysphasia are the direct consequence of defective processing of rapidly changing acoustic information and an associated, possibly consequential reduced memory span for auditory sequence.[*]

We only know what we know, which is not enough

Although considerable controversy exists as to the centrality of auditory processing disruptions to child language disorders, our perspective is that study of this relationship is fundamental to understanding child language disorders, some disorders more than others. The search for auditory processes and their relationship to child language disorders is not over.

Auditory processing disruptions, disruptions of the processing stage within the Speech to Language segment of our processing unit on the CLPM, are not language dis-

[*]From Tallal, P., and Piercy, M., Defects of auditory perception in children with developmental dysphasia. In M.A. Wyke (Ed.), *Developmental Dysphasia*. New York: Academic Press, 82 (1978). Copyright by Academic Press Inc. (London) Ltd.

orders. However, evidence exists that disruptions of these processes bear a causal relationship to child language disorders. In the conductive and sensorineural hearing losses this relationship is somewhat stronger than in the case of the auditory perceptual operations. It is only through a careful study of the literature, continued research, and careful clinical documentation that we will grasp the contribution of auditory processing as prelinguistic analysis of speech input to child language disorders. In the meantime we offer a set of precautions for speech-language pathologists to use in their efforts to understand, assess, and treat auditory processing disorders.

All child language disorders do not stem from auditory processing disruptions. This precaution is basically a reiteration of material presented throughout this book. It is clear that we do not view child language disorders from such a perspective. Instead, we present them as stemming from a variety of intrinsic and extrinsic causal interactions that develop over time.

It must be kept in mind that the information presented in this chapter on auditory processing in relationship to child language disorders has mostly derived from research done on learning disabled or aphasic children. Thus the assumption that pervades this material is that there is a direct processing deficit related to neurologic disruption.

It may well be that future research will demonstrate the validity of Eisenson's (1972) position rather than Rees' (1973) position. However, we, unlike Eisenson (1972) and more in keeping with workers such as Morley (1972) and Rapin and Wilson (1978), believe that child language disorders including those stemming from processing disruptions are not homogeneous. Some may stem from disrupted auditory processing, but others may stem from processing disruptions in other parts of the language processing system. We do not believe that we have the data or the theoretic support for the view that the primary basis of child language disorders, even aphasia in children, stems from auditory processing disruptions.

Considerable evidence demonstrates that some children with language disorders do not have difficulty with processing speech input. Instead, their problems arise from central language processing or language output processing deficits (Aram and Nation, 1975; Johnson and Myklebust, 1967; Morley, 1972). Even Tallal and Piercy (1974, 1978), who have done some of the most careful and systematic research devoted to prelinguistic processing in dysphasic children, found that on many of their auditory perceptual tasks the children did not all perform in a like manner. For example, in examining the relationship between speech perception and speech production impairment in children with developmental dysphasia, Tallal, Stark, and Curtiss (1976) reported that 7 of the 12 dysphasic children presented more difficulty discriminating stop vowel syllables presented with a 43 millisecond formant transition than when either the steady state vowel or the transitions were extended to 95 milliseconds. Yet five of the dysphasic children reached criterion on the 43 millisecond formant transition. They referred to the former group as "perceptually impaired" and the latter group as "perceptually unimpaired." What too often is overlooked in discussion of such findings is the fact that all children did not perform in a uniform manner. Therefore while prelinguistic processing deficits may be found to explain linguistic processing breakdowns in some dysphasic children, such findings are in no way universal for all dysphasic children.

Children may fail auditory processing tasks because of the task rather than because of an auditory processing deficit. Numerous auditory processes (operations) have been specified and defined operationally by the tasks required to carry them out. Children with language disorders given these tasks may fail in terms of age expectations and then be labeled as having an auditory processing dysfunction.

However, as we have discussed, language disordered children may fail these tasks for a variety of reasons, including the fact that they are language disordered and therefore for one reason or another fail to accomplish the task. Every speech-language pathologist could create an auditory processing task that his or her language disordered children would fail.

For example, many language disordered children have difficulty with the same-different concept; yet having this concept is a requisite of several auditory discrimination tests. Failures on auditory discrimination assessed in this manner may or may not be real, depending on whether there is independent evidence that the child can reliably indicate this difference. In effect what such tasks often demonstrate is that the children present metalinguistic difficulties, that is problems with awareness of the languages as a rule-based system, rather than more primary problems with auditory operations. Or, when giving a child a discrimination task, unless one has independently demonstrated that the child knows the meaning of the words being discriminated, we may find that the child cannot perform acceptably on the discrimination test. However, we cannot conclude from this that he has a discrimination deficit. Some auditory processing tasks require that a child learn and then operate within a complex teaching paradigm, for example associating colored blocks with different phonemes to demonstrate that he can discriminate and/or sequence sounds by pointing to or aligning same or different colored blocks. This task therefore requires that a child not only form sound-block associations, but that he be able to act on a metalinguistic concept of same-different. Children may have a semantic problem, visual problem, peripheral hearing problem, pointing problem, or a cooperation problem—the possitilities are many for explaining their failure on discrimination tasks, many of which may or may not have anything directly to do with discrimination. The precaution that we hope speech-language pathologists incorporate is to critically evaluate whether auditory processing problems exist or are merely reflective of task difficulty.

We must maintain alternative perspectives on the causal relationship of auditory processing disruptions and child language disorders. Given all the uncertainties in understanding the role of auditory processing in child language disorders, we caution the speech-language pathologist not to draw premature conclusions that auditory processing disruptions do or do not have anything to do with language disorders. Until clear evidence is obtained, we suggest viewing the relationships among auditory processing disruptions and child language disorders from several causal perspectives similar to those explored by Tallal and Piercy (1978). These perspectives simply stated are:

1. Auditory processing deficits cause language disorders.

2. Language disorders cause auditory processing deficits.

3. An X factor causes both an auditory processing deficit and a language disorder.

This precaution can perhaps best be exemplified through reference to auditory memory. Frequently children with language disorders are described as having problems with recognition, storage, and/or retrieval of auditory information, all of which may be viewed as memory tasks. The causal assumption sometimes made is that the memory deficit caused the language disorder. Others would argue persuasively that the language problem caused the memory problem, since the language disordered children do not have a ready, automatic means by which information can be chunked for more accessible storage and retrieval. A third alternative is equally tenable: that memory and language are not causally related to each other, but rather both deficits are related to a third factor, for example, a more general failure for hierarchical abstraction and storage. Thus a child may have both language and auditory memory deficits, not because one causes the other but because another causal factor is operating on the speech and language system.

chapter 6

Language to thought to language processing

In Chapter 5 the discussion centered around auditory processes and operations assumed to underlie certain child language disorders. Breakdowns in these processes are presumed to prevent the child from effectively using auditory information for language processing. In this chapter we turn to language processing, those processing stages essential for understanding the structure of the message, interpreting the complexities of meaning within the message, creating a response to messages within communicative contexts, and formulating the structure of the message to be produced.

DOMAIN OF LANGUAGE TO THOUGHT TO LANGUAGE PROCESSING

The Language to Thought to Language Processing Segment of the CLPM presented in Chapter 3 (Fig. 3-2) defines the domain of this chapter. This segment incorporates four language processing stages: (1) language comprehension, (2) language integration, (3) language formulation, and (4) speech and language repetition.

Depending on the nature of the communi-cative act, the normal language user involves various processing stages. The usual flow of information is from comprehension to integration to formulation, with meaningful repetition coming into play as needed. It is assumed that children with language disorders also use a similar flow of information; however, disruptions of one or more of the language processes will affect the others, giving rise to disordered language and performance. In some instances some processes are nonfunctioning, as when a child may only be able to echo a stimulus with no evident meaning.

Language disordered children present a variety of disordered language performance based on the difficulties they have at each or all of the processing stages. The majority of children with language disorders appear to have disruptions of these central language processes.

In Chapter 3 we suggested that variable patterns of language performance occur. These patterns, based on previous work (Aram and Nation, 1975), revealed that language disordered children present differential performance depending on which processes are most affected.

Observations of a child's response to or use

of language as discussed in the CLPM provide the basis from which inferences as to loci of processing breakdown are made. Difficulty with the understanding of syntax and semantics implicates a comprehension disruption. If a child was observed to have difficulty either responding to or using the pragmatic aspects of his language, we suggest that his language processing disruption centers on the process of language integration. Similarly, if his major difficulties lie in expressive semantics and syntax, we locate the processing disruptions as language formulation. Description of the child's response to language input and his language output, therefore, provides the performance data base from which processing breakdowns are inferred.

With the understanding that child language disorders are usually revealed as patterns of performance across processes and language levels, we will go on in this chapter to discuss each processing stage somewhat independently of the others. We will provide a definitional viewpoint of each stage raising issues of concern and then provide a review of the literature that reveals information about the language disorders that occur if the processing stage is disrupted.

COMPREHENSION PROCESSING STAGE
What do we mean by comprehension?

Comprehension is a term that calls up a variety of meanings among speech-language pathologists. Rees and Shulman (1978) in their critical article, "I Don't Understand What You Mean By Comprehension," state that the profession has taken a limited view of comprehension. They point out that most of the tests and tasks used clinically and in research with language disordered children are limited to measures of lexical and syntactic comprehension, what they term the literal meaning of messages. They go on to suggest that

A more comprehensive approach would go beyond measuring the child's ability to comprehend the literal meaning of sentences to include two other aspects of obtaining information from spoken utterances: presupposition and inference and illocutionary acts.[*]

They see these aspects of comprehension as requiring more complex linguistic integration and inference.

How do we view language comprehension in the CLPM? Certain aspects of language that Rees and Shulman (1978) consider as more complex language comprehension (including presupposition and illocutionary acts) are what many authors, for example Bates (1976b), treat as the pragmatic level of language. Although Rees and Shulman (1978) would not disagree with that position, we feel a distinction needs to be made between language comprehension and language integration.

In the CLPM we take the more literal view of language comprehension that was criticized by Rees and Shulman (1978) as the processing stage whereby the child understands the words and grammar of what he has heard but does not necessarily fully interpret the complexities of meaning embedded in the message. This is a function we view more in line with the language integration processing stage. Thus language comprehension in our sense will be confined to the understanding of the semantic and syntactic aspects of language. Semantic comprehension includes the child's ability to understand both lexical meaning and semantic relations. Syntactic comprehension incorporates the complexity of syntax as well as the length of the utterance.

---

[*]From Rees, N.S., and Shulman, M., I don't understand what you mean by comprehension. *Journal of Speech and Hearing Disorders,* **43,** 208 (1978).

Semantic comprehension disruptions

Disruptions of semantic comprehension are a pervasive characteristic of children with language disorders. All but a very few can be shown to have some limitations in this ability. At times these deficits are not obvious to the observer and can be demonstrated only on subtle comprehension tasks such as understanding spatial or temporal relational words. In the following discussion of semantic comprehension we will examine the literature addressed to (1) the lexicon and (2) semantic relations.

Lexicon. Comprehension of the lexicon in language disordered children ranges from little to no ability, as occasionally is apparent in children with severe auditory agnosias (Chappell, 1972; Stein and Curry, 1968) to apparently normal performance when the children are given standardized tests such as the Peabody Picture Vocabulary Test (Dunn, 1965) or the Boehm Test of Basic Concepts (Boehm, 1971).

◻ **A question that could be pursued here is whether auditory agnosia, either congenital or acquired, is primarily a problem within the Speech to Language Processing Segment (speech perception) or in the Language to Thought to Language Processing Segment (semantic comprehension). Review the positions taken by Rapin and Wilson (1978), Stein and Curry (1968), and Worster-Drought (1971).**

The most prevalent work directed toward describing comprehension of lexical items has been to document and describe vocabulary development against normative data in children with language disorders stemming from some other primary deficit, for example mental retardation. There is research that addresses development of vocabulary comprehension in the retarded (Harrison, 1958; Jordan, 1967; Spreen, 1965; Taylor, Thurow, and Turner, 1977), in the autistic (Balaxe and Simmons, 1975; Pronovost, 1961), in the hearing impaired (Myklebust, 1964),

and so forth. Although a wide range of lexical disabilities have been reported, we must point out that certain tests of lexical comprehension can lead to erroneous conclusions about a language disordered child's level of comprehension, particularly if used alone. Frequently a child's best ability is brought out when he is required to attend to only short, single-word stimuli, such as are employed on the usual vocabulary comprehension task (Peabody Picture Vocabulary Test, Dunn, 1965; and the Assessment of Children's Language Comprehension: Vocabulary, Foster, Giddan, and Stark, 1972). In addition, lexical comprehension tests tend to draw from relatively concrete, picturable items, again an area of relatively good performance for many language disordered children. For example, the Peabody Picture Vocabulary Test (Dunn, 1965) includes noun and a few verb forms, leaving untapped comprehension of any adjectives, adverbs, or prepositions—word types that are often more difficult for these children to comprehend.

Typically for the children with whom we have worked, comprehension of noun forms is the easiest. Language disordered children frequently correctly indicate nouns on the Peabody Picture Vocabulary Test (Dunn, 1965), Carrow Test of Auditory Comprehension of Language (Carrow, 1973), or the Assessment of Children's Language Comprehension (Foster, Giddan, and Stark, 1972), but fail when other parts of speech are presented, for example, verbs on the Peabody Picture Vocabulary Test and verbs, prepositions, and adjectives on the Assessment of Children's Language Comprehension.

◻ **Studies done with the Peabody Picture Vocabulary Test (Dunn, 1965) have been numerous. Explore the manual to this test and review the studies presented there on groups of children who might have language disorders.**

Going beyond studying the degree of vocabulary comprehension deficits in language disordered children, investigators are now looking at underlying reasons for these deficits, particularly investigating the conceptual and semantic structure underlying the lexical deficit. Several of these studies have been undertaken with mentally retarded children. For example, Sperber, Ragain, and McCauley (1976) found that semantic relatedness (that is, eagle and robin are more closely related than eagle and chair) affects the rate of information processing in the mentally retarded and concluded that there is an organized structure of semantic memory in the retarded that is based partly on categoric relationships. Similarly, Blount (1968) concluded after a comprehensive review of concept formation in the retarded that retardates do have concepts available to them but are less able to use these concepts than normal children when they are required to produce verbal labels. When attention is called to the relevant cues in a situation, the retardate does as well as or better than his mental-age matched control. Semantic organization has also been studied in deaf and hearing impaired subjects (Tweney, Hoemann, and Andrews, 1975). Tweney et al. (1975) found that deaf subjects manifested abstract hierarchial relations among the meaning of words that were not dependent on "visual mediators" or hindered by the absence of "acoustic mediators." In short, these investigators have suggested that the organization of the lexicon of the deaf is comparable to that of hearing persons and that the central language and cognitive processes are not modality (visual or auditory) dependent.

Semantic relations. One of the few studies documenting comprehension of semantic relations in a disordered population is that of Duchan and Erickson (1976). These investigators compared normal and retarded subjects' comprehension of four semantic relations (agent-action, action-object, possessive and locative) in three different verbal contexts: the expanded (including inflections and function words); telegraphic (deleting articles, prepositions, and auxiliaries); and nonsense forms (nonsense syllables, replaced functions, and inflectional morphemes). No difference was found between the mentally retarded and the normal subjects (all of whose MLU was between 1 and 2.5 morphemes) and as might be expected, all found the expanded context to be easiest, followed by the telegraphic and lastly the nonsense form. Overall, the subjects responded differently to the four semantic relations presented. The possessives were the easiest, followed by the action-object, the agent-action, and the locative relations.

It is clear from the preceding that little information exists about the nature of the semantic comprehension deficit in children with language disorders. The primary information comes from vocabulary studies on children grouped by a primary deficit; for example, mental retardation, hearing impaired, autistic, and so forth. In these studies the children score below the expected norms. Beyond this information we see that studies demonstrating underlying semantic structural difference for semantic deficits and comprehension of semantic relations are few. The limited evidence available has not demonstrated differences in the organization of semantics between impaired (retarded and hearing impaired) and normal groups. So far we know that many language disordered children do not understand lexical items as well as do their normal peers, but we do not know if this deficit represents a mere reduction in diversity, a delay, or a different development in semantic comprehension abilities. For example, do children with severe motor restrictions that limit their ability to explore their en vironment develop the same early lexicon as do normally active children? How do visual impairments seen in blind children affect the meaning of their early words? Questions such as these, tying etiology or resulting processing deficits to semantic development, remain for the most part unanswered.

Syntactic comprehension disruptions

Studies of language disordered children's ability to comprehend syntax have not always taken into account two important stimulus parameters that could confound the results, namely syntactic complexity and length of the stimulus. Studies are only beginning to unravel the relative contribution of both these parameters to comprehension of connected sentences. The discussion here will first address findings relative to language disordered children's performance on syntactic complexity measures, then it will turn to an examination of the effect of length of stimuli on comprehension of sentences.

Syntax complexity. Although it can be demonstrated quite convincingly that many, possibly most language disordered children do show limitations in comprehension of syntactic complexity (much the same as comprehension deficits), cautions need to be raised against overgeneralization. In approaching the research findings, the reader must first consider on what basis or criteria the language disordered children were grouped. Were syntactic complexity limitations found for all children classified as language disordered? Or were simply mean scores reported? Are the language disordered children studied a homogeneous group in terms of their ability to understand syntax? As we (Aram and Nation, 1975) have pointed out, all language disordered children are not comparable in their performance on measures of comprehension of syntactic complexity. Therefore, can we justifiably talk about com-

prehension of syntactic complexity for language disordered children as if they are a single identifiable group?

As in the measurement of any behavior, one must question as well if the findings may actually be attributed to the stated variable, or if other factors may be accounting for the findings. For example, Marquardt and Saxman (1972) examined the language comprehension of a group of 30 articulation deficient and 30 articulation-proficient kindergarten children using the Test for Auditory Comprehension of Language (Carrow, 1973). These authors found the articulation-deficient children to be deficient on this test. They suggested that children with numerous misarticulations present syntactic deficits in performance because of underdeveloped syntactic knowledge. However, when one examines the selection criteria for both the articulation deficient and proficient groups, the contribution of other, noncontrolled factors arises.

The two groups were matched on the basis of chronologic age, sex, race, father's occupational level, and level of education, but no intellectual data were available except that all children were "not considered by the classroom teacher to have significant intellectual deficits." Certainly, the omission of IQ as a criterion raises the possibility that the two groups were not compatible and that syntactic comprehension findings are as related to IQ level as to articulatory skill. Although subsequent study may find articulation-deficient children to be inferior in syntactic comprehension, the Marquardt and Saxman (1972) study allows for alternate explanations.

Despite these cautions, considerable evidence has documented disruptions of comprehension of syntactic complexity for many language disordered children. We (Aram and Nation, 1975) demonstrated that many but not all of the language disordered preschoolers in our study presented some difficulty with comprehension of syntactic complexity as measured by the Receptive Subtest of the Northwestern Syntax Screening Test (Lee, 1969). The exceptions were children who fell into the Phonologic Deficit Pattern and the Formulation-Repetition Deficit Pattern (see Chapter 3). These findings indicate one of the preceding cautions—that you cannot generalize findings regarding syntactic comprehension deficits across all language disordered children.

Similarly, Liles, Shulman, and Bartlett (1977) reported that their group of 15 language disordered children were inferior to normal children in their ability to recognize rule violations concerned with syntactic agreement and word order. However, the language disordered children and the normal children did not differ in their ability to recognize rule violations concerned with lexical choices.

Most of the documentation for reduced syntactic comprehension has come from case study reports or analysis of relatively small groups of children. For example, in children with traumatically acquired aphasia, Yeni-Komshian (1977) has documented the improvement in language abilities, including comprehension tasks, and has related improvement to performance on a dichotic listening task. Other case studies, such as Landau, Goldstein, and Kleffner (1960) and Oelschlaeger and Scarborough (1976) also have documented difficulties in comprehension of syntactic complexity in children with acquired language disorders.

Several studies have compared children with right or left hemispheric involvement in their ability to handle syntactic comprehension tasks. Rankin, Aram, and Horwitz (1980) reported findings for three right hemiplegic and three left hemiplegic children between the ages of 6 and 8 years old. All the children had incurred unilateral hemisphere insults

prenatally or perinatally as confirmed by a CAT (Computerized Axial Tomography) scan. The right hemiplegics (left hemisphere lesions) were markedly inferior to the left hemiplegics on both measures of syntactic complexity employed, including the Northwestern Syntax Screening Test (Lee, 1969) and Part 5 of the Token Test (DeRenzi and Vignolo, 1962), which primarily measures syntactic complexity. The right hemiplegics demonstrated difficulty with word order (such as in passive sentences and sentences containing before and after) as well as with inflectional endings (such as subject-verb agreement and contrasting tense markers).

Similarly, Dennis and Kohn (1975) have presented evidence suggesting that subtle syntactic problems exist in hemispherectomized children who only have the right hemisphere remaining. They contrasted the syntax of five right hemidecorticates (left hemisphere remaining) and four left hemidecorticates (right hemisphere remaining) who had lateralized cortical pathology dating from age 1, which eventually lead to removal of the diseased brain half. On a syntax test of active and passive, affirmative and negative sentences, the right hemidecorticates showed superior comprehension of passive negative sentences (The boy is not pushed by the girl), but equivalent comprehension relative to the left hemidecorticates on active affirmative and active negative sentences. The authors conclude that after perinatal cerebral pathology and subsequent hemispherectomy, syntactic skills are not mediated equivalently by left and right remaining hemispheres.

Another study comparing syntactic skills of children with only a right or a left hemisphere is that of Dennis and Whitaker (1976, 1977), who reported language development data for three children who underwent hemidecortication, one with a remaining left hemisphere and two with remaining right hemispheres.

These authors presented results for 21 different language tests, including both standardized and experimental tests that were either devised for the investigation or adapted from tests for adults with acquired language disorders. These authors concluded that syntactic skills were developed asymmetrically in the two isolated hemispheres, although phonemic and semantic abilities were similar. These studies, taken together, not only demonstrate syntactic disorders in children who are processing language in the right hemisphere, but also suggest that syntactic tests may be very sensitive indicators of subtle language disorders.

Length of stimulus. In addition to having difficulty comprehending syntactically complex sentences, some language disordered children have been shown to have increased difficulty with comprehension of sentences as a function of increased length of the input. Although the length of a sentence is independent from its syntactic complexity, length and syntactic complexity have been confounded in some tasks purporting to measure syntax. Therefore we are including consideration of length in the present section. We have found that some language impaired children fail to understand connected language because of the syntactic complexity, while others fail because of the length of the stimulus sentence.

Two standardized measures have been widely employed to examine children's ability to respond appropriately to utterances of increasing length. The first of these, the Assessment of Children's Language Comprehension (Foster, Giddan, and Stark, 1973) includes the four following parts: (A) Vocabulary (single word stimuli that will be used in the following three parts), (B) Two Critical Elements (horse standing/horse running), (C) Three Critical Elements (ball under the table/ball on the table), and (D) Four Critical Ele-

ments (boy standing in the house/boy sitting in the house/boy standing on the house).

The second measure, The Token Test, which was originally developed for use with adult aphasics (DeRenzi and Vignolo, 1962), has been adapted for children (Token Test for Children, DiSimoni, 1978), and comprises 5 parts. Parts 1 to 4 require comprehension and, importantly, retention of increasing amounts of information. However, the syntactic patterns remain unchanged. Part 5 is primarily a test of syntactic complexity. Examples of the commands for each part of the Token Test (DeRenzi and Vignolo, 1962) are as follows:

Part 1. Point to the red circle.
Part 2. Point to the small green circle.
Part 3. Point to the yellow circle and the blue circle.
Part 4. Point to the small white square and the large white circle.
Part 5. Together with the yellow circle, take the blue circle.

☐ **We have included this discussion of length of the stimulus in this section on syntactic comprehension. When language disordered children fail on tasks that are of increasing length, the question arises whether comprehension is faulty or whether there is a disruption of auditory memory for lexical information. We addressed this issue in Chapter 5. Review that information and determine your view of the relationship of length of stimulus to comprehension of syntax.**

Numerous studies have found language disordered children to have increased difficulty as sentences increase in length. For example, Tallal (1975) found that a group of 12 dysphasics performed significantly poorer than the matched control group on Parts 2 to 5 of the Token Test (DeRenzi and Vignolo, 1962). As the information load increased on Parts 2 through 4, creating greater demands for auditory retention of information, the performance of these children progressively deteriorated. Although still inferior to the control group on Part 5 of the Token Test (DeRenzi and Vignolo, 1962), the dysphasic children's ability improved somewhat when complexity rather than length was primarily under test on Part 5. In analyzing the errors made by the dysphasics in Part 5, Tallal (1975) concluded that the errors were characterized predominantly by a recency memory effect rather than a specific difficulty related to the degree of grammatic complexity.

Further, in the Rankin, Aram, and Horwitz (1980) study, comparing right and left hemiplegic children cited earlier, the right hemiplegics (left hemisphere lesions) were found to have increasing difficulty on the Token Test as a function of length and, similar to the children in the Tallal (1975) and Aram and Glasson (1979) studies, improved somewhat in their performance when syntactic complexity was the prime object of test.

These studies, along with other literature, demonstrate that many language disordered children do present difficulty with syntactic comprehension, although findings must be carefully considered in relationship to the criteria employed for selection of subjects. Further, we have pointed out the necessity for distinguishing between syntactic complexity and length of presented information when describing syntactic comprehension in language impaired children.

INTEGRATION PROCESSING STAGE
A view of language integration

From time to time we encounter children whose chief difficulty with language seems to be the manner in which they relate incoming language to the store of information they possess. These children may perform relatively well on structured semantic and syntactic comprehension tasks, particularly when the auditory stimulus is coupled with some form of visual representation, either in pictures or in written form. Also, when they initiate the

communication, these children speak in well-formed sentences, where again syntax and semantics appear appropriate. When talking about something that interests them, or when they are in charge of the idea and conversation, their use of phonology, syntax, and semantics seems quite appropriate.

Where these children often encounter problems is in grasping the subtle points of what is being said or in modifying what they have to say to the particular situation. Stated differently, these children seem to have difficulty integrating the incoming language with their past experiences and knowledge and in connecting the language with a verbal response that fits with the context. At times it seems as if a mismatch between comprehension and formulation occurs and that what comes out is only obliquely or tangentially related to the language that has gone in.

In the CLPM we have developed the language processing stage of integration that is viewed as an indispensable link between comprehension and formulation. Although dependent on language comprehension and formulation, which are acting more or less literally on the message, language integration goes beyond language structure itself. The process of integration, then, is that process through which the language code is related to the child's past experience and knowledge, other sensory experience, and his cognitive representational abilities and strategies. Language development is tied to cognitive development, as was presented in our working definition of child language disorders in Chapter 3. Language and cognition (thought-representation) are interrelated for interpretation and creation of the complexities embedded in the message that is heard or in the message that has been created.

The process of integration allows the listener to apprehend the pragmatics of the language to which he is exposed, allowing him to be aware of the intentions involved in communication directed toward him, and aids in interpreting the communicative context. Similarly, it is from integration, or a juxtaposition of language and thought, that a speaker arrives at the intentions for his own communication and the contextual modifications required to make his message appropriate to the time, place, and persons present.

Although integration in our view handles the pragmatic component of language, the development of this process also allows for increased interpretations of complex aspects of language. Thus a 10-year-old might understand that the concept of "grandfather" requires a reciprocal relationship between a grandfather and grandchild, yet a 5-year-old may only understand grandfather as a particular person related to him. Similarly, a normally developing 10-year-old child may well be on his way to understanding what is implied by "Republican," while this may be beyond the ability of a retarded 10-year-old. Or a nonlanguage impaired 8-year-old will be able to figure out "if you worked right along every day, would you accomplish more work in a week or a month," while an 8-year-old language impaired child may seem puzzled.

Integration, therefore, requires an interpretation of language against what else the listener or speaker knows. Through the process of integration, the significance of language is apprehended, and abstract meanings are understood for purposes of communication. The following discussion of integration will center on two aspects of language that may be disordered following breakdowns in integration: pragmatic disruptions and complex meaning disruptions. We will first turn to pragmatic disruptions, where a discussion of intentions/functions and communicative competence will be followed by suggestions for future work. Disruptions in complex meaning will be approached from the level of abstraction

involved, the number and type of comparisons required, and the number and type of rearrangements required.

Language integration and pragmatic disruptions

Even though few systematic studies of pragmatic disruptions in language disordered children have yet appeared, and even though no single agreed upon theory or list of pragmatic functions is available to guide the speech-language pathologist, our field is beginning to recognize that pragmatic disorders do occur and to apply the available information to assessment and treatment of these children. The literature regarding normal pragmatic development, which has guided the work of the speech-language pathologist, centers around the study of (1) language intentions/functions and (2) communicative competence.

The study of the functions of language in disordered populations has been impeded by the lack of a generally embraced set of universal functions, although those provided by Dore (1975) or Halliday (1975) have received considerable attention.

Several writers have suggested that some groups of language disordered and/or retarded children may be restricted in the diversity and relative frequency of functions of language available to them, particularly restricting their use of language to question or as an information-seeking tool (Bates, 1976b; Morehead and Ingram, 1973). They do not seem to understand what language is for and what purposes it serves for them in both intrapersonal and interpersonal aspects.

Similarly, autistic children have been described as deviant in their functional use of language (Baltaxe and Simmons, 1975; Kanner, 1943; and Vetter, 1969). Language disordered children, unspecified etiologically, likewise have been found to be restricted in the frequency of questions they ask (Morehead and Ingram, 1973).

Blank, Gessner, and Esposito (1979) provided a detailed case study of a child who had language without communication. To them their case study indicates a separation of language as a system for expressing syntactic-semantic relations from language as a system for interpersonal communication. In this sense their case presentation reinforces the position we take in the CLPM of distinguishing between language comprehension-formulation and language integration. They state:

It is suggested that the structural and communicative aspects of language are based upon different sets of skills (processes) which particularly in cases of language disorder may function independently of one another.*

Communicative competence. Another thrust in normal pragmatic development has been toward growing awareness of modifications that are and must be made to meet the "communicative context," sometimes referred to as the tactics of communication (Bates, 1976a,b; Ervin-Tripp and Michell-Kernan, 1977; Gleason, 1973; Hymes, 1971; Sachs and Devin, 1976; Shatz and Gelman, 1973). Or, as Hymes (1971) has stated, acquiring the knowledge of who can say what, in what way, where, when, by what means, and to whom. Some researchers have directed their study specifically to explicating turn taking in conversational interactions or discourse (Bloom, Rocissano, and Hood, 1976; Bruner, 1975) and to the assumptions or presuppositions underlying communication (Bates, 1976a,b).

Studying communicative interactions has aided our understanding of the role the environment plays in language development, particularly in mother-child interactions, so-

cial discourse, and in the study of dialectic differences. A frequent hallmark of language disordered children, which becomes more apparent as their phonologic, syntactic, and semantic abilities improve, is their ineptness in the social use of their language. They often present an inability to grasp the subtleties of the communicative context or to adapt what they want to say to the demands of the situation they are in. In short, they are impaired in what Hymes (1971) has called "communicative competence" or what Wiig and Semel (1976) have referred to as the "social perceptions" related to language.

Although there have been few systematic studies of language impaired children's awareness of contextual demands of communication, it has been our experience that the majority of language impaired children present some limitations in this area. Wood (1976) provided a very readable account of the development of verbal and nonverbal communication, much of which concerned the pragmatic aspects of communication. Gallagher and Darnton (1978) documented the limitations that language disordered children have when required to revise their conversation. Bedrosian and Prutting (1978) noted similarities between mentally retarded and normal adults in the types of control exercised in conversational settings. The more impaired the child, the more obvious is his failure to adapt his language to his listeners and the context in which he finds himself. The inability to take into account the other person's perspective when speaking has been described for some time in groups of psychotic and retarded individuals (Kanner, 1946).

As language disordered children reach the latter elementary grade levels and their teenage years, often the syntactic and semantic problems so obvious when they were younger now appear secondary to the obvious inability to adapt their language to the communicative

---

*From Blank, M., Gessner, M., and Esposito, A., Language without communication: A case study. *Journal of Child Language*, **6**, 329 (1979), Cambridge University Press.

and social requirements of the situation. Wiig and Semel (1976), in describing language and learning disordered children and adolescents, were forerunners in describing these children's difficulties in acquiring and grasping the significance of the nonverbal cues in communication that provide information about people's attitudes, feelings, and intentions. The following vignettes demonstrate some of the problems that these language disordered young people present in using the tactics of pragmatics.

Adrian, 11 years old, after years of treatment for autism, now goes for the phone when it rings. After lifting up the receiver and putting it to her ear, she waits speechless. Only prompting, "say hello" gets her to respond verbally.

Larry, 20 years old, has recently returned to language therapy because he feels his social ostracism is related to his long-standing communication problem. Although his speech is readily intelligible and for the most part is syntactically appropriate, he is seen as a naive, not-with-it young man who has painfully learned that he cannot say whatever is on his mind, but has not figured out what is and is not acceptable.

Edgar, 16 years old, says as little as possible, hoping to minimize the blunder his comments always seem to bring about. He has learned from the faces of others that what he says often strikes them as weird. When he does not talk, people do not react that way to him.

George, 9 years old, is a case in point. Although during his early history, George gathered a variety of diagnoses, including "autism," "dysphasia," "specific learning disability," by 9 years old he was reading, spelling, and doing math at grade level, although in no way did he appear to be a "normal" third grader. Formal vocabulary and syntactic comprehension and formulation tests found him to be functioning within normal limits, yet his use of language appeared peculiar to all who knew him. One might characterize his use of language as "raw intentions" unmodified by the setting. For example, George would not hesitate to stand up in his reading group and announce unself-consciously that he had "to go pee." Or if he was curious about his examiner ("How old are you?" "What kind of a car do you have?"), no inhibitions or pressure toward social conformity held his tactless, immature questions in check. Although reported to have a crush on his classmate, Alice, he was at a loss for how to approach her and talk to her. Rather, George would go up to Alice and gently stroke her hair in a tender manner, reminiscent of how he might stroke a pet cat. The concrete mechanics of George's speech and language were quite adequate, yet he utterly and miserably failed at using his language in a manner appropriate to the setting.

These vignettes describe only a few of the ways in which language disordered children struggle with the difficulty of learning how to adapt their language to contextual demands.

Future directions. The pragmatics of children with language disorders is not yet described extensively, but it is a rich and multifaceted arena for study. Since we have very little large-scale descriptive information from which we might address questions of future directions, it is both improbable and illogical to search for unitary descriptive patterns of pragmatics that will describe the functions of language for all language disordered children. Different patterns will likely emerge across different groups of language disordered children, similar to the findings of other levels of language.

Areas in which future research will hopefully be forthcoming concern the following questions: Can pragmatics of language be disordered in isolation from disorders on other levels of language? Do language disordered children present a delay in the development of pragmatics, or is their use of the functions of language qualitatively different from that of normal children? Do pragmatically disordered children present an across-the-board reduction in the frequency with which they use various functions of language, or do they use language for some functions at the exclusion of other functions?

It may well be that the spectrum of child language disorders begins and ends with pragmatic concerns. For the very young and/or severely impaired child the primary functions of communication are of focal interest. Signaling in whatever way possible may be all that the severely retarded, motorically handicapped, or autistic child may be able to achieve. For other children who are less impaired yet nonverbal, language development may well begin with prelinguistic, functional use of vocalizations.

On the other end of the spectrum are the "high level" language impaired children, whose only remaining language deficits are confined to learning the contextual and largely social cues to language use. Although these individuals may speak in well-formed, semantically rich, clearly intelligible speech, they may be viewed as insensitive or socially inept by their peers, teachers, and parents. For them, a pragmatics "finishing school" may be in order.

Language integration and complex meaning disruptions

The other major aspect of language we are suggesting is handled by the process of language integration is ascertaining and abstracting complex meanings from messages, an operation that is closely tied to the child's cognitive abilities and experiences. In order to understand complex meanings, a child is required to relate what he hears with what he knows, which in turn depends on his cognitive level and his past and current experience. He must integrate language with what he knows about the world, but he can only do this to the limit of his cognitive capability. We are suggesting that complex meanings are understood through the process of being integrated with past experience and knowledge, other ongoing sensory experience, and cognitive abilities. For example, a 4-year-old may know "grandmother" as a particular white-haired woman whom he visits occasionally and who reads stories and makes cookies for him. His understanding of "grandmother" will be determined largely by his experience with a particular woman or women who he may even know as "Mommy's mommy" or "Daddy's mommy" or "Grandma Worzella." Yet he has little understanding of "grandmother" beyond the perceptual attributes of these few women and the contact he has had with them. By 7 or 8 years old, he undoubtedly will have a broader view of categoric "grandmother" and will understand the reciprocal relationships involved. This understanding, however, cannot develop until a higher level of cognitive ability has been obtained (Clark, 1973; Piaget, 1955).

Wiig and Semel (1976) and Blank (1978) have suggested two views of children's abilities and disabilities in understanding complex meanings. Wiig and Semel (1976) have listed six levels of cognitive-semantic processing abilities (processing of semantic units, classes, relations, systems, transformations, and implications), and they operationally discuss each of these abilities through specific tasks that might be used to measure each level.

Blank, Rose, and Berlin (1978) have suggested that language complexity is a function of the distance between the experience (perception) being considered and the language through which the experience is being discussed. When the distance between language and perception is minimal, the language demands are simple; however, as distance increases, the language demands become increasingly complex. Blank, Rose, and Berlin (1978) have suggested a four-tiered hierarchy of complexity: (1) matching perception, in which the language demands essentially match the salient perceptual features ("Find one like this"); (2) selective analysis of perception in which the children must begin to extract selected features of the material ("Name two things that are rectangles"); (3) reordering perception, where the children must use the language so as to restructure or reorder the way they view the material before them ("What was that story about"); and (4) reasoning about perception, which requires the children to deal with the realm of problem solving and reasoning ("Why is it a good idea to take turns").

☐ **Compare and contrast Wiig and Semel's (1976) six levels of cognitive-semantic processing with Blank's (1978) levels of language complexity.**

Our view of complex meaning is that a continuum exists, becoming increasingly complex along the dimensions of (1) abstraction, from a one-to-one concrete instance of a word to no external reference, (2) the number of comparisons that need to be made to integrate the information, and (3) the number of rearrangements or transformations of information that need to be made to relate incoming language with past information and experience. Therefore, tasks that present a rather close one-to-one correspondence between the language and the visual stimulus call for less integration than tasks that provide no visual representation. However, they require complete interpretation based on past experience or cognitive manipulation of the data. Similarly, tasks that require comparisons along only one dimension are simpler than those requiring multiple comparisons. Finally, tasks that require fewer mental manipulations or transformations will be integrated more readily than those with multiple, interrelated rearrangements of elements.

Before providing further examples of the abstraction, comparison, and rearrangement continuum, we want to point out that aspects of integration of complex meanings overlap with the process of comprehension of semantics, and no clear demarcation divides the two. Semantic comprehension in our view tends to focus on the understanding of the language code, whereas integration goes beyond the language code to interpret the language code

in active reference to other perceptual, cognitive, and experiential parameters. It may be that when new semantic information is being acquired, the process of integration is active, whereas when the word-concept relationship has been established, a more automatic process of comprehension takes over. For example, when a child is learning what the word *cat* means, he is active in integrating his sensory information of "catness" with his motor exploration and experience of "catness." When his knowledge of *cat* is firmly established, he may then understand the spoken word *cat,* through the process of comprehension. However, if he encounters a nonexpected use of *cat,* for example in reference to "catting around" or to nondomesticated felines, he may rely more heavily on the process of integration to augment his understanding of *cat.*

Abstraction. On the abstraction continuum, items requiring a close one-to-one match with some representation of the concept require less integration than those concepts for which no representation is possible. For example, understanding *chair, apple,* and *shoe* all provide possible one-to-one examples when these words are used. Going up the abstraction continuum, adjectives such as *happy* and *dirty* seem to be much less complex and more readily understood than *anxious* or *stingy,* partially because fairly readily represented aspects of the former words may be portrayed, for example the smile associated with *happy* and the smudged aspect associated with *dirty.*

Verb forms (such as walking and eating) and prepositions often are found to be more difficult to understand for language disordered children than are noun forms. One possible factor contributing to this difficulty is that the verb and preposition forms have to be abstracted from whatever is represented in the picture, the object, or the people acting in relation to one another from which these concepts derive.

At the high abstraction level of the continuum one may place concepts that have no representation (and for that matter whose meaning is relative to the user's experience), for example, *justice, nice,* and *honor.* Also at the high abstraction level fall words and concepts that can only be defined in terms of some symbol system, for example a mathematical formula. Thus high abstraction can be defined as either having no concrete representation with meaning evolving from experience and social consensus, or as concepts and words that are only defined in terms of some symbol system.

Comparison. Using and comparing information is much less complex if only a few, rather than multiple, comparisons are being made. For example, in indicating the bigger of two objects, the comparison required is limited to one dimension, that is, the size. Such a task requires much less language integration than a task that does not limit the dimension by which the comparison must be made (for example, how are an egg and an apple alike), or if it requires comparisons to be made against accumulated past experience (for example, what is silly about a one-armed man holding a banana and combing his hair). In the former case, where the dimensions to be compared are not specified, the child must bring up images of the two things to be compared and sort through the possible comparisons. Frequently, the comparisons given by language disordered children on such tasks relate to the most obvious physical attributes, for example, an egg and an apple are alike because they are both round. Functional comparisons that are not physically depictable require a more advanced basis on which to compare.

More difficult still are the language integration tasks that call on the child to compare

what is said to past experience, frequently requiring multiple comparisons. For example, in the Detroit Test of Learning Aptitude (Baker and Leland, 1967), for items on which the child is required to tell what is silly about a one-armed man holding a banana and combing his hair, the child must compare this statement with the usual circumstance, that is being two-armed, and needing to have two arms to perform the stated tasks. Such tasks seem to make particular demands on a child's ability to integrate information together with past experience in order to go from language to thought and then back to language again. Often it has been our experience that children can give evidence of understanding all the single components of a statement, such as that of the one-armed man, but that they cannot relate this information to what they know about the real world. The number and concreteness of the comparisons to be made would seem to be one useful way of viewing this breakdown.

Rearrangement. A third manner in which the difficulty of integration items may be viewed is in terms of the number of rearrangements of information necessary to understand the statement and solve the stated problem. Many of the language tasks that pose problems for older language impaired children require transformations of information in order to comprehend what is said, to answer questions, and to solve problems. What Wiig and Semel (1976) refer to as "cognition of semantic implications," (such abilities as comprehending implied cause-effect relationships, predicting outcomes, noting inconsistencies, recognizing absurdities, and understanding puns, proverbs, and idioms) would seem to require transformations of thought. Wiig and Semel's (1973, 1976) logico-grammatical sentences not only require comparisons of stored information, but equally important, they require rearrangements or transformations of the incoming language information.

For example, to respond correctly to the temporal relationship, "Does noon come after morning?" the child must refer to what he knows about the usual course of the day, that is, that morning comes first, then noon. He also must mentally rearrange the elements of the stimulus sentence into their temporal occurrence, and only then he must match what was said to the real-world parallel to respond affirmatively that noon does come after morning. Such a task not only requires comparison of information but also transformation of the presented information and concepts.

Probably some of the tasks requiring the most continuous transformations of language are proverbs, where words are used metaphorically throughout. Thus "a stitch in time saves nine" has very little to do with sewing, although this is not apparent directly from the statement. To interpret such a proverb, the listener must know not to take the statement literally but to undergo semantic transformations in order to grasp the complexities within the message. Such metaphoric transformations often fly over the heads of adolescents with language disorders who do not realize that the message is not to be decoded literally, or if they are aware of the nonliteralness implied, seem unable to understand the connection between the statement and the figurative meaning.

Ascertaining complexity, then, may be seen to represent several dimensions. The level of abstraction, number of comparisons required, and number of rearrangements of information provide one perspective from which to view integration as a continuum of meaning complexity. It is not enough for children to understand the words in a message; they must be able to use this information in reference to the stored experience and learning that constitutes their thought. Integration, then, implies language to thought interactions, integrating the language code with past experience and knowledge.

☐ **Working Part IV of our definition of child language disorders addressed the issue of cognitive development in relationship to language development and disorders. Leonard (1979) has reviewed certain research studies that have addressed the issue of language impaired children's performance on representational nonlinguistic tasks from a Piagetian orientation. What conclusions does he draw from his review? What do Morehead and Morehead (1974) and Kamhi (in press) add to our understanding of this relationship?**

FORMULATION PROCESSING STAGE

The bulk of the literature in child language disorders centers around measures of language output usually presented in terms of deficits in semantics, syntax, and phonology with less information available about the pragmatic level of language. Not all language output disorders, however, are a direct result of formulation processing disruptions. Therefore before proceeding with a discussion of formulation disruptions in child language disorders, it is important to draw a distinction between language output disorders and formulation processing disorders.

Defining language formulation and output disruptions

Language formulation on the CLPM is defined as the ability to select and retrieve words and the organization of these words into a logically acceptable and syntactically appropriate form. Formulation translates the speaker's intentions and messages (language integration) into language structure. We see language formulation principally concerned with the semantic and syntactic aspects of expression rather than initiation of intentions (attributed to the process of integration) and phonology (relegated primarily to speech programming). *Retrieval* and *selection* are key aspects of formulation. A child may understand a given lexical word or syntactic contrast as demonstrated on comprehension tasks. Formulation requires retrieval or selection of what he understands. Thus a child with a formulation disorder may be able to point to the correct picture of "the boy writes" and "the boys write," yet be unable to mark noun plurality or inflectional endings on verbs. Such a child appears not to be able to use what he has demonstrated that he understands on passive comprehension tasks. Similarly, one 3½-year-old child clearly could identify *mommy, daddy, doctor, teacher,* and *grandma* by pointing to the real persons or pictures of these persons, but when she spoke she used the word "dada" to refer to all five of these adults. This child apparently did not have available different names to refer to these adults, yet she had no difficulty indicating that she understood the difference. In sum, we see formulation disorders as the inability to retrieve or select correctly syntactic and semantic aspects for expression.

This distinction will be taken up further by presenting three issues revolving around language formulation disorders: (1) the existence of language formulation disruptions in isolation from other processing disruptions, (2) postulating the basis for the formulation processing disruption as an isolated phenomenon, and (3) considering the relationships among the levels of language output disorders.

Isolation of formulation disruptions. Many questions arise as to whether formulation processing disorders can exist in isolation from other language processing disruptions, particularly comprehension. This issue is difficult if not impossible to resolve at this time since it depends on the available information about language output disorders. The primary resource for an attempt to do this would be to unravel the literature that has been written on aphasia in children, particularly the issue of "expressive aphasia."

Virtually all of the early writers (see Chapter 2) in child language disorders included an expressive form of the disorder (Myklebust, 1954; McGinnis, 1963; and Morley, 1957, 1965, 1972). Thus for example, McGinnis (1963) listed contrasting language characteristics for expressive and receptive aphasic children. The expressive aphasics that she felt were quite rare were described as lacking expressive speech but as having understanding of language comparable to a normal child. McGinnis' (1963) criteria for classifying children as motorically or expressively aphasic included IQ within normal limits, normal hearing and understanding of language, inability to imitate words, and inability or limited ability to imitate speech sounds.

Myklebust (1954) included a "predominantly expressive" group of aphasic children, which he considered to be essentially normal children except for their limited use of speech. He described them as a rather homogeneous group that was relatively easy to differentiate and diagnose. The behavioral characteristics these children presented were not as significantly disturbed as those in children defined as having receptive aphasia. He concluded that the child with pure expressive aphasia demonstrated little if any auditory problems, although there were some who presented minimal difficulty in auditory discrimination. These children appeared to have a good relationship to their environment, including their auditory environment. They generally demonstrated basic comprehension, followed directions, and presented normal nonverbal behavior; however, they were relatively "mute," emotionally phlegmatic, quiet, and complacent children.

Later, Johnson and Myklebust (1967) differentiated three subgroups within their broad category of expressive aphasia: (1)

those whose primary deficit was in word selection because of difficulties in "reauditorization," a group that appeared to present primarily lexical formulation disorders; (2) those with defective syntax who could not plan or organize words for expression of ideas in complete sentences; and (3) those who could not execute the motor patterns necessary for speaking, classified as an apraxic group.

We gain more information about children with expressive language disorders from Morley in the three editions of her book, *The Development and Disorders of Speech in Childhood* (1957, 1965, 1972). She presented case histories and descriptions of 74 aphasic children of which she classified 72 as mainly executive. (Note: this distribution seems at odds with many others who feel "receptive" aphasia occurred with greater frequency.) She described these children as falling into two primary groups. The first group consisted of those with transitional developmental aphasia who "come out of it" at some later age. Fifty of the children fell into this group. The second group included children with prolonged developmental aphasia, who do not "come out of it." Of this group, 16 had normal IQs, whereas 8 had IQs from 80 to 90.

Morley noted that these children often used little or no vocal play or babbling, frequently were confined to one or two isolated words during the first 2 or 3 years of life, had word finding difficulties resulting in omission or substitution of words, demonstrated a limited auditory memory, (particularly for mastering language rules), and developed concomitant reading difficulties.

More direct evidence comes from Aram and Nation's (1975) description of children falling into their Specific Formulation-Repetition Deficit Pattern. The language disordered children who fell into this pattern of performance demonstrated essentially normal comprehension but had formulation disorders apart from any difficulties with motor speech production. It is important to note, however, that at the time this study was conducted we had not postulated a specific language integration processing stage as part of the study. Therefore, some of these children's formulation deficits may have stemmed from integration disruptions. Two children will exemplify these findings.

Edward was born to a 40-year-old woman whose pregnancy was without difficulty except for mild anemia. At 7 months old, he was hospitalized for a hernia and during the surgery went into cardiac arrest followed by temporary blindness. Although the blindness resolved, Edward was notably late in beginning to speak. When initially tested at 3 years and 9 months old, Edward's level of language comprehension was well within normal limits as demonstrated by the following test results. On the Peabody Picture Vocabulary Test (Dunn, 1965) his IQ score was 112. He only missed 2 items on the entire 2 to 4 critical elements on the Assessment of Children's Language Comprehension (Foster, Giddan, and Stark, 1973). He scored above the 90th percentile on the receptive portion of the Northwestern Syntax Screening Test (Lee, 1969). Despite this very good comprehension, coupled with a performance IQ of 122 on the Leiter International Performance Scale (Arthur, 1952), Edward could only name four pictures on the Vocabulary Usage Test (Nation, 1972) and could use no connected language. Thus he was unable to score on any measure of connected syntax. Except for a minor difficulty with tongue elevation to the upper lip, Edward presented no difficulties with his articulators, yet he could only produce (spontaneously or in imitation) 8 different phonemes.

Melissa's medical and developmental histories were unremarkable except for the notable limitations in speech. When first evaluated at 3 years and 3 months old, Melissa's Peabody Picture Vocabulary Test (Dunn, 1965) and Assessment of Children's Language Comprehension (Foster, Giddan, and Stark, 1973) were at age level, while her performance on the receptive portion of the Northwestern Syntax Screening Test (Lee, 1969) was at the 25th percentile for children her age. Despite a nonverbal performance IQ of 121 on the Leiter International Performance Scale (Arthur, 1952), Melissa could only name 8 items on the Vocabulary Usage Test (Nation, 1972) and could provide no correct answers on the expressive portion of the North-western Syntax Screening Test (Lee, 1969). Her phonemic repertoire was restricted to 9 correct responses on a 52-item articulation test, and in imitation she correctly repeated only 4 of 19 phonemes acceptably.

The issue expressed at the beginning of this section remains: Do children have isolated formulation disorders without comprehension disorders or other language processing deficits? From the early writers in childhood aphasia, it would appear that some children have isolated formulation disorders, since each writer has an "expressive" type aphasia. In addition, our experience with children like Edward and Melissa provides evidence of children with no concomitant comprehension deficits. However, these are seldom pure and often are coupled with integration disorders, auditory processing disorders, and/or apraxia of speech. It may be that isolated formulation disorders may exist but more commonly are only part of multiprocessing disruptions.

Processing basis for isolated formulation disruptions. How can children comprehend language but not use the same language for formulated speech? First, we could postulate a psychologic-emotional mechanism for the lack of language formulation. Some children are seen who withhold speech and language; that is, they appear to comprehend but simply do not use language to express their needs, wants, and desires. We believe this causal explanation should be used only very infrequently to explain isolated formulation disorders. "Elective mutism" on the part of a child is rare and likely to be accompanied by other severe behavioral and emotional disorders. However, it might be that some children withhold language because they know they have difficulty talking and may not feel emotionally secure enough to reveal these difficulties to others. BUT is this truly a formulation disorder?

Second, we could postulate a maturational problem. It is difficult to define exactly what is meant by this; however, it is quite likely that some children do not begin to talk with any degree of facility until later in childhood. We have all heard the parent who has said, "Johnny did not begin to talk until he was 4 years old, and then he began talking in sentences." These children may reflect a genetic basis for delayed maturation of the neurologic substrate of formulation. Many have familial histories of late-talking fathers and grandfathers. Morley (1965) talks of them as "late bloomers"—some children simply do talk later than others. If this maturational lag has a genetic basis, we need to discover more about it and its transmission.

Third, if we postulate that the underlying mechanisms for language comprehension and formulation can be discretely disrupted, we will need to develop and test models to demonstrate these theories. Processes that can be disrupted singly must have some distinct developmental basis during language learning.

In order to demonstrate this distinction in child language disorders, we would have to differentiate a child's ability to comprehend the same material that he is not able to formulate and express. To do this requires careful task design and analysis, and it may never be completely successful, since the language processes are continuous and interactive. However, we must strive for this in the tasks we use. For example, if we are interested in a child's ability to comprehend and formulate plural markers, we must be sure the task for plurality does not get lost in other variables, such as vocabulary, the qualities of the pictorial stimuli, and so forth.

Benedict (1979) has reported a study whereby she compared the first 50 words comprehended and "produced" by eight normal infants between the ages of 9 months and 1 year, 8 months. Her information confirmed that comprehension preceded production and that analysis of word classes used in comprehension and production differed in terms of proportion and types of action words. This comprehension precedes production paradigm might be useful in designing studies in language disordered children to view distinctions among the language processes. Our study (Aram and Nation, 1975) represents one of the few studies comparing comprehension-repetition-formulation of language disordered children.

☐ **What insights does Ingram (1974) provide that might assist in developing tasks to measure comprehension and formulation?**

Levels of disordered language output. For the most part, all language disordered children will have disorders of language output at one or more of the language levels, and it is this topic that receives the most attention in the literature on child language disorders. For example, Leonard's (1979) major review of the literature focuses on language output or, as he states it, "the speech of language impaired children." His review covers (1) syntactic output, (2) semantic output, (3) pragmatic output, (4) phonologic output, and (5) output that reflects other representation abilities, that is, cognitive development. Much of this literature, however, does not attempt to address the issue of the underlying processing reason for the language output disorders.

Not all these output disorders are a direct result of disruption of language formulation. Many of the output disorders stem from disruptions of other processing stages: sensation, perception, comprehension, integration, and repetition. In these instances the language formulation process can only perform in relation to what has been processed by earlier stages. Thus children might well present output problems that reflect their ability to formulate language; however, not all of these are from direct disruptions of language formulation. Since the language formulation processing stage follows the earlier processing stages, we will see language disordered children with output problems of two basic types: (1) those whose output disorder reflects earlier processing disruptions and (2) those whose output disorder is a direct result of language formulation disruptions.

If we are to understand language formulation disruptions, we must also consider the relationship among the levels of language output that are disordered. Is there a hierarchical arrangement to pragmatics, semantics, and syntactics? If so, what is the arrangement and the effects of one level on another? Can it be expected that if the pragmatic level is affected, all other levels will be similarly affected?

Some evidence exists for both views: the interrelated and the independent. For example, many inner-city children demonstrate adequate syntax but have a limited vocabulary. Certain anomic children seem to do the same. However, it is also evident that children, particularly mentally retarded children, demonstrate deficits at all levels. The assumption here might be that the integrative, cognitive base from which language proceeds is inadequate; thus all levels of language are also inadequate.

A number of researchers have examined the relationship between "articulation" disorders and language disorders (Shriner, Holloway, and Daniloff, 1969; Vandemark and Mann, 1965), generally demonstrating that children with defective articulation also were deficient on measures of syntax. These studies, however, did not clearly differentiate between articulation (motor speech production) and phonology. Thus these articulation problems may well have represented phonologic rather than purely articulatory disorders. Menyuk and Looney (1972), however, through use of a repetition task, examined the accuracy of repetition of both syntactic and phonologic structures by language disordered children. These investigators found syntactic structure and phonologic sequence errors to be significantly correlated, suggesting that the two disorders tend to go hand in hand. However, these were repetition tasks, a different process from formulation.

What has not been clearly documented is children who present multiple phonologic problems that are restricted to only the phonologic or morphophonemic level. Although researchers at times select for study children for inclusion who are said to present only articulatory or phonologic problems, often the inclusion criteria are suspect in that the "language measure" used was a comprehension-based measure such as the Peabody Picture Vocabulary Test (Dunn, 1965), or a global language measure such as the Utah Inventory of Language Development (Mecham, Jex, and Jones, 1967). And although designated phonologic or articulatory impaired children may "pass" such tests, no measures of expressive (formulated) syntax or semantics may have been included.

We (Aram and Nation, 1975) have suggested that formulation disorders may be hierarchical in that when "higher" language levels are impaired, so also are the lower levels disordered. For example, a child may present only a phonologic problem, but a syntactic problem will also be accompanied by some degree of a phonologic problem. A semantic formulation problem will include a syntactic *and* phonologic formulation problem. Such a position, however, is speculative and is not supported by recent research (Healy, 1980).

In the following sections we will discuss the literature that best reveals language output disorders resulting from disruption of the language formulation process. However, one of the major problems in discussing such formulation disruptions is that little descriptive data is available that isolates language formulation from other processing disruptions. Although much attention has been given to selecting children with a particular mean length of utterance (MLU), almost no attention has been given to selecting children with a particular processing breakdown with the exception of sensation disorders. The assumption apparently has been that language disorder X resulting in an MLU of 2.5 is the same as language disorder Y resulting in an MLU of 2.5. Thus the literature describing language disordered children's expressive syntax and semantics has focused upon groups with heterogeneous processing breakdowns. Hopefully the coming years will contribute more descriptive information of circumscribed formulation disorders; now we can only extrapolate from these more heterogeneous groups.

Semantic formulation disruptions

Semantic formulation disruptions will be viewed here in terms of disorders of the lexicon and of semantic relations paralleling the discussion in semantic comprehension disruptions. As is true for the other levels of language, the study of semantic disorders has been heavily influenced by developments in normal language acquisition. Therefore, an understanding of the normal acquisition of the lexicon and semantic relations is basic to work concerning disordered semantics in children. (See Chapters 2 and 3.)

Lexicon. Just as word retrieval problems are associated with many adult aphasic syndromes, lexical problems are a very frequently encountered clinical problem in many children presenting language disorders. In describing the lexical problems of language disordered children, six characteristics may be noted: (1) estimate of breadth of available vocabulary, (2) level of naming, (3) latency of response, (4) word class asymmetries, (5) misnaming, and (6) conceptual structure breakdown.

Leonard (1979), in his review of semantics in language impaired children as he has defined them, found little information related to lexical factors other than the very early work of Nice (1925) and Weeks' (1974) longitudinal study of a single child. In both those works the children studied were extremely slow in acquiring a basic 50-word vocabulary.

Various attempts toward word counts have been employed in order to estimate vocabulary size in certain groups of children with language problems. Among these are cleft palate children (Nation, 1970), the retarded (Papania, 1954; Winters and Brzoska, 1975) and the deaf (Griswold and Commings, 1974). Generally these word counts are compared to normative data, and age-level extrapolations are given. These and other similar studies indicate that children with language disorders have reduced abilities when compared to norms or normal control groups.

In learning disabled adolescents, Wiig and Semel (1975) reported that on six subtests used to measure semantic production, learning disabled children scored less well than did normally achieving children. Denckla and Rudel (1976) compared dyslexics and other learning disabled children's naming ability on the Oldfield-Wingfield Picture Naming Test (Oldfield and Wingfield, 1965). These investigators found that the dyslexics had longer latencies in naming than did the nondyslexics, but that the nondyslexic minimal brain dysfunction group produced a higher percentage of wrong names. Interestingly, Jansky and deHirsch (1972) reported that kindergarteners' performance on a picture naming test was the most powerful predictor of later reading failure.

Children with language disorders will often present misnaming or what are often de-

scribed as anomic responses. For example, an 8-year-old may say "toothbrush" for "hairbrush." Eisenson (1972) feels that some of the anomic responses seen in aphasic children are a result of syntactic formulation difficulties. He states:

> When the aphasic child attempts syntactic formulations, he sometimes appears to be suffering from anomia, apparently hunting for the word he needs for his utterance to be conventional and acceptable. We believe that the appearance of anomic difficulty is really an indication that he is striving, however belatedly, to express himself in a sentence unit, that he is working out a complete verbal formulation and is no longer satisfied with asyntactic utterance.*

If a child presents what appears to be an anomic response, that is, if he calls up the wrong word when asked to name something, we need to keep in mind how his response is related to parts of speech and to word class asymmetry. Is his ability to recall nouns different than verbs, than adjectives, and so forth? Is the child using words of one type disproportionately to other types of words? Is his symmetry of use balanced and reasonable? For example, we have found that some autistic children can give very specific noun categories in response to a stimulus but provide very few, if any, verb forms.

Anomic responses might be better viewed in terms of latency of response as well as part of speech affected. A focus on latency of response could provide information about the child's retrieval processes. He may have the word available but require a longer processing time for retrieval; thus latency of response can help tell us whether the child really has the word to retrieve or whether he simply takes longer to gain access to it. Latency of naming has also been used to assess knowledge of conceptual categories in different groups of

---

*From Eisenson, J., *Aphasia in Children*. New York: Harper & Row, Publishers, 196 (1972).

children (Sperber, Ragain, and McCauley, 1976).

As well as looking at the types of words a child might be retrieving and using, we can look at the underlying conceptual structure of the words being used. This view relates to how words are learned, what basis accounts for their learning, how cognitive information and sensory information play a role in what the words mean, and how they might be recalled and used.

Rosch (1973) has performed a series of studies based on the idea that individuals have images for things and that categories of words have prototypes. People have a central prototype for various words. For example, if people are asked to respond to *red,* the degree of difficulty in using the word depends on how far removed the stimulus is from their prototype, from their central tendency for "redness." Rosch (1973) has looked into how people develop these prototypes and has explored how normal children use commonalities for certain words such as *vegetable, furniture,* and *clothes*. From these results, Rosch (1973) concludes that people have greater difficulty calling up words that are less prototypic than others.

From this information questions arise about the nature of semantic formulation difficulties. Are they problems of retrieving a word, linguistic problems, or problems with underlying concepts for the word, that is, language integration problems?

Semantic relations. Several studies have examined the semantic relations of language disordered children in order to ascertain whether or not their semantic systems represent delayed or disordered language systems. In general these studies have found that when language disordered children are matched by MLU to their normal control groups, few differences are found between groups, suggesting that the language disor-

dered children's semantic relations are delayed rather than disordered. When language disordered children are matched by chronologic age to their normal control groups, differences are found between the two groups.

For example, Freedman and Carpenter (1976) compared the semantic relations of four normal and four language impaired children at Brown's Stage I. Although all eight children were at Stage I with a mean length of utterance between 1.7 and 2.0 words and were matched for IQ, the mean chronologic age of the normal children was 25 months (2 years and 1 month) and the mean chronologic age of the disordered group was 51.75 months (4 years and 3+ months). Thus the chronologic ages of these children were well over 2 years apart. For the 10 basic semantic relations compared, Freedman and Carpenter (1976) found only a significant difference for one relation, with the language impaired group demonstrating greater diversity in the use of the introducer + entity relation than the normal group. In discussing their findings, Freedman and Carpenter (1976) conclude that their language impaired children possess the necessary nonlinguistic cognitive precursors for linguistic development. They suggest that the children are impaired in their ability to acquire the various syntactic devices and operations they need in order to relate the basic semantic relations they perceive to the syntactic structure of sentences.

A second study examining semantic relations is that of Leonard, Bolders, and Miller (1976), who matched 20 language defective children to normal control groups, one group with equal MLU and the other group with equal chronologic age. Fifty utterances were analyzed using a modification of Fillmore's (1968, 1971) case grammar. The only overall subject group difference was in the disordered group's lack of use of the dative (animate being affected by action or state identified by verb). This difference in the use of the dative, as well as the frequency of use of the semantic relations, distinguished the normal and disordered groups when matched by chronologic age. However, when matched by MLU, the semantic relations used by both normal and disordered groups were the same and did not differ in frequency of use. Leonard et al. (1976) suggest that these findings support the theory that the disordered language usage reflected in semantic relations is consistent with an earlier level of development rather than a deviantly developing system. These authors also conclude that frequency data are more useful in examining comparisons between normal and disordered children's use of different structures than a mere listing of structure types.

Whereas the Freedman and Carpenter (1976) and the Leonard et al. (1976) groups of language disordered children were of essentially normal intelligence and etiologically nondefined (although obvious emotional and neurologic disorders were eliminated), Coggins (1979) studied the relational meaning used by four Down's syndrome children. Using nine semantic relation categories based on the work of Bloom (1970) and Brown (1973), Coggins (1979) found that Down's syndrome children demonstrate as much diversity in their use of relational meanings as do normal children at the same linguistic stage.

From these studies we can conclude that, at least for the groups of language disordered children studied, when compared with children of similar linguistic development (matched by MLU), language disordered children show few differences in their use of semantic relations. However, when matched by chronologic age, differences in the use of semantic relations are more apparent, particularly when frequency of use is taken into account.

The very significant chronologic age differences between the normal and disordered children in these studies cannot be ignored, however. Even when the nonverbal intelligence of language disordered children is normal, as in the Freedman and Carpenter (1976) and Leonard et al. (1976) studies, very significant age differences are apparent. When retarded children are studied, as in the Coggins (1979) study, the chronologic age differences understandably are even more pronounced.

As of yet the semantic relations of only very limited groups of language disordered children have been studied. Therefore it may be premature to conclude that no language disordered children present a different system of semantic relations. It would be interesting, for example, to have reports of the semantic relations used by deaf, blind, and autistic children, since these groups may be critical extensions of the disorder-delay issue.

Syntactic formulation disruptions

The hallmark of child language disorders to date has been the study of syntactic disorders that ushered in the era of linguistic and psycholinguistic description. The literature in child language disorders is filled with descriptions of language impaired children's syntax. A multitude of assessment approaches and procedures are available as are a vast selection of intervention techniques and programs. At times these syntactic disorders are subtle and not readily apparent in conversational speech. In other cases they may be more prominent at one point in development than at another. Most language disordered children will at one time in their developmental course evidence some difficulty in syntactic expression. Again, although we have chosen to summarize this vast literature on expressive syntax disorders here, the majority of the data presently available has not clearly specified where processing has gone awry. Thus these data derive from heterogeneously grouped children, only some of whom truly present formulation disorders.

We have studies that have examined the syntax of mentally retarded children (Graham and Graham, 1971; Lozar, Wepman, and Haas, 1973; Naremore and Dever, 1975), of hearing impaired and deaf children (Brannon and Murry, 1966; Ivimey, 1976; Quigley, Power and Steinkamp, 1977; West and Weber, 1974), of autistic children (Pierce and Bartolucci, 1977), and so forth. However, most of the literature on syntactic disorders in language impaired children has been descriptive and centered on the issue of whether the output response was delayed or deviant—a quantitative or qualitative issue.

Delayed or deviant? Menyuk (1964) was one of the first to suggest that language impaired children presented deviant rather than delayed language. Menyuk (1964) matched 10 normal and 10 "infantile speech" children by sex, age, IQ (determined by Full-Range Picture Vocabulary Test (Ammons and Ammons, 1958), and socioeconomic status. In addition, she observed one "infantile speech" child from 2 to 3 years old.

Menyuk (1964) concluded that the term *infantile* was a misnomer, since the grammatic production of the oldest infantile speech children did not match or closely match the grammatic production of the youngest children with normal speech. For example, the 3-year-old infantile speech child used both more transformations and more restricted forms than the 2-year-old with normal speech, but at the same time used restricted forms that were never used by the normal speech children. A very striking characteristic of the infantile speech children was that they seemed to use the most general rules, with many

more omitted forms than normal children and with very limited or deviant use of transformations. Menyuk (1964) suggested that the deviant syntax perhaps could be viewed as a basically useful grammar in English, that is, one that conveys sufficient meaning. However, grammar was oversimplified, and the sentences seemed to be reflections of a basic unmarked grammar.

Similarly, Lee (1966) suggested that language disordered children may well present a qualitative rather than a delayed pattern of development. Unlike Menyuk (1964), Lee (1966) compared children at approximately the same stage of linguistic development. In exemplifying the use of the original form of her Developmental Sentence Types, Lee (1966) compared a 4-year, 7-month old language disordered child to a 3-year, 1-month old normal child. Although these children used the same length of utterances, striking differences were noted. The language disordered child used no designative or predicative two-word constructions, used only one noun phrase, and generated only verb phrase constructions and actor-agent sentences. In addition, the language impaired child used no questions and used unusual pivots, such as "be." On the basis of this illustrative comparison, Lee (1966) suggested that at least some language disordered children developed language in a manner different from that of normal children.

Leonard (1972) carried the debate of deviant versus disordered language one step farther. He matched nine normal and nine language defective children by chronologic age, Peabody Picture Vocabulary Test (Dunn, 1965) scores, socioeconomic status, and level of education (all attended normal kindergarten). He analyzed 50 spontaneous utterances from each child in terms of phrase structure rules, transformations, and morphologic markers. Leonard (1972) suggested that any blanket statement about how a particular structure is used by "normal" children and not by deviant language users is quite inaccurate because both groups use some of the structures some of the time.

Leonard (1972) suggested that the differences in use of each syntactic and morphologic structure can best be described in terms of frequency of usage. If a frequency of usage criterion is maintained, it appears that many deviant speakers exhibit the following: (1) use of indefinite pronouns, personal pronouns, main verbs, and secondary verbs with a lower frequency than their normal peers; (2) use of negation, contraction, auxiliary "be," and adjectival transformations less frequently than their peers; and (3) more frequent use of deviant forms charcterized by verb phrase omissions, noun phrase omissions, and article omissions.

Leonard (1972) also suggested that the Developmental Sentence Scoring (DSS) system developed by Lee and Canter (1971) might provide an effective means of distinguishing between deviant language users requiring treatment and "slow" language developers, because frequency is credited in the DSS system in weighted scores. It is important in Leonard's (1972) study to note that when a comparison was made of the number of structures used, there was no difference between normal and deviant speakers; only when frequency of usage was compared did significant differences between the two groups arise.

Finally, Morehead and Ingram (1973) matched 15 normal and 15 linguistically deviant children by MLU and compared five aspects of their syntactic development: phrase structure rules, transformations, construction types, inflectional morphology, and minor lexical categories. In contrast to Lee (1966) and Menyuk (1964), Morehead and Ingram

(1973) concluded that the linguistically deviant children do not develop different linguistic systems but rather develop similar systems with a marked delay (mean age difference between the two groups was over 4 years) in onset and acquisition time. When matched by MLU, results suggest that language impaired children are not seriously deficient in the organization of phrase structure rules, types of transformations, number of transformations used in a given utterance, minor lexical items, or inflectional morphology. However, they appear to be restricted in their ability to develop and select grammatic and semantic features that allow existent and new major lexical categories to be assigned to larger sets of syntactic frames. Morehead and Ingram (1973) supported the observation of Menyuk (1964) that on the whole, the utterances produced by deviant children are less well formed than that of normal children.

Other investigators addressing the delay versus deviant issue have examined grammatic morphemes of language impaired children. In general, these studies have shown that language disordered children appear to acquire grammatic morphemes in the same order as normal children, although some variations in the stage at which they appear have been noted. These investigators have approached the study of morphologic development in two primary ways: the first, employing Berko-like (1958) tests whereby children have to generate the appropriate inflectional ending for various nonsense names, and the second, through an approach fashioned after Brown's (1973) longitudinal study of the appearance of various morphologic markers.

For example, Newfield and Schlanger (1968) adopted a Berko (1958) approach to testing morphology in retarded children and concluded that the retarded children learned English morphology in a manner comparable to normal children but at a significantly slower pace. Johnston and Schery (1976), in a cross-sectional study of 287 language disordered children where some of the children were also studied longitudinally, reported that these children developed the 14 morphemes listed by Brown in much the same order as found for normal children (Brown, 1973; de Villiers and de Villiers, 1973). However, Johnston and Schery (1976) also called attention to the very pronounced difference between normal and deficient children in the age at which they acquire these morphemes (for example, the mean age of the deficient children at levels 1 and 2 was 81 months versus Brown's normal children whose mean age at these levels was 28 months). They also noted that the deficient group reached 90% criterion level of correct usage one or two levels later than normal children, and that the course for morphologic acquisition seemed to be abnormally protracted in the deficient population.

In his review of much of this same literature around the issue of delayed or deviant syntax in language impaired children, Leonard (1979) criticizes the studies that concluded that syntax is deviant and entrenches the view that it is delayed. He states:

> A close examination reveals that, contrary to earlier impressions, the particular syntactic features evidenced in the speech of these children are not unique to this population. Rather, these features seem to be the same as those used by younger children.*

We, however, do not believe that the issue has been settled and perhaps is just a "straw man" issue, in that it is quite likely that some language disordered children will be delayed and others will be deviant as well as delayed. Ruling out deviancy of syntactic formulation

during language development appears arbitrary, is not yet warranted by the literature available, and might well lessen interest in future research in this important area of investigation. Here we will raise some of the considerations we believe are important for continued evaluation of this issue.

First, in the studies where children were matched by age, they were also matched by either IQ or some measures of receptive vocabulary. The fact that same aged children with comparable IQ or receptive vocabulary scores were chosen suggests that these language impaired children were functioning at a relatively high level in comparison to the total population of language impaired children. Even so, differences were found between the groups when matched by chronologic age (Menyuk, 1964), particularly when frequency of usage of a particular structure was taken into consideration (Leonard, 1972).

Second, the more refined the specific measure of syntax, the more likely were differences between normal and disordered groups to appear. For example, when the measure employed generalized phrase structure rules or frequently appearing transformation rules (Morehead and Ingram, 1973), differences were not reported when children were matched by linguistic level. However, minor lexical categories and less frequently occurring transformations did reveal differences, meaning that these later measures were possibly more sensitive indicators of linguistic impairment.

Third, virtually all investigators who did not select subjects by chronologic age stressed the marked difference in age at which the language disordered and normal children acquired various structures. Frequently these differences were as great as 4-year differences between the groups. At what point do delays of such magnitude become qualitative and

---

*From Leonard, L.B., Language impairment in children. *Merrill-Palmer Quarterly*, **25**, 212 (1979).

present a difference in kind rather than degree?

Fourth, there is no longitudinal evidence that these language impaired children actually do "catch up," and there is considerable evidence that many language impaired children present language and learning problems well into or throughout their school years (Aram and Nation, 1980; Hall and Tomblin, 1978; Wolpaw, Nation, and Aram, 1977). Therefore, suggesting that syntactic development is delayed may be somewhat misleading, since the implication is that the process is essentially the same as normal acquisition only slowed down.

Fifth and very important from our view of child language disorders is an issue that stems from the definition used for language impaired children. Most of the studies center around children who are defined in terms of output responses. We do not have literature that relates output responses specifically to differing process disruptions. The children in the previous studies represent only one portion of the population of language disordered children as presented in detail in Chapter 3. Children who form subgroups of the language disordered population, for example the aphasic child, the mentally retarded child, and so forth, may well present patterns of deviancy within delayed development, based on differences in processing.

Therefore although we conclude that many language disordered children may well present delayed syntactic development, we cannot conclude that all language disordered children present simply delayed development. At least some would appear to present a deviant system of syntactic acquisition.

☐ **What does Weiner's (1974) case study of Art and the studies by Naremore and Dever (1975), Steckol and Leonard (1979), and Moran and Byrne (1977) add to the delayed versus deviant issue?**

REPETITION PROCESSING STAGE

The repetition processing stage on the CLPM is considered a low level language process. Unlike the other language processes, repetition requires study of both an external auditory input and an external spoken response.

Repetition-imitation-echolalia

The terms *repetition, imitation,* and *echolalia* have been used somewhat synonymously in the literature, and clarification for purposes of the following discussion is in order.

Repetition. According to the concepts presented in the CLPM, speech and language repetition implies that a stimulus is reproduced verbally with no assumptions made regarding the meaningfulness or purposefulness of the response. In the CLPM we suggest that repetition may occur in at least two ways. First, repetition may proceed through the usual comprehension-integration-formulation sequence that would involve all central language processes, in which case the stimulus would be comprehended as well as purposefully reproduced. Such repetition may be termed *meaningful repetition.* Second, repetition may result via a shortcut whereby information is shunted from speech perception directly to speech programming, thus bypassing the processes of comprehension, integration, and formulation and resulting in nonmeaningful repetition. In either of these cases, the meaningful or nonmeaningful, there is an utterance that resembles to some degree the language (auditory) stimulus that has been presented.

Imitation. Imitation is a term often used interchangeably with repetition. However, the term has gained a distinctive use in both normal and disordered child language literature. It has been described in language development as a strategy by which parents and others respond to children to assist them in language development. In addition, imitation has also been used to refer to a particular technique to elicit language. Thus one may read that a researcher employed an "imitation task" or that he gained "elicited imitations."

□ **Prutting and Connolly (1976) and Rees (1975) have considered the terminologic confusions surrounding the use of the term *imitation*. How have Prutting and Connolly contrasted use of this term depending on the theoretic viewpoint of the researcher?**

IMITATION AND NORMAL LANGUAGE DEVELOPMENT. A major issue that developed in normal child language development centered around the role that imitation played in the process. Relatively early in the era of psycholinguistic description, Brown and Bellugi (1964) noted the striking frequency with which children imitated their parents and in turn parents imitated their children. This led Brown and Bellugi (1964) to suggest three processes in the acquisition of language that they termed imitation with reduction (the child reducing the adult model, for example, Fraser will be unhappy → Fraser unhappy), imitation with expansion (the parental expansion of the child's telegraphic utterances, for example, baby highchair → baby is in the highchair), and induction of the latent structure (the process whereby the child induces the rules of regularity in his language). Although Brown and Bellugi hypothesized that imitation played an important role in language acquisition, what that role is has been the subject of considerable controversy and research.

Early writers suggested that a child's repetitions of adult speech were nonprogressive, that they imitated no better than they produced language spontaneously. Ervin-Tripp (1964) studied the naturally occurring imitations of young children between age 1 and 2 and concluded that these children imitated structures at the same level as their spontaneous speech; in other words, their imitations were not advanced or progressive. Similarly, Menyuk (1969) suggested that normal children's imitations are not significantly better than their spontaneous speech and noted that length and complexity of the stimulus sentences were important factors related to imitation. Some investigators, however, have found children to be able to imitate some grammatic structures not found in their spontaneous language (Lackner, 1968; Menyuk, 1963; and Smith, 1970), although the converse, spontaneously using structures not imitated has also been reported (Prutting, Gallagher, and Mulac, 1975).

Certain investigations have revealed that imitation is highly variable among children and influenced significantly by the context in which the imitation occurs. Bloom, Hood, and Lightbrown (1974) studied the spontaneous imitations of six children as part of a longitudinal study of language acquisition. Spontaneous imitations for their children ranged from under 6% to as high as 33%. Kemp and Dale (1973) studied 30 children between MLU of 1.5 and 3.5, inserting 40 model sentences into conversation with their children. Their children varied from as low as imitating no sentences to as high as imitating 14 sentences. Similarly, Ramer (1976) demonstrated that normal children differ in the extent to which they use imitations, noting that a child's dependence on imitation is related to the function of imitation.

That context influences imitation has also been demonstrated by Bloom (1974), who reported that children were more able to produce longer and more accurate imitations when the context paralleled the imitation. Finally, several writers (Bloom, Hood, and Lightbrown, 1974; Dale, 1976; and Ramer, 1976) have suggested that young, normally developing children generally imitate newly acquired features in their language:

Imitation is a selective process that represents the 'growing edge' of language; it may serve a useful function in firmly establishing new aspects of language, but it is not the means by which the child picks up new features.*

Although the literature on the role of imitations in normal language acquisition has evidenced considerable variability among children, the use of elicited imitation tasks has been employed widely in the study of both normal and disordered language.

☐ **What does Clark (1977) conclude about the role of imitation in development of syntax?**

Echolalia. Echolalia typically has been used descriptively to refer to a particular type of language response. For example, some children may be described as echolalic or their language characterized as echolalia, but seldom are children characterized as repetitious or their language termed repetitious. Schuler (1979), in a very comprehensive discussion of echolalia, points out that echolalia is commonly thought of as meaningless repetitions of the speech of others. She goes on to comment, however, that in spite of the amount of information about echolalia, terminology and etiology are unclear and used loosely.

In this section, we will view repetition, imitation, and echolalia as arising from the repetition processing stage of the CLPM as either meaningful or nonmeaningful repetitions. When used, the terms repetition and imitation need specification in terms of meaningfulness. However, echolalia will always be treated essentially as a nonmeaningful response. Thus imitation will generally imply a

repeated, elicited, meaningful response and echolalia an abnormal response most often not formally elicited.

Lacking in much of the literature addressing these repetition behaviors is specification of a number of parameters, including the following: How accurate must the response be to be considered an imitation or echolalia? What aspects of language must be repeated with the greatest degree of accuracy (a phonologic copy, a syntactic copy)? What degree of intentionality or context sensitivity may be present to qualify as imitated or echolalic speech?

Repetition disruptions

Elicited imitations. Normal children's use of imitation is varied, and this variability hinders the validity and reliability of elicited imitation procedures for gaining estimates of language behavior. This problem is even more exacerbated in children who have language disorders. Imitation and echolalia in some groups of language disordered children may be quite different from that of children developing language normally. These aberrant imitations may be viewed as signals of language pathology and have important diagnostic significance.

First of all, language disordered children's ability to repeat does not necessarily closely parallel their spontaneous language productivity. Some language disordered children may not imitate as well as they spontaneously produce language, while others imitate at a level far exceeding their ability to comprehend or meaningfully use similar structures.

Menyuk (1964) was one of the first to call attention to the observation that some language impaired children failed to imitate at the level of their spontaneous syntactic production or to imitate at a later time spontaneous utterances they themselves produced. Furthermore, she found that sentence length correlated significantly with the accuracy of

---

*From Dale, P.S., *Language Development: Structure and Function* (2nd Ed.). Copyright © 1972 by the Dryden Press Inc. Copyright © 1976 by Holt, Rinehart and Winston. All rights reserved. Reprinted by permission of Holt, Rinehart and Winston.

repetition for the language disordered children but not for the normal children in her study. Menyuk attributed this inability to reduced short-term memory that made it difficult for the language impaired children to retain the complete stimulus sentence. She suggested that length was a particularly crucial variable affecting language impaired children's repetitions.

Menyuk and Looney (1972), as discussed in Chapter 5, further examined language disordered children's ability to repeat sentences depending on the length and structure of the sentences. These investigators presented normal and dysphasic children four different sentence types (active-declarative, imperative, negative, and question), each three, four, and five words long. The language disordered children's performance when sentences were held to three to five words long was found to be more affected by structure than by length. The normal children showed no difference in their repetition of sentences varying by length or by structure.

Echolalia. Although Menyuk's (1964) findings apply to some groups of language disordered children, for other groups of child language disorders, the excessive, exceptional, and for the most part nonmeaningful repetition has been a notable and dominant characteristic of their language disorder. When children repeat excessively, they are often termed echolalic, a characteristic not infrequently seen in retarded and psychotic children. Often echolalia is regarded as a sign of a child's noncomprehension. For example, some retarded children echo the last word or two of whatever is said to them while evidencing no understanding or integration of the message. More dramatic are the autistic children who echo verbatim whatever is said to them, coupled with little evidence of comprehension or spontaneous use of the same structures.

In Chapter 3 we described a group of language disordered children termed "echoers" in that their repetition skills were superior to both comprehension and spontaneous formulation, unlike other children in the study whose repetition skills generally paralleled their spontaneous formulation (Aram and Nation, 1975). Included in this group of children were some who were clearly retarded and others who were later diagnosed as psychotic.

Exceptional repetition skills or echolalia have been described by a number of writers, and echolalia subtypes have been identified. Kanner (1943), in his original description of childhood autism, commented on the excellent "rote memory" of these children in the absence of other uses of language. Kanner went on to distinguish between immediate echolalia, which occurred at the time the child heard the stimulus, and delayed echolalia, in which the child seemed to store the information heard and repeat it at a later time. Since Kanner's early (1943) description, these characteristics of the language of the autistic child have received considerable attention (Baltaxe and Simmons, 1975; Fay and Schuler, in press; Lovaas, 1977; Prizant and Ferraro, 1979; Rutter and Schopler, 1978).

The consensus among the writers seems to be that autistic children present serious difficulties in comprehension of language. Their echolalia appears to reflect this failure to comprehend and abstract the meaning and structure of the language code (Rutter, 1968). As implied by the CLPM, the language input appears to be shunted directly through the system to output.

Although children who are significantly retarded or autistic present some of the most frequent and notable echolalia, exceptional repetition ability can hold for at least some other language disordered children. Therefore, echolalia is not confined to retarded and autistic children but may be associated with other types of language disorders in children, characteristically those with comprehension disorders.

□ **In Schuler's (1979) review, in what groups of language disordered children does she feel echolalia plays a major part?**

Most clinicians at one time or another work with echolalic children. Erwin and Ricky are examples of two such children.

Erwin at age 4 could not be tested on the Leiter International Performance Scale (Arthur, 1952) because he could not be taught to match, a task required to perform this test. He scored very low on all comprehension and formulation tasks but was exceptional in his ability to repeat what was said to him. For example, he was unable to understand or formulate any of the items on the Northwestern Syntax Screening Test (Lee, 1969). However, he correctly repeated 37 of the 40 items on the expressive portion of the test. Not only was he unable to correctly formulate any of the items required on the expressive portion of the Northwestern Syntax Screening Test (Lee, 1969), but his spontaneous language included only 2- and 3-word telegraphic utterances. Erwin excelled in repetition, although it in no way paralleled language competence. Five years later Erwin was functioning in a low EMR class. Although the echolalia was no longer a prominent feature, he continued to be severely deficient in language skills.

Similarly **Ricky,** another echoer who later was diagnosed as autistic and who demonstrated the major characteristics associated with autism, demonstrated a high average nonverbal intelligence, receiving an IQ of 118 on the Leiter International Performance Scale (Arthur, 1952) at age 3 years, 9 months. In contrast to his very good nonverbal intelligence, Ricky was unable to achieve a basal score on the Peabody Picture Vocabulary Test (Dunn, 1965), nor could he correctly identify any of the vocabulary items on the Assessment of Children's Language Comprehension (Foster, Giddan, and Stark, 1972) other than *shoe*. Despite his complete failure on all language comprehension and formulation tasks, Ricky accurately imitated 8 of 40 items on the expressive portion of the Northwestern Syntax Screening Test (Lee, 1969).

Most clinicians working with language disordered children can report similar case studies of children whose ability to repeat far exceeds their useful comprehension and formulation of language.

Fay and his colleagues have made an extensive study of echolalia, extending the information beyond the study of autistic children. Their thrust has been toward understanding the use of echolalia by a variety of children. Fay (1967) and Fay and Butler (1968) studied developmentally a group of echolalic 3-year-old children matched to nonecholalic control subjects. Fay (1967a) compared three 3-year-old echolalic children to an older echolalic group drawn from a clinic population, noting that both groups exhibited a similar percentage of echoic responses. One year later, assessment of these two echolalic groups revealed that only the younger, nonclinical children had abated their echolalic behavior to be within the range of the control subjects. In comparing the echolalic and normal 3-year-olds, it was found that the echolalic subjects performed more poorly on all verbal comprehension and expression tasks other than articulation (Fay and Butler, 1968). Furthermore, Fay and Butler (1968) identified two groups of echolalic children, the *pure echoers* who repeat the stimulus sentences essentially unchanged, and the *mitigated echoers* who produce slightly modified echoic responses characterized by either pronominal reciprocation ("Where do you sleep?"/"I sleep.") or by a supplement to a pure echoic segment ("Are you a boy or girl?"/"Huh? Boy or girl."). The mitigated echoers had a higher verbal performance than the pure echoers and a significantly higher mean IQ.

Fay and Butler (1968) discussed echolalic behavior according to the relationship between repetition and comprehension during language development, suggesting that the audio-motor system can function relatively independent from the syntactic-semantic system. They suggest that a convergence of the audio-motor and the syntactic-semantic system is beginning to occur in the mitigated echoer and thus mitigated echolalia reflects a developmental progress in spontaneous speech. Fay (1973) has drawn parallels between the echolalia of autistic and blind children. He sees language comprehension as deficient in both groups of children. Because of the deficient semantic-syntactic systems, he suggests these children overdeveloped their audio-vocal system in an effort to communicate. He states:

> Now: if such a drive to communication develops to a given level beyond which it cannot proceed into the normal acquisition of the symbols and structure of language, then the result would be an ever-increasing facility with echolalia. The desire to communicate would not necessarily diminish, but the requisite tools and skills to do so would be unavailable.*

Thus echolalia may be viewed as the highest verbal achievement for groups of children with severe comprehension problems, and echolalia or exaggerated repetition skills may signal comprehension deficits.

It is tempting to draw a parallel between the echolalia of some groups of language disordered children and a similar pattern of language response in adult aphasics. Adult aphasics characterized as sensory transcortical aphasics typically have exceptional repetition abilities coupled with severely deficient comprehension skills. Such a language pattern in acquired aphasics is suggested to arise from a disconnection of the more anterior audio-motor system from the posterior temporal-parietal language areas (Geschwind,

Segarra, and Quadfasel, 1968). Some investigators have suggested similar neurologic mechanisms that could explain the echolalic language observed in autistic children (DaMasio and Maurer, 1978; Simon, 1975).

Pneumoencephalographic findings in autistic children (Delong, 1978; Hauser, Delong, and Rosman, 1975) have documented left temporal lobe anatomic defects in many autistic children. Discussing the implications of these findings, Delong states:

> A particularly attractive hypothesis is drawn from the work of Milner [1972], who has found that the memory function of the temporal lobe is specific for each hemisphere and that specific cortical functions are not transferred to the contralateral hemisphere unless there is a lesion in the cortical area involved. This leads naturally to the suggestion that in autism the function of the left hemisphere may be uniquely impaired by the failure of the hemispheral memory or integrative learning function, without takeover of the critical functions by the opposite hemisphere. Such a formulation can explain in a satisfying fashion some of the most striking phenomena of the autistic syndrome.*

An understanding of the process of repetition-imitation-echolalia in child language disorders is beginning to be unraveled. Many unresolved issues, however, remain, including (1) the role of imitation and echolalia in normal language development, (2) differentiating pathologic echolalia from the imitations of normally developing children, (3) clarifying the communicative intent and functions underlying echolalia, (4) discovering the etiologic basis for exaggerated and reduced repetition ability, and (5) arriving at an understanding of the appropriate role of both imita-

---

*From Fay, W.H., On the echolalia of the blind end of the autistic child. *J. Speech Hearing Dis.* **38,** 483 (1973).

*From Delong, G.R., A neuropsychologic interpretation of infantile autism. In M. Rutter and E. Schopler (Eds.) *Autism: A Reappraisal of Concepts and Treatment.* New York: Plenum Press, 217 (1978).

tion procedures and spontaneous echolalia in the therapeutic process.

We maintain that a language disordered child's repetition ability contrasted against his comprehension, integration, and spontaneous formulation abilities provides a very fundamental avenue toward differentiating among types of language disordered children. In addition, such a contrast among processing abilities points toward more carefully designed treatment approaches tailor-made for each language disordered child's processing strengths and limitations.

chapter 7

Language to speech processing

DOMAIN OF LANGUAGE TO SPEECH PROCESSING

After a speaker has developed his intentions for communication and has formulated the semantics and syntax of his message, that message must be translated into a speech event. As a speech event the message is finally actualized as a series of sequential motor movements resulting in an output response through: (1) selection and ordering of speech sounds that represent the words and sentences of the message, (2) transduction of this representation into motor commands, and (3) innervation and movement of the speech musculature. The domain of language to speech processing as viewed in the CLPM takes into account two postlinguistic processing stages. These two processing stages have been described in Chapter 3 as (1) speech programming and (2) speech production.

We maintain that distinctions can be made in output responses between disorders related to each of these two postlinguistic processing stages. We are suggesting that phonologic disorders and developmental verbal apraxia result from speech programming disruptions, and that articulatory (phonetic) and motor speech disorders result from disruptions of speech production.

Whether or not these disorders fall legitimately within the realm of child language disorders or are more appropriately viewed as part of motor speech disorders has been questioned. Speech disorders such as dysarthria result from disruptions of the neuromotor system. The basis for phonologic disorders and developmental verbal apraxia is less clear. Many phonologic disorders in young children may stem from disruptions in other processing stages, particularly in speech perception, as was discussed in the speech to language processing segment. Therefore the distinction between phonologic disorders stemming from disrupted auditory operations versus speech programming processes is at this time difficult to make. At any rate, phonology and phonologic disorders have generally been classified as a level of language and language disorders.

The questions that arise about verbal apraxia often revolve around its relationship to childhood aphasia: Is it a part of or separate from childhood aphasia? If separate from childhood aphasia, is it a part of motor speech disorders? These are only some of the questions that make the boundaries of language to speech processing less than clear. These issues and appropriate literature will be discussed in this chapter.

SPEECH PROGRAMMING DISRUPTIONS

Speech programming on the CLPM stands at the junction between the language to thought to language segment and the language to speech segment, since it is considered both a language-based and a motorically based process. As a language-based process, it receives the pragmatic, semantic, and syntactic message that has been intended and formulated. To this message a phonologic representation is added through one aspect of the process of speech programming. Thus speech programming draws from and contributes to available phonemic categories and applies phonologic processes. It therefore is an active process involved in the development, selection, and ordering of phonologic categories and processes. Speech programming also is considered a speech-based process, responsible for turning phonologic sequences into motor commands for execution.

Disruptions of the speech programming processing stage therefore take into account a wide range of the phonologic disorders seen in young children. Our emphasis in this chapter, however, will be developmental verbal apraxia, since most phonologic disorders in children are considered a somewhat separate domain for study in speech-language pathology.

Phonologic disorders in children

As diagrammed in Fig. 3-2, observations of a child's use of phonology provide information about the process of speech programming. From the extent of phonemic categories and phonologic processes used by the child, we can make inferences regarding certain aspects of speech programming. But because the effects of other processing disruptions may be cumulative throughout the processing system, not all phonologic impairments will be the result of speech programming disrup-

tions. Others may arise from sensation or speech perception breakdowns, the other processes primarily responsible for phonologic information coming into the system (see Chapter 5).

Until the past decade, children's disordered sound systems were primarily viewed as articulatory disorders. With the outpouring of theories of phonology and phonologic development, interests became focused on the disordered phonologic (language-based) systems that these children often present. Whereas earlier the emphasis had been in evaluating the "substitutions, omissions, and distortions" in reference to normative data, investigators began seeing the phonologically impaired child as presenting his own rule-observing phonologic system where features and processes could be described, both in reference to the child's unique system as well as to phonologic development in normal children. Thus investigators including Compton (1970), Crocker (1969), Ingram (1976), McReynolds and Engmann (1975), McReynolds and Huston (1971), Panagos (1974, 1978), Panagos, Quine and Klich (1979), and Pollack and Rees (1972) have been instrumental in changing the direction from description of speech sound errors toward recognition of distinctive feature systems and phonologic processes underlying phonologic disorders in children. Typically, however, investigators describing phonology in language disordered children do not specify or speculate where processing has gone awry. Therefore we cannot directly relate work such as that of Panagos (1974, 1978) and Compton (1970) to any specific processing disorder.

Even in the mentally retarded where some work has been done, mostly studies of "articulation disorders" (Everhart, 1960; Massengill, 1970; Sommers, 1970; and Wilson, 1966), controversy exists as to the pattern of phonologic development. For example, Bangs

(1942) feels the error pattern reflects a simple delay, whereas Wilson (1966) believes the pattern is deviant. Ingram (1976) falls somewhere in between, believing that mentally retarded children show patterns of delay but often do not develop a number of normal aspects of phonology.

☐ **In his review of phonologic difficulties in language impaired children, Leonard (1979) states that the phonologic processes are for the most part the same as those seen in young children. What literature did he review and how did he arrive at this conclusion?**

Since the role of phonology is paramount in intelligible communication, the issue of phonologic development and disorders in child language disorders must be addressed directly in terms of processing disruptions if we are to develop appropriate assessment and treatment programs for them. Their language is limited as it is, and they do not need the extra burden of limited intelligibility.

☐ **Vahcic, Nation, and Sugarman (1977) proposed a phonologic disorder in an adult mentally retarded woman. How did they justify this disorder to be other than a disorder of articulation?**

Developmental verbal apraxia

The classic disorder attributed to disruptions of the speech programming process has been acquired apraxia of speech in mature speakers following central nervous system lesions. In children, a developmental form termed *developmental verbal apraxia* has been described and has similarly been attributed to a breakdown in speech programming. At the outset, however, it must be stated that as much is not known as is known about developmental verbal apraxia. Thus, although we are suggesting that at least some aspects of verbal apraxia represent speech programming deficits, a clearer description and processing explanation must await further research. The following material will develop the concept of developmental verbal apraxia rather extensively, since we feel a need to bring together in a single source the diversity of information that exists pertaining to this little understood disorder in children.

Heritage in acquired apraxia of speech. Far antedating recognition of the developmental form, acquired apraxia in adults following cortical insults has been described at least since Broca (1961a,b). The aphasiology and neurolinguistic literature is filled with discussion and controversy pertaining to various aspects of the disorder. A principal theoretic division has been to view apraxia as a motor speech disorder, or alternately as a linguistic-based, phonologic disorder—a distinction that may be less than real.

The first of these perspectives is exemplified by Darley, Aronson, and Brown (1975), who treat apraxia of speech as a motor speech disorder. They state:

> When certain brain circuits devoted specifically to the programming of articulatory movements are impaired the resulting articulatory disorder is called *apraxia o speech.*[*]

Investigators and clinicians working from this perspective stress the absence of paresis or weakness of musculature, the variability of phonemic production, and the groping gestures and disturbances in prosody (Darley Aronson, and Brown, 1975; Deal and Darley 1972). These investigators tend to view acquired apraxia as a disruption restricted to motor programming for speech and to implicate phonetic or articulatory error types.

The second group of investigators has viewed acquired apraxia as a linguistic encoding disruption primarily but not exclusively of phonology (Blumstein, 1973; Lesser, 1978

---

[*]From Darley, F.L., Aronson, A.E., and Brown, J.R *Motor Speech Disorders.* Philadelphia: W.B. Saunder Co., 2, (1975).

Martin and Rigrodsky, 1974; and Martin, 1974).

Irrespective of the controversies in approaching acquired apraxia in adults, most clinicians and investigators have come to view apraxia of speech as (1) predominantly a phonetic or phonemic disorder and (2) the result of demonstrable central nervous system dysfunction, usually stemming from anteriorly located lesions, although variable forms have been ascribed to alternately placed lesions.

The study of developmental verbal apraxia has been approached with the assumption that (1) this disorder likewise was one predominantly of the sound system, either as an articulatory or phonologic disorder attributed to a motor porgramming deficit, and (2) the disorder was a result of a neurologic, presumably anterior, cortical dysfunction. For example, Rosenbek, Hansen, Baughman, and Lemme (1974) state:

> Like apraxia of speech in adults, developmental apraxia of speech has often been confused with aphasia. This is unfortunate because developmental apraxia of speech is an articulation disorder subsequent to brain damage. Characterized by impaired ability to accomplish the volitional production of speech sounds and sound sequences, it is not a disorder of language, although it may coexist with language deficits and learning disability.[*]

State of the art in developmental verbal apraxia. Although similar disorders have been described since at least the late 1800s (Hadden, 1891), Morley (1967) is one of the first to have provided a comprehensive description of developmental apraxia in a group of 12 children. To date, her study stands as the only incidence study of developmental apraxia that has been reported in the literature. Others

---

[*]From Rosenbek, J., Hansen, R., Baughman, C., and Lemme, M., Treatment of developmental apraxia of speech: A case study. *Language, Speech and Hearing Services in Schools,* **5,** 13 (1974).

have reported about apraxic children (Ferry, Hall, and Hicks, 1975; Rosenbek and Wertz, 1972); however, only a single systematic research study has of yet appeared in the literature (Yoss and Darley, 1974).

The Ferry et al. (1975) study described 60 patients between ages of 4 and 30 seen at the University of Oregon Health Science Center for delayed speech or poor response to speech therapy, along with 20 ambulatory, nonverbal residents of a state institution. Rosenbek and Wertz (1972) described a group of 50 children between ages of 2 years 9 months and 14 years, 45 of whom were seen at the Mayo Clinic and five of whom were from the University of Colorado Speech and Hearing Clinic. Yoss and Darley (1974) studied a group of 30 children with defective articulation who were drawn from a public school system, identifying 15 of whom they considered to be developmental apraxic children. Recently, Aram and Glasson (1979) have reported detailed phonologic, phonetic, language, and neurologic findings for a group of eight children with normal nonverbal intelligence and language comprehension.

Beyond these few studies, the remainder of the reports have concerned theoretic or non-data-based discussions of the nature of developmental apraxia (Edwards, 1973; Eisenson, 1972); case studies or studies with small numbers of children (Dabul, 1971; Logue and McClumpha, 1970; Prichard, Tekieli, and Kozup, 1979); a report of a familially based verbal dyspraxia where 34 of 66 family members had defective speech, 12 of whom were extensively tested (Saleeby, Hadjian, Martinkosky, and Swift, 1978); and articles principally concerning therapy with apraxic children (Chappell, 1973; Daly, Cantrell, Cantrell, and Aman, 1972; Rosenbek, Hansen, Baughman, and Lemme, 1974; Yoss, 1974).

The few case studies, reports, and research studies available are plagued by a number of problems that make it difficult to arrive at conclusions or cross-comparisons between studies. Probably the most serious of these problems center on criteria for classification as developmental verbal apraxia. Furthermore, studies vary enormously in the degree of homogeneity (Aram and Glasson, 1979; Yoss and Darley, 1974) or heterogeneity (Ferry et al., 1975; Rosenbek and Wertz, 1972) in the group described. Often children with significant retardation are included (Ferry et al., 1975), and frequently no details are given relevant to language abilities beyond the phonologic level (Ferry, Hall, and Hicks, 1975; Rosenbek and Wertz, 1972; Yoss and Darley, 1974) or the sensory, particularly tactile and kinesthetic, abilities of the described group (Aram and Glasson, 1979; Rosenbek and Wertz, 1972; Yoss and Darley, 1974). In addition, studies are mixed as to the age range described and the severity of apraxia included which may range from relatively mild (Yoss and Darley, 1974) to profound disorders rendering a child essentially nonverbal (Logue and McClumpha, 1970).

Because of the variability among populations studied, we have summarized some of the important variables of the major studies of developmental apraxic children in Table 7-1. In the discussion that follows, we must keep in mind the lack of comparability among studies and the absence of unanimity of thought in the study of developmental verbal apraxia.

Definition and criteria for developmental verbal apraxia. A variety of terms have been used to refer to this condition we are describing, including developmental articulatory dyspraxia (Morley, 1967); verbal dyspraxia (Edwards, 1973; Ferry, Hall, and Hicks, 1975; Saleeby, Hadjian, Martinkosky, and Swift, 1978); childhood verbal apraxia (Chappell, 1973); "dilapidated" speech (Ferry, Hall,

and Hicks, 1975); and developmental apraxia of speech (Logue and McClumpha, 1970; Macaluso-Haynes, 1978; Rosenbek, Hansen, Baughman, and Lemme, 1974; Rosenbek and Wertz, 1972; Yoss and Darley, 1974). Here we will use the term developmental verbal apraxia to signify that the disorder may be more comprehensive than the term *speech* implies.

Most definitions of developmental verbal apraxia have stressed the inability to carry out the voluntary movements required for speech in the absence of a paresis in the speech musculature. Similarly, most definitions have focused on the articulatory aspects and the inability to sequence speech movements. For example, Morley (1967) has stated:

Developmental articulatory apraxia, or dyspraxia in its less severe form, has been described as an inability to perform voluntary movements of the muscles involved in articulation although automatic movements of the same muscles are preserved.[*]

Similarly, Eisenson (1972) describes apraxia as a restriction in

. . . the child's ability to organize and produce the appropriate movements for the production of certain phonemes or sequences of phonemes, and is likely to include those phonemes related to consonant sounds requiring movements of the lips and/or movements of the tongue tip or tongue blade.[†]

Or, as Edwards (1973) has stated:

. . . an impairment of the ability to carry out purposeful movement of the organs of articulation for speech.[‡]

---

[*]From Morley, M., *Development and Disorders of Speech in Childhood*, Edinburgh: Churchill Livingstone, 274 (1972).
[†]From Eisenson, J., *Aphasia in Children*. New York: Harper & Row, Publishers, 191 (1972).
[‡]From Edwards, M., Developmental verbal dyspraxia. *British Journal of Disorders of Communication*, **8,** 64 (1973).

TABLE 7-1. *Population data from selected studies of developmental verbal apraxia*

Study	Number	Institutions drawn from	Age range	IQ range	Language abilities	Neurologic
Yoss and Darley (1974)	16—apraxic 14—non-apraxic defective articulation	Hospital clinic	5-1 to 9-10 (median: 6-4)	90 to 122 (median: 103)	No more than 6 months below CA on Utah Test of Language Development	All seen by neurologist for clincial examination
Ferry, Hall, and Hicks (1975)	60	40—hospital clinic 20—nonverbal residents of state institutions	4 to 30 years (majority between 4 and 10 years)	40 to 120	No data reported	All seen by neurologist for clinical examination 20—state residents had EEGs
Rosenbek and Wertz (1972)	50	45—hospital clinic 1—university clinic	2-9 to 14 years (median: 4,9)	No data except no effort to exclude mental retardation	No data reported, except no effort to exclude language delay	36—Pediatric neurology examination 26—EEGs
Morley (1967)	12	Hospital clinic and school	4 to 17 years	Performance IQ 105 to 130 (mean: 114)	5—delayed, some with language disorders 3—dyslexia 1—spelling disability	No data reported
Aram and Glasson (1979)	8	Hospital clinic	4-7 to 14-4 young group median: 5 years older group median: 10 years	80+ to 136	Extensively studied	7—clinical examination 5—EEG 6—CT scan

Beyond agreement that the predominant problem in developmental apraxia centers on the phonologic and phonetic levels and that these children present a contrast in voluntary versus involuntary production, the boundaries of developmental apraxia are not well defined. This lack of agreement on who is and who is not a developmental apraxic child may at least partially derive from the limited research attention given this group of children. Macaluso-Haynes (1978) has characterized developmental apraxia of speech as "hard-core" articulation disorders that are extremely resistant to treatment by traditional methods, a theme echoed by Jaffe (1979).

In addition to the specification of developmental verbal apraxia as a disorder of voluntary movement of the articulators for speech that is resistant to remediation, most writers have required that two additional conditions be met in order to classify a disorder as developmental verbal apraxia: (1) receptive language abilities far superior to expressive abilities and (2) a presumed neurologic basis

TABLE 7-2. *Differential diagnosis summary for dysarthria, dyspraxia, and dyslalia*

	Isolated developmental dysarthria	Articulatory dyspraxia	Dyslalia
Family history	Often positive	Often positive	Infrequent
Movements of tongue, lips and palate	Movements of one or more muscle groups obviously affected. There may be excessive dribbling, or sucking, swallowing or chewing difficulties. Movements are limited, slow and clumsy.	No spasticity, normal movements of tongue, etc., except for articulation. These movements are not well directed and may appear awkward and clumsy during speech.	No obvious difficulties in the movements of the muscles for speech.
Development of speech	May occur at the normal time, but there is usually some delay which may be developmental aphasia or anarthria.	Often a little retarded, but usually within the normal range.	Normal age for speech development. Fluent.
Articulation	May be normal in isolation, in single words or syllables or at a slow speed in speech according to the degree of dysarthria. Consonants often omitted. Substitutions may be consistent and determined by the group of muscles chiefly affected. Consonant combinations often defective.	The imitation and use of single sounds, syllables, or words is better than their use in long sequences. Use of consonants and substitutions often erratic. There may be faulty pronunciation of whole words, transposition of sounds, reversals and perseveration.	Consonant substitutions usually consistent, sounds rarely omitted except in mental deficiency.
Vowels and diphthongs	Usually normal, but sometimes defective, particularly diphthongs.	Usually normal, but are affected in some severe cases.	Normal
Ability to imitate the sounds of speech	Normal on auditory stimulus alone within, the limits of muscular movement.	Auditory stimulus may be insufficient. Imitation is assisted by visual stimulus and may be normal when the child is watching the therapist's movements. Seeing the word in print helps the older child.	Normal
Phonation	There may be incoordination, of phonation and articulation, or of both with respiration.	Usually normal.	Normal
Rate of speech	Increased rate, anxiety, or excitement causes deterioration in muscle movements and articulation. Such relapses persist so long as neuromuscular control is inadequate.	Speech can be rapid without deterioration in muscle movements, but use of consonants may deteriorate with stress. Periods of relapse occur until new habits of articulation are fully stabilised.	Normal speed, but some relapsing articulation occurs until normal articulation is stabilised.
Associated disabilities	Aphasia, which may be persistent, dyslexia, spelling disability, or dysgraphia may occur in association with this condition.	Aphasia is rare, but there may be verbal paraphasia, or difficulties in the use of words, rather than a severe delay in the onset of speech. Dyslexia, especially if visual discrimination and visual memory for printed symbols is not well developed. Spelling disability. Dysgraphia.	Rare
Lateral dominance	Left-sidedness is found more commonly than in the normal population, or there may be left-handedness in association with a preferred right eye.	Cross laterality occurs more frequently than in the normal population—usually right-handedness in association with a preferred left eye.	The majority right sided, the proportion of left-sidedness and cross laterality being similar to that in the normal population.

evident in gross motor behavior, an accompanying oral apraxia, and/or other subtle neurologic findings.

DIFFERENTIATION FROM OTHER ARTICULATORY AND LANGUAGE DISORDERS. Many writers have stressed that developmental apraxia of speech is not a dysarthria (Morley, 1967) or a language disorder (Hansen, Baughman, and Lemme, 1974; Morley, 1967), while most have stated that these conditions frequently co-occur (Ferry, Hall, and Hicks, 1975; Greene, 1967; Morley, 1967; Rosenbek and Wertz, 1972).

Efforts to differentiate apraxia from other functional articulatory disorders have been offered by Rosenbek and Wertz (1972) who suggested the four following symptoms that differentiated developmental apraxia from a functional articulation disorder with a high degree of probability: (1) the presence of vowel errors, (2) an increased number of errors in longer response, (3) an oral apraxia, and (4) groping postures of the speech muscles. Morley (1967) has contrasted developmental apraxia with developmental dysarthria and dyslalia in a tabular form that has been reproduced in Table 7-2.

Despite the attempt to differentiate developmental apraxia from dysarthria or a neuromuscular weakness, distinctions become blurred, and it is often questionable whether or not a clear demarcation can be made. For example, although a "pure" apraxic child when tested will not present an observable dysarthria, frequently his history as an infant or young child included excessive drooling or difficulty learning to suck, both symptoms often associated with neuromuscular weakness.

Although Rosenbek, Wertz, Baughman, and Lemme (1974) have stressed that developmental apraxia of speech is an articulatory disorder and *not* a language disorder, we take exception to such a dichotomy, based on information to be presented later. Since all the answers are far from conclusive, we maintain that a less than arbitrary position should be taken, including the theory that developmental apraxia may be a part of rather than apart from a child's language disorder.

We shall be examining the phonologic/phonetic, language, and neurologic findings in detail in the following sections. Following this expanded treatment of the data, we shall revisit the issue of criteria for developmental verbal apraxia.

Phonologic and phonetic findings in developmental verbal apraxia

With two exceptions (Aram and Glasson, 1979; Yoss and Darley, 1974), most investigators have not differentiated between phonologic and phonetic characteristics of developmental verbal apraxia. Ferry, Hall, and Hicks (1975), Ingram and Reid (1956), Morley (1967), Rosenbek and Wertz (1972), and Yoss and Darley (1974) have reported group characteristics for their children while Aram and Glasson (1979) have differentiated between younger and older children and phonologic and phonetic findings. No attempt has been given by any of these writers to differentiate between levels of severity and the phonologic and phonetic findings. The characteristics reported by these various investigators follow:

Morley (1967)

1. May be able to imitate sounds in isolation, but not used in speech.
2. May not be able to imitate speech sounds.
3. Increased difficulty as length of word increases.
4. Some are consistent in use of consonants and substitutions; in others the use is erratic.
5. Consonant sounds frequently are transposed with reversal in order.
6. Vowels and diphthongs often normal, but may be affected in some cases, especially diphthongs.

McClumpha and Logue (1972)

1. Difficulty in sequencing sounds.
2. Difficulty with phonetic synthesis.
3. Variability of articulation in response to stimulation versus spontaneous speech.
4. Severely disintegrated articulation that cannot be explained on the basis of peripheral breakdowns.
5. Multiple place, manner, and voicing errors.

Rosenbek and Wertz (1972)

1. Prominent phonemic errors: omissions (errors are more from omission of sounds and syllables than substitution of sounds and syllables), substitutions, distortions, additions, repetitions, and prolongations.
2. Frequent metathetic errors, (for example, sound and syllable reversals.
3. Errors increase as words increase in length.
4. Repetition of sounds in isolation is often adequate; connected speech is more unintelligible than would be expected on the bases of single-word articulation test results.
5. Errors vary with the complexity of articulatory adjustment; most frequently, errors are on fricatives, affricates, and consonant clusters.
6. Errors are highly inconsistent.
7. Prosodic disturbances: slower rate, even stress, and even spacing, perhaps in compensation for the problem.

Yoss and Darley (1974)

1. Greater difficulty with polysyllabic words.
2. In repetition tasks: two- and three-feature errors, prolongations and repetitions of sounds or syllables, distortions (e.g., nasal assimilation and subtle voicing and unvoicing errors), and additions.
3. In spontaneous speech: distortions, one-place feature errors, additions, and omissions.
4. Prosodic features may be altered, especially in older children, slow rate, and equalized stress.

Ferry, Hall, and Hicks (1975)

1. Speech varies from nonexistent to partially intelligible.

Aram and Glasson (1979)
Phonologic characteristics of young children

1. High vowel to consonant ratio.
2. Simplification errors.
3. Individual children use different strategies that indicate some regularity in their products, that is, reduplications, only final consonant inclusion.

4. May be able to imitate single sounds, but not use them in sequencing.
5. Unable to repeat multisyllabic words.
6. Omissions and substitutions predominate.

Aram and Glasson (1979)
Phonologic characteristics of older children

1. Speech intelligibility varies according to the length and complexity of utterances, with conversational speech being the least intelligible. There is no variation in production in terms of automatic and more representational utterances.
2. Children make frequent metathetic errors in multisyllable words.
3. Consonant blends are simplified following typical patterns of omitting one of the consonants, substituting a simpler sound for the entire blend, or producing one target consonant and one substituted sound.
4. There are no unusual substitution patterns for single sounds in children with the full phonemic repertoire.
5. Most older children have a full phonemic repertoire. In the group of four older children, only one (a 10-year-old) was still operating with significant limitations.
6. Prosodic difficulties are present in all older children, including slow rate and trial and error groping kinds of repetitions.
7. Imitation improves errors of phonemic selection and combination but not phonemic distortions.
8. Multisyllable word errors involve syllable omissions, often of the final syllable or substitution of a vowel for CV or VC syllable.
9. Distortions are more obvious in older than in younger children.

Aram and Glasson (1979)
Phonetic characteristics for younger and older children

1. Voicing errors are variable with prevocalic voiceless consonants often voiced and final voiced stops devoiced.
2. Nasal resonance errors are not simply the result of the substitutions of a homogenic stop. Some present assimilation nasality. Some add oral stop after nasals resulting in /ŋg/.
3. When produced, medial consonants are often imprecise.
4. Glottal plosives and bilabial fricatives are common nonphonemic sounds.
5. Consonant blends are often aided by intrusive vowel.
6. Vowels are often lengthened before some omitted medial consonants.

Although some discrepancies appear in the descriptions, many commonalities exist:

1. Apraxic children may be able to produce sounds in imitation that they do not use in connected speech.
2. Severity increases as the length of the word or utterance increases. (For example, a child may use /k/ in cup but omit all /k's/ in cupcake producing /ʌʔæ/.
3. Metathctic errors are frequent (efelant/ elefant).
4. Errors may be highly inconsistent (especially for older children) upon repetition of the same multisyllabic word (hopital, hostipal/hospital).
5. Intrusion of a vowel often is present in consonant blends (balue/blue, galass/ glass).
6. Simplification (omission) errors predominate in young children who often present a high vowel/consonant ratio.
7. Prosodic disturbances, especially of rate and stress, are frequently observed, especially with older children.
8. Various phonetic adjustments, such as voicing errors (big/pig), nasal resonance errors, use of nonphonemic sounds, and lengthening vowels before omitted consonants, are present.

In evaluating these findings, we suggest that at least three variables be kept in mind that may influence interpretation for any given child:

1. *Age of the child*. Our experience has been that young apraxic children tend to present markedly restricted repertoires of speech sounds. Older children tend to develop a greater phonologic diversity, but having connected speech often reveals additional difficulties such as difficulty with prosodic features and sequencing of syllables in multisyllabic words.
2. *Severity of the disorder*. Children can range from presenting relatively mild disorders to being nonverbal and unable to acquire useful speech.
3. *Differentiation between phonologic and phonetic disorders*. Aram and Glasson (1979) concluded that children with developmental apraxia of speech present both phonologic and phonetic errors, although this is an area in need of more complete and precise description.

Several writers have documented the marked difficulty apraxic children have in repeating sequences of speech sounds, such as /pʌtəkə/. Yoss and Darley (1974) reported that oral diadochokinesis rates, especially for /kʌ/ and /pʌtəkə/, were slower in apraxic children than in nonapraxic children with defective articulation and they commented that repetitions of the combined /pʌtəkə/ are often produced with intrusion of incorrect syllables. In the Aram and Glasson study (1979), five of the eight children were abnormal in their repetition of /pʌ/, and all eight of the children were unable to successfully repeat sequences of /pʌtəkə/. In our experience, the adequacy of repetitions of /pʌtəkə/ is almost pathognomonic of developmental apraxia, except for children who have learned this task through concerted training.

Language findings in developmental verbal apraxia

Although investigators have suggested that apraxia is not a language disorder (Rosenbek, Hansen, Baughman, and Lemme, 1974), most investigators have not described language behavior of these children beyond some general statement regarding the high level of receptive abilities. Table 7-3, reproduced from Morley (1967), indicated that 8 of 12 of their apraxic children demonstrated some associated language or learning difficulty.

TABLE 7-3. *Details concerning 12 children with developmental articulatory apraxia*

	Sex	Position in family	Age period of observed years	Development of speech		Articulation defects	Associated language disorders	Family history	General remarks
				Words	Phrases				
B.A.	M	1	5½ to 7½	10/12	14/12	Erratic, e.g., [θ (th)] = [f] or [p] [k] = [t] initial position, but = [k] in final position.	Dyslexia and dysgraphia.	+	Speech was normal at 7½ years.
J.B.	M	2	4½ to 7	2	4	[j (y)], [v] [s] [ʃ (sh)] [θ (th)] = [d] [f] = [p] [tʃ (ch)] =[t] [dʒ (j)] = [d].	Some delay in the development of language. No dyslexia.	+	Speech normal at 7 years.
M.B.	F	3	28 to 29	?	about 2	[p] [b] [t] [d] and [w] were the only consonants used. Consistent throughout.	No dyslexia. Spelling disability. She spelt as she spoke.	–	Some improvement, but she ceased to attend before speech was normal.
M.C.	M	2	4½ to 8½	18/12	2	Plosives used normally, but all fricatives defective.	Dyslexia. Reading age at 8½ = 6½.	–	Some difficulty in the use of consonants persisted to 8½ years.
G.C.	M	3	4 to 5½	1	18/12	Many substitutions, omits final sounds, transposes sounds.	Nil.	+	[s] not quite normal at 5½ years.
L.L.	F	2	4 4/12 to 5½	11/12	4	All consonants defective except [p] [b] [t] [d] [l] [w]. Omits final sounds	Some delay in the use of sentences.	+	Speech almost normal at 5½ years.

						Erratic use of consonants in speech.			
J.N.	F	1	5³/₁₂ to 7½	¹⁸/₁₂	2	[p] [b] [t] [d] [l] [w] only consonants used. Substitutions used consistently.	Nil.	+	lack of easy control of movements for articulation at 17 years.
R.P.	M	2	4²/₁₂ to 7½	¹⁸/₁₂	2	[p] [b] [l] [w] only sounds used. Mostly consistent, but many consonants omitted in speech.	Nil.	−	
F.S.	M	3	6 to 10	2	4	[p][b][w][j (y)] only. Most consonants omitted with use of glottal stop.	Dyslexia. Reading age at 9 = 6 years at 10 = 9 years.	−	Slow improvement. Consonants rarely defective at 8½, but not used easily. Normal at 10 years.
E.W.	F	2 Has a twin brother	5³/₁₂ to 10	2	4+	Few defective consonants in simple words, but had great difficulty in their use in speech.	Some delay in speech development.	+	Articulation better in reading than in speech, which is still unintelligible at 10 years.
P.W.	F	2	4²/₁₂ to 7	3	4		Some delay in speech development.		

From Morley, M., *Development and Disorders of Speech in Childhood*. Edinburgh: Churchill Livingstone, 284-285 (1972).

Ferry, Hall, and Hicks (1975) stated that their patients presented normal or near-normal auditory and visual receptive ability, but provide no supportive data. These findings seem surprising given that 20 of their 60 children were institutionalized and nonverbal. Rosenbek and Wertz (1972) stated that 40% of their group had both aphasic and apraxic disorders and that 18% presented isolated apraxia. These investigators qualify their findings by stating that the incidence of isolated apraxia may be spuriously high due to

. . . difficulty in measuring aphasic involvement in children, both because the behaviors to be called aphasia in children are not agreed upon by all speech pathologists and because language testing is difficult in children with severe output disturbances.*

Despite such incidence statements, however, Rosenbek and Wertz (1972) provide no specific data regarding language, commenting that the children had been seen over a period of years by three different speech pathologists, and thus no standard speech and language findings were available.

Yoss and Darley (1974), on the other hand, set performance within 6 months of a child's chronologic age on the Utah Test of Language Development (Mecham, Jex, and Jones, 1967) as a criterion for inclusion in the study. Beyond stating the criterion, however, no other language data are provided. The general nature of the Utah test and the absence of syntactic analyses on this test again raises questions as to whether these children's abilities were as adequate as the investigators assumed.

In their discussion of disorders of speech output, Rapin and Wilson (1978) differentiate between "defective phonemic and syntactic programming" and "defective phonemic pro-

gramming"; in the second condition syntax is intact but phonologic programming is inadequate. They cite Yoss and Darley's (1974) work in support of this disorder. However, they go on to state:

It is not certain whether it is legitimate to separate this syndrome from [defective phonemic and syntactic programming], as it may represent only a milder variant. . . Some of these children may represent no more than a subgroup at the extreme of phonemic immaturity which characterizes so many otherwise normal preschool children.*

Because of the limited data available regarding language abilities in developmental apraxic children, Aram (1979) undertook a detailed study of the language abilities of a group of eight apraxic children. The findings of this study follow and will be discussed together with what little related information can be gleaned from other investigators.

Since we will be drawing heavily from the Aram (1979) and Aram and Glasson (1979) study in the following pages, we have summarized the age and intelligence characteristics of the group described so that the reader can refer to this information in interpreting subsequent findings (Table 7-4).

The intent of the selection criteria for the study was to restrict the group to those presenting relatively "clean" disorders of developmental apraxia. Thus we accepted only children who presented nonverbal IQ's as assessed by the Leiter International Performance Scale (Arthur, 1952) of 80 or greater, who had normal hearing, and who had no observable dysarthria. In addition, we required that all children demonstrate normal performance on at least some language comprehension tasks, present persistent and relatively static phonologic/articulatory disorders, and

---

*From Rosenbek, J., and Wertz, R., A reivew of 50 cases of developmental apraxia of speech. *Language, Speech and Hearing Services in Schools,* **3,** 27 (1972).

*From Rapin, I., and Wilson, B.C., Children with developmental language disability: Neurological aspects and assessment. In M. Wyke (Ed.), *Developmental Dysphasia.* N.Y.: Academic Press, Inc., 28 (1978).

TABLE 7-4. *Age and intelligence characteristics of eight children with developmental verbal apraxia*

Subjects	Age		Nonverbal IQ
	Year	Month	
J.P.	4	7	136
A.S.	4	10	83
M.N.	5	2	100+
J.S.	5	6	97
S.C.	10	0	131
P.B.	10	0	86+
P.O.	10	9	96+
J.K.	14	4	63 to 77

TABLE 7-5. *Language acquisition milestones of eight children with developmental verbal apraxia*

Child	Single words	Two-word phrases	Comment
J.P.	3.5 years	4.5 years	Reduced babbling Never imitated sounds
A.S.	2.5	4.0	After 6 months, no babbling
M.N.	2.0	3.0	
J.S.	4.0	5.0	
S.C.	1.5	6.0	Quiet infant
P.B.	4.0	4.0+	Reduced babbling
P.O.	2.5	3.5	
J.K.	3.0	3.5	
RANGE	1.5 to 4.0 years	3.0 to 6.0 years	
MEAN	2.9 years	4.2 years	

show notably slow progress in speech therapy. By concentrating on a small but select group of relatively "pure" apraxics, we felt we could better understand apraxia without introducing confounding variables. When referring to Table 7-4, a number of comments can be made. First, the children conveniently fell into a younger age group, ranging from approximately 4½ to 5½ years old and an older group with three 10-year-olds and one 14-year-old. This two-part grouping by age allowed us to compare younger and older children's performances. Second, although we had set our IQ criterion at 80, J.K., our 14-year-old, did not reach this criterion but was included because his verbal IQ based on the Peabody Picture Vocabulary Test (Dunn, 1965) was within normal limits, and his Leiter performance seemed to be adversely affected by what appeared to be a constructional apraxia. We now turn to language findings with this and other groups of apraxic children.

Language development milestones. Reports in the literature regarding language development milestones are equivocal. Morley (1965) reported that 4 of her 12 apraxic children were delayed in onset of speech.

Rosenbek and Wertz (1972) reported that all 50 of their apraxics were delayed. In addition, several writers have commented on the absence of normal babbling during infancy in children who later would be diagnosed as apraxic (Eisenson, 1972). In the Aram and Glasson (1979) group, all children were notably delayed in both onset of single words and two-word phrases as indicated by parental report. Referring to Table 7-5, onset of single words ranged from 1.5 to 4.0 years with a mean of 2.9 years, and onset of two-word phrases ranged from 3.0 to 6.0 years with a mean of 4.2 years. Four of the eight children were described as unusually quiet babies who did not babble as expected.

Language comprehension. As noted earlier, the literature provides virtually no specific findings documenting language comprehension abilities in children with developmental verbal apraxia. The children in the Aram and Glasson study (1979) all demonstrated essentially normal semantic and syntactic compre-

TABLE 7-6. *Comprehension of connected speech in eight children with developmental verbal apraxia*

Child	ACLC (% correct)			NSST (percentile)	Token test (SD)				
	Two elements	Three elements	Four elements		I	II	III	IV	V
J.P.				50th					
A.S.	90/93.2	60/74.9	70/63.4						
M.N.				>50th	OK	OK	−1SD		+1SD
J.S.	90/94.3	80/90.1	40/83.6						
S.C.	100%	100%	100%						
P.B.				30/40	OK	OK	OK	−2SD	−1SD
P.O.					OK	OK	−2SD	−3SD	−1SD
J.K.	100%	100%	100%		OK	OK	−1SD	−1SD	−3SD

hension abilities when length of the input stimuli was not a factor. These children's vocabulary comprehension as assessed by the Peabody Picture Vocabulary Test (Dunn, 1965) ranged between an IQ of 81 and 104 with a mean of 92. Their ability to understand connected speech generally was age appropriate when items presented were short. However, when length increased, so did their difficulty in handling these items.

Table 7-6 summarizes these children's performance on various tests of comprehension of connected language, including the Assessment of Children's Language Comprehension (ACLC) (Foster, Giddan, and Stark, 1972), the Northwestern Syntax Screening Test (NSST) (Lee, 1969), and the Token Test (DiSimoni, 1978). These data indicate that when items were short, as on the two-element portion of the ACLC, the NSST, or Parts I and II of the Token Test, all children performed quite adequately. However, several of the children demonstrated marked difficulty as the length increased, for example **J.S.** on the ACLC and **M.N., P.B., P.O.** and **J.K.** on the Token Test. It is interesting to note that several children had more difficulty with the demands of increased length than with syntactic

complexity. For example, **P.B., M.N.,** and **P.O.** all improved their performance on Part V of the Token Test, which is primarily a test of syntactic complexity, as opposed to Part IV, which presents commands of invariant syntactic form but requires maximal retention of information.

Overall, then, the apraxic children studied by Aram and Glasson (1979) presented essentially normal vocabulary comprehension and syntactic complexity comprehension, but they experienced difficulty when they were required to retain information of increasing length.

Language formulation. In marked contrast to these children's language comprehension and to much of what has been reported in the literature, all children studied by Aram and Glasson presented difficulties with language formulation encompassing both vocabulary and syntax.

SEMANTIC FORMULATION. Information gathered relevant to semantic formulation was based on the children's spontaneous speech as well as a number of vocabulary tests, including the Bankson Language Screening Test: Semantic Subtest (Bankson, 1977), the Vocabulary Usage Test (Nation, 1972), and the Verbal Fluency Subtest of the Boston Diagnostic Aphasia Examination (Goodglass and Kaplan, 1972).

Based on the data gathered, the following summary statements can be made:

1. None of the children had normal expressive vocabularies. Their deficits ranged from mild to severe. For example, one of the young children called all women figures "mama," while for another, all animals were "dodi" (doggie).

2. Several of the young children used gestures to convey their intended meanings, along with onomatopoetic sounds, such as the r-r-r-rhum of a motor to indicate a car or truck.

3. Two of the young children used almost no verb forms. For example, **J.S.** had only six verbs at age 4, including run, go, walk, eat, snore, and stop.

4. Virtually all the children had difficulty with words denoting spatial relationships, that is prepositions, as seen by one of the 10-year-olds who said "on top of" for a variety of relations including above, over, and on.

5. Several of the children were anomic, occasionally calling up the wrong but associated word, or notably searching for a word that could not be "remembered." One child, **J.K.,** who was given the Reporter's Test (DeRenzi and Ferrari, 1978), an expressive form of the Token Test in which he was asked to describe what the examiner had done with the tokens, frequently substituted "square" for "circle" or gave the wrong color name, although able to name all the colors and shapes on command. In short, he "called up" the wrong word.

SYNTACTIC FORMULATION. Developmental Sentence Scores (DSS) were computed for six of the eight children and are summarized on

TABLE 7-7. *Developmental sentence scores on six children with developmental verbal apraxia*

Child	DSS score	DSS 50th percentile for age	Standard deviation
J.P.	3.70	8.04	1.64
A.S.	2.45	8.04	1.64
M.N.	4.78	8.04	1.64
J.S.	6.58	9.19	1.90
S.C.	1.54	10.94+	2.26
P.O.	6.41	10.94+	2.26

Table 7-7. DSSs were not computed for two children, since one spoke only in one- and two-word spontaneous phrases and the other almost always spoke in a stereotyped noun + verb + object syntactic pattern with few inflectional endings marked. When compared to the DSS norms for the 50th percentile for same-aged children, these developmental apraxics are markedly below the norms. Although these children had difficulty with inflectional endings, they also had notable difficulty with word order, pronoun number and case, use of clauses, and so forth.

Some spontaneous sentences are provided on p. 160 for **M.N.** and **S.C.,** and some examples of the sentence stimuli and responses for a repetition task are provided for **P.B.** and **P.O.** Examples such as these demonstrate that these children presented syntactic formulation problems that went beyond inflectional omissions, evidencing selection and ordering difficulties of syntactic elements.

Accompanying learning difficulties. In addition to the language formulation disorders presented by all the apraxic children studied by Aram and Glasson (1979), all children of school age also presented learning difficulties beyond those of spoken language. Despite normal nonverbal intelligence and essentially

---

**SPONTANEOUS AND REQUESTED
SYNTAX EXAMPLES FOR FOUR
SELECTED CHILDREN WITH
DEVELOPMENTAL VERBAL
APRAXIA**

M.N. (5-2)

> When we going do this.
> I not see the fire inside.
> Him makes a Kiss costume at home.

S.C. (10-0)

> The boys is doing the ball.
> Men ask money is that candy/men ask for
> money for the candy.

P.B. (10-1)

> Have you been gone? → You been you
> gone?

P.O. (10-9)

> Couldn't Daddy have been coming? →
> Have Daddy been coming?
> She would have liked to go. → She have
> like to go.
> She showed the girl the boy. → The girl
> showed the boy.

---

normal language comprehension, all four of
the older children had reading and writing
problems beyond those related to articulation
or the mechanics of writing.

Of the four older children, one **(P.B.)** was
being educated in a regular classroom coupled with tutoring in reading and writing.
P.O. spent half-days in an LD classroom.
S.C. was in a multihandicapped classroom,
while **J.K.,** who formerly had been in an LD
class, had recently been transferred to an
EMR program. All of the 10-year-olds, if functioning at a normal level, should have been

achieving at the fourth grade level. None read
higher than a second grade level on either
word recognition or reading comprehension
tests. Spelling presented problems for all older
children. For example, **J.K.** produced the following words to dictation: strong → graer;
science → seanes; valley → faley; dust →
dase. Written expression gave the children as
much difficulty as did verbal expression. For
example, **J.K.** wrote: "When i was walk hone
to school in my hose gosh on fies" (loosely
translated, this means: When I was walking
home from school, my house got on fire).

Morley (1967) reported that 4 of her 12
apraxic children had learning difficulties described as dyslexias, dysgraphias, and spelling
difficulties (Table 7-3). Apart from this, the
only other report of learning disabilities accompanying developmental apraxia is that of
Yoss and Darley (1974), who reported that 5
of their 16 apraxic children had received remedial help and were having difficulty in
school achievement, whereas no children
needed remedial help in the comparison
group of 16 nonapraxic children with defective articulation.

Data such as the above suggests that apraxic children's language difficulties go beyond
verbal expression and typically include reading, writing, and spelling as well.

Summary of language findings. To summarize the language difficulties presented by
the apraxic children in the Aram and Glasson
(1979) study as well as scattered reports from
other investigators, we conclude that:

1. Most if not all apraxic children are delayed in the onset of single words and
   two-word combinations.
2. Comprehension of semantics and syntax
   often are normal, if nonverbal mental
   age is normal.
3. Length of sentences negatively affects
   sentence comprehension.

4. Limitations in semantic formulation, ranging from mild to severe, are usually present.

5. Formulated syntax is disordered, presenting deficiencies in inflectional markers as well as selection and sequencing of syntactic elements.

6. Reading, writing, and spelling difficulties are typically apparent at school age.

These data lead us to conclude that developmental verbal apraxia is not confined to the phonologic and articulatory aspects of speech. Rather, all levels of formulated language may be affected, including the lexical, syntactic, and phonologic aspects. As well, the disorder goes beyond one of verbal expression, involving reading and written expression as well. In short, we see developmental verbal apraxia as a disorder that is as much language-based as articulatory.

Neurologic findings in developmental verbal apraxia

As noted earlier, developmental verbal apraxia, like its adult counterpart, is generally thought to arise from a neurologic disruption. Despite such a view, neurologic findings with developmentally apraxic children are equivocal at best.

Clinicial examination, EEG, and CT scan. Besides case study descriptions, three studies of groups of apraxics have reported neurologic findings for the apraxic children they described (Ferry, Hall, and Hicks, 1975; Rosenbek and Wertz, 1972; Yoss and Darley, 1974). The findings of these studies are summarized in Table 7-8. Yoss and Darley (1974) reported that 15 out of 16 apraxic children as opposed to 4 out of 16 nonapraxic children with defective articulation presented "soft" neurologic findings, including difficulties with fine motor coordination, gait, and alternate movements of the extremities and tongue. Of the 60 apraxics in the Ferry, Hall, and Hicks (1975) study seen by a neurologist for a clinical examination, 27 incidences of "hard"* neurologic findings were reported, including 13 with spastic diplegia and 2 with hand tremors. Because of the manner in which these findings were reported, it is unclear how many of these findings coexisted in the same individual. Ferry et al. (1975) also reported EEG findings for their 20 institutionalized subjects, all of which showed mild generalized slowing, a finding that may well be a result of the retardation and may not be associated with the apraxic condition.

Finally, the Rosenbek and Wertz (1972) group of apraxics included 36 who were seen for a neurologic examination. Of these, 14 presented positive "hard" findings, including hyperreflexia and spasticity in 8, muscle weakness in 3, hyporeflexia and weakness in 1, and hyperkinesia in 2. Rosenbek and Wertz (1972) also reported EEG findings for this group of 26 children, 15 of whom were abnormal. Again, it should be pointed out that mentally retarded children may have been included in this group since the authors made no attempt to exclude such children from their study. Therefore the 10 abnormal EEGs showing a generalized cortical disturbance may have been related to retardation, although this is not clear from the reported data. Of the five focal EEG abnormalities, two were bilateral, one indicating bilateral motor strip abnormalities and one Sylvian-parietal abnormalities. It may be noted that this one case of bilateral motor strip findings is the only documented finding suggesting anterior dysfunction for developmentally

---

*"Hard" neurologic findings denote findings that indicate pathology regardless of age, such as paralysis and movement disorders, whereas "soft signs" such as clumsiness characterized by synergism and associated movements may occur normally in younger children.

TABLE 7-8. *Neurologic findings from selected studies of developmental verbal apraxia*

Study	Clinical examination	EEG	CT scan
Yoss and Darley (1972)	15 of 16 Children evidencing "soft" findings		
Ferry, Hall, and Hicks (1975)	N = 60; 27 incidences of "hard" neurologic findings	20 of 20 institutionalized retardates; mild generalized slowing; no focal findings	

Rosenbek and Wertz (1972)	14 of 36 positive findings
	11 of 50 excessive drooling
		15 of 26 abnormal
		10 generalized cortical disturbance
		5 focal abnormalities
		2 bilateral
		  1 motor strip
		  1 Sylvian-parietal area
		3 right hemisphere, all temporal or temporoparietal	

Aram and Glasson (1979)	2 completely normal A.S.—intermittent left esophoria; parietal area wider than frontal area J.S.—head circumference >98% P.O.—strabismus; slightly hypotonic; hyperextensible ankles P.B.—difficulty with walking on heels and toes and tandem walking J.K.—problems with coordinated movements	5 of 5 normal	4 normal 1(?) bilateral parietal-occipital temporal atrophy 1 posterior expansion of quadrigeminal cistern and prominence of vermion cistern

apraxic children. The remainder of the focal abnormalities were all unilateral, implicating either the temporal or temporoparietal region of the right hemispheres.

The children in the Aram and Glasson (1979) series were seen by pediatric neurologists for clinical examination. Five had EEGs, and six had CT scan findings. Beyond gait and coordination problems, only three presented positive, somewhat idiosyncratic clinical findings that do not lend themselves to any one general characterization. One observation, however, is that these children demonstrated very little evidence for focal cortical problems and in particular not for anteriorly placed cortical lesions. As can be seen

in Table 7-8, the EEG results were all negative. That these normal findings contrast with what has been reported by Ferry, Hall, and Hicks (1975) and Rosenbek and Wertz (1972) may be explained by the exclusion of retarded children in the Aram and Glasson (1979) study. Again, the CT scan findings reported by Aram and Glasson also do not for the most part implicate focal cortical lesions, with the one exception where there was a question of bilateral parietal-occipital-temporal atrophy.

In summary, then, the clinical examinations, EEG, and CT scan findings that had been reported provide very minimal evidence for focal cortical pathology associated with developmental verbal apraxia, with only one incidence of documented evidence suggestive of focal anterior pathology.

Gross motor and hand coordination. Many writers have described developmentally apraxic children as clumsy and poorly coordinated. For example, Gubbay (1975) has written a book entitled *The Clumsy Child: A Study of Developmental Apraxia and Agnostic Ataxia,* which concerns bodily apraxias rather than verbal apraxia. Or as McGinnis (1963) has commented, these children are "capable of stumbling over a chalk line." In the Aram and Glasson (1979) group of apraxic children, six of the seven tested had difficulty standing on one foot, hopping on one foot, or skipping. Three of the seven had difficulty with coordinating alternate hand movements such as finger tapping and alternately slapping thighs with the front or back of the hand.

Hand preference. Theories of mixed laterality have been implicated in developmental apraxia of speech as well as in many other developmental speech and language disorders. Although findings reported are somewhat equivocal (see summary in Table 7-9), our experience has been that apraxic children generally do not show as early or clearly established hand dominance as do normally developing children. We agree with Eisenson's (1972) observation that many apraxic children show "ambi-nonlaterality," that is, they are equally inept with both hands, as opposed to ambidextrous, being equally good with both hands.

Accompanying oral apraxia. As with adults with acquired apraxias of speech, a nonspeech oral apraxia is a condition that may, but does not necessarily, accompany verbal apraxia (Ferry, Hall, and Hicks, 1975; Morley, 1967; Rosenbek and Wertz, 1972; Yoss and Darley, 1974). Yoss and Darley (1974) state that difficulty with volitional oral movements of the tongue and lips is usually present. Ferry

TABLE 7-9. *Hand preference and developmental verbal apraxia from selected studies*

Study	R	L	Mixed or questionable
Rosenbek and Wertz (1972)	21	4	6
Yoss and Darley (1974)	11	1	3
Aram and Glasson (1979)	2	0	5

TABLE 7-10. *Sex ratio of children with developmental verbal apraxia: selected studies*

Study	Boys	Girls	
Morley (1967)	7	5	
Rosenbek and Wertz (1972)	38	12	
Yoss and Darley (1974)	26	4	(In entire group of apraxic and nonapraxic children with defective articulation)
Ferry, Hall, and Hicks (1975)	40	20	
Aram and Glasson (1979)	8	0	

et al. (1975) reported that 36 of their 60 apraxics had an orofacial dyspraxia, and Aram and Glasson (1979) found four of their eight children to have difficulty with production of single, nonspeech movements, although this number increased to five when the children were required to sequence nonspeech volitional movements.

Sex ratio. Although the literature is equivocal in respect to the ratio of boys to girls who have developmental apraxia, our experience is that developmental apraxia is predominantly, although not exclusively, a disorder of boys. Table 7-10 reports the ratio of boys to girls.

Familial history. A final finding that appears to be significant in children with developmental verbal apraxia is the frequent positive family history for speech, language, and learning disorders. We have been repeatedly impressed by both the frequency and the severity of other speech disorders in these children's families. In the Aram and Glasson (1979) group of eight apraxics, all but three had striking family histories of speech, language, and learning disorders including the following: one child with several male cousins with delayed speech and a paternal aunt with delayed speech and articulation; one child whose father began talking at age 5 and who as an adult continues to have a reading and writing disorder, whose maternal aunt also did not begin talking until after age 5, and whose two paternal aunts had reading and speaking problems; one child whose identical twin also was late to begin talking and continues to have mild articulation and reading problems; one child whose mother is a severe stutterer, whose brother had a mild articulation disorder, and whose paternal grandmother has an articulation disorder; and finally, one child whose brother has speech and learning difficulties.

Morley (1967) reported that 6 out of 12 of her apraxic children had histories of speech disorders in parents, siblings, or close relatives, including one child where five out of eight family members presented speech disorders as adults. Ferry, Hall, and Hicks (1975) also commented on the positive family histories in developmental apraxia, noting that 17 of their 60 children had positive family histories, usually of male relatives (fathers or brothers). The Ferry et al. (1975) study included two sets of brothers with almost identical patterns of apraxic speech. Finally, Saleeby, Hadjian, Martinkosky, and Swift (1978) reported a study in which 34 of 66 family members were reported to have had defective speech, 12 of whom were tested. These authors suggested that this condition is inherited in an autosomal dominant fashion based on its distribution within the family. Likewise, Ferry et al. (1975) as well as Aram and Glasson (1979) have suggested that the preponderance of males and strong family histories suggest a genetic basis for developmental apraxia at least in some children.

Summary of neurologic findings. The neurologic status of verbal apraxic children can be summarized as follows. A majority of the children present positive although generally nonlocalizing findings on clinical examination. Findings may include evidence of overt neurologic disorders (hard signs) or indications of more subtle (soft) findings. Although frequent generalized slowing has been reported for EEG results with many apraxics, it appears that at least some of these may be attributed to retardation rather than apraxia. A few incidences of EEG findings suggestive of localized pathology have been reported, although there is only one documented EEG report implicating anterior pathology. Very few CT scan studies have been reported; most do not point to localized cortical pathology.

Many, if not most, apraxic children have some difficulty with gross motor coordination, and some have difficulty with fine motor coordination. Many apraxic children do not have a clear hand preference. Furthermore, an oral apraxia for nonspeech movement generally, but not invariably, accompanies developmental verbal apraxia. Finally, developmental apraxia is much more frequent in boys than in girls, many of whom present significant family histories for speech, language, and learning disorders.

Explanatory hypotheses for developmental verbal apraxia

The "why" of developmental verbal apraxia is still unknown, although several investigators have offered hypotheses to explain the basis of this condition. Hypotheses have tended to address either the neurologic bases or a language processing base.

Neurologic explanations have generally been extrapolated from findings with adults. Ferry et al. (1975), drawing from Geschwind's (1964) work with adults, have suggested that these children have a developmental disruption in the cerebral association pathways such as the arcuate fasciculus from the parietal operculum to the motor cortex. Rosenbek and Wertz (1972), on the other hand, trying to reconcile the limited evidence for cortical focal pathology in apraxic children, have suggested that the praxic centers in children may be more diffusely represented than in adults, involving large cortical centers in both hemispheres. These investigators go on to hypothesize that with maturation, the praxic centers may lateralize and become more focal. Closely akin to the neurologic explanations are the genetic explanations that have already been mentioned by Aram and Glasson (1979), Ferry et al. (1975) and Saleeby et al. (1978), which are in keeping with Morley's (1967) hypothesis that there may be delay in the maturation of association pathways resulting in faulty laying down of articulatory patterns, which, if persistent, continues into adulthood.

At the beginning of this chapter we stated that many investigators including ourselves consider developmental apraxia of speech to represent a processing breakdown in speech programming, and thus we have here viewed developmental verbal apraxia as the chief exemplar of a breakdown in this process. Or as Edwards (1973) has stated:

Production too may be coded in neural stretches. Output involves unified sequences of movement and it is most probable at the programme planning stage of these movements that breakdown is likely to occur.*

*From Edwards, M., Developmental verbal dyspraxia. *British Journal of Disorders of Communication*, **8,** 67 (1973).

Although most investigators have emphasized the breakdowns in programming for the articulatory aspects of speech, Aram and Glasson (1979) have suggested that programming breakdowns underlie both the language and articulatory disorders that are seen to coexist in developmental verbal apraxics. They have suggested in contrast to other investigators that the articulatory and language disorders do not simply coexist, but that both stem from a common breakdown in the selection and sequencing of both language and articulatory elements.

As it stands, we are left with hypotheses for developmental verbal apraxia that must incorporate language processes of both formulation and speech programming. Speech programming is responsible for selection and sequencing of the sound system and also is responsible for transducing this information into a motor code for initiation as an articulatory response. Thus, if words, sentences, and sequential speech sounds are not appropriately formulated and programmed, they will not be transduced appropriately into a motor code, resulting in a variety of output responses described as developmental verbal apraxia.

Criteria for developmental verbal apraxia revisited

Having laid out the data, we now return to and expand our criteria for developmental verbal apraxia. We suggest that children with developmental verbal apraxia generally present the following characteristics, keeping in mind the variability presented by age and severity:

1. They demonstrate a contrast in their voluntary versus their nonvoluntary use of the speech articulators.
2. Their disorder is notably one of selection and sequencing of both phonologic and articulatory movements, typically

exemplified in difficulties in repetition of multisyllabic words or /pʌtəkə/.

3. They have essentially normal (if mental age is normal) language comprehension abilities but disordered lexical and syntactic formulation.
4. They present learning difficulties in some instances, particularly in reading, written expression, and spelling.
5. Their condition improves slowly and is often highly resistant to therapy used for other articulatory disorders.
6. They present some positive neurologic findings, including difficulties with fine and gross motor coordination, although neurologic findings are usually nonfocal.
7. They usually, but not always, have an accompanying oral apraxia of nonspeech movements.
8. They often fail to show a clear hand perference.
9. They typically are boys.
10. They often have a strong family history of speech, language, and learning problems.

SPEECH PRODUCTION DISRUPTIONS

The final processing stage in the Language to Speech Segment of the CLPM is speech production. This processing stage takes into account the systems whereby neuromuscular responses are initiated, coordinated, transmitted, and ultimately actualized through the structures of the speech mechanism—those responsible for breathing for speech, phonation, resonation, and articulation.

From this action of the speech mechanisms an output response occurs. Observations of the results of speech production help the speech-language pathologist to determine if the disordered output response is due to a speech-to-language, a language-to-thought-to-language, or a language-to-speech processing disruption, singly or in some combination.

A speech not a language process

The speech production process is not one of language per se, and disruptions in structure and function are typically considered to result in disorders of speech, not language. However, the process of speech production becomes implicated in language disorders in several ways.

First, any earlier processing disruptions are fed through the process of speech production to gain final verbal expression. Because the speech production process is the terminal process, it becomes the most direct process to which disordered output responses can be tied. Often speech production is the first process implicated when expressed speech is disordered. Therefore, for example, if an /s/ is distorted, this may be most immediately attributed to a speech production disruption, in which it would represent a phonetic, or articulatory, disorder rather than a language-based phonologic problem. On the other hand, the distorted /s/ may be the result of a mild high-frequency hearing loss, a disruption of sensation, or a failure to discriminate or appropriately categorize the /s/ phoneme from other phonemes, a disruption in speech perception.

The speech production process is the ultimate culprit, that is, it is the tongue that occludes the oral cavity rather than merely restricting its diameter, thus giving rise to a stoplike consonant rather than the appropriate fricative sound. However, the responsibility for the error lies with the faulty instructions received from other processes. Thus the breakdown is not one in speech production; rather, speech production acts in an inadequate manner because of inappropriate instructions.

The second manner in which speech production becomes implicated in language disorders is in "guilt by association," whereby whatever caused the language problem also caused the disordered output response. Thus Rh incompatibility may cause a sensorineural hearing loss (a breakdown in the process of sensation), but it also may result in motor control problems, causing a speech production breakdown. Or, alternatively, Down's syndrome includes mental retardation, significantly disturbing all processes in the language-to-thought-to-language segment, but it also may include a number of motor and structural problems manifested as disruptions in speech production.

Finally, as will be discussed in the remainder of this section, there may exist some as yet not well understood interdependence between various language processes and the process of speech production. Because such relationships are not yet well described, these interrelationships are speculative and will only be treated briefly here. Three such interrelationships will be mentioned:

1. The relationship between certain problems of prosody and language (Here we will refer to the often commented upon but little described coexistence of language disorders and cluttering and stuttering symptoms.)
2. Motor speech disorders, importantly cerebral palsy and the speculative back-up effect between motor limitations and the development of language
3. The influence of structural abnormalities on language (Here the discussion will include children with cleft lip and palate and children who have had tracheotomies for sustained periods of time.)

Relationship between prosody and language disorders

Both cluttering and stuttering have been viewed as fluency (prosody) disorders in which concomitant language disorders are also implicated.

Whether or not a cluttering disorder distinct from other speech and language disorders exists has been a matter of controversy, yet the condition is described by a number of writers (Perkins, 1977, 1978; Rieber and Brubaker, 1966; Weiss, 1964). Weiss (1964), who is one of the few Americans to have treated cluttering extensively, has described the disorder as follows:

Cluttering is a speech disorder characterized by the clutterer's unawareness of his disorder, by a short attention span, by disturbances in perception and formulation of speech and often by excessive speed of delivery. It is a disorder of the thought processes preparatory to speech and based on a hereditary disposition. Cluttering is the verbal manifestation of Central Language Imbalance, which affects all channels of communication (e.g., reading, writing, rhythm and musicality) and behavior in general.[*]

Later, Weiss more specifically outlines both the speech and language aspects of cluttering in the following statement:

The excessive speed and the articulatory deviations, as well as the restlessness, in general, can be considered as motoric (expressive) failings. The repetitions, drawling, and interjections are the manifestations of difficulty in word finding. The weakness of perception and unawareness of disturbance, along with the reading and writing difficulties, belong to the sensory (receptive) side of the ledger. The grammatical difficulties seem to stand astride the line which separates (or unites) the expressive and receptive realms of speech. The poorly integrated thought processes and the gaps of inner language can be paralleled with transcortical aphasia. Lack of rhythm and of musicality bear resemblance to amusia.[†]

---

[*]From Weiss, D.A., *Cluttering*. Englewood Cliffs, N.J.: Prentice-Hall, Inc. 1 (1964).
[†]From Weiss, p. 61.

In this description Weiss seems to imply that the fluency disorder either stems from the language disorder or that the fluency and language disorders are coexisting disorders, symptoms of a common hereditary neurologic dysfunction.

An overlap between language and disfluent behavior has also been described for young stutterers. Considerable attention has been directed toward describing the linguistic context of disfluencies in children who present stuttering problems (Bloodstein, 1974; Bloodstein and Gantwerk, 1967; Muma, 1971; Soderberg, 1967).

It is not uncommon for children who have had delayed language problems to become markedly disfluent during the course of therapy, sometimes developing considerable struggle behavior and secondary symptoms (Hall, 1977; Lee, 1974). The development of disfluent speech in such children is frequently attributed to the "pressures" of therapy, including the therapist's and parents' expectations. Or, alternatively, the disfluencies are seen to arise from the same neurologic dysfunctions that caused the language disorder. Others have viewed the disfluencies as the children's struggle to cope with the acquisition of increased language skills (Hall, 1977).

Some investigators have suggested that at least some disfluent children present anomic-like word finding problems that create pauses, giving rise to disfluencies in their speech. Others, however, have suggested that grammatic aspects are not present in the initial phases of stuttering but emerge only later in the course of development of the problem (Bloodstein and Gantwerk, 1967).

Apraxic children also have been seen to have disfluent speech along with the language and articulatory problems previously described (Ingram and Reid, 1956). Apraxic children are frequently observed to repeat phonemes or syllables, to effortfully grope for

positioning of their articulators, to prolong sound elements, and to slow the rate of delivery (Ferry, Hall, and Hicks, 1975; Morley, 1967; Rosenbek and Wertz, 1972). Some have suggested that the groping trial and error behaviors and the prosodic disruptions tend to be present only in older children (Yoss and Darley, 1974), and the relationship to years of speech therapy has been questioned. However, we have observed notably disfluent speech in preschool-aged apraxic children. Although it is generally assumed that these disfluencies stem from the apraxic's language and articulatory difficulties, such a relationship lacks empirical evidence.

Although concomitant difficulties with language and speech fluency have been described, the relationship between these children's disfluencies and their language disorders is as yet unclear. It has been suggested that either the two types of disorders arise from a common causal basis or that the language disorders cause the fluency disorders, either as a result of therapy or because language has not been formulated in a sufficiently fluent flow as to feed ongoing speech.

☐ **St. Louis (1979) has prepared a major review of the stuttering literature, focusing on linguistic and motor aspects of stuttering. What support does this review offer for viewing stuttering as a linguistic and/or speech programming disruption? What future research directions does St. Louis suggest will be occurring?**

Relationships between motor speech and language disorders

That the language abilities in children with significant motor speech disorders has not been studied to a greater extent is an unanswered paradox. These children are often classified as having cerebral palsy and commonly have very significant communication disorders. Typically, however, these disorders have been viewed as motor speech disorders or stemming from hearing disorders with a notable scarcity of description directed to their language abilities. Most writers have concentrated on the motor aspects of speech, making only limited statements and descriptions of the language disorders of these children (Boone, 1975; Hartman and Hood, 1973; Irwin, 1972; McDonald and Chance, 1964; Mysak, 1968; and Westlake and Rutherford, 1961).

Some of this lack of language description undoubtedly arises from the assumption that any limitations are the result of motor execution; the language that is "there" just cannot be expressed. There is evidence that this is the case for some severely motorically involved individuals, as described by Lenneberg (1962) or as eloquently presented by Richard Boydell (Fourcin, 1975), a 38-year-old man with congenital spastic quadriplegia and severe athetosis who was aided by a specially designed foot-controlled electric typewriter.

Thus it often has been assumed that any language disorders presented by motorically handicapped children result from a failure to get the language out, and if one could find an appropriate modality for expression (for example, typing or communication boards), the language would be intact if language comprehension were intact. However, we have already seen in apraxic children how language comprehension abilities are not necessarily mirrored in expressed language and that a unitary language "competence" need not underlie both comprehension and expression.

If they are not the result of neuromotor blocking of expression, often language disorders in children with cerebral palsy are seen as the result of mental retardation, which frequently accompanies the motor impairments (Hartman and Hood, 1973; Mecham, Berko, Berko, and Palmer, 1966). Furthermore, hearing loss is common in at least some types of cerebral palsied children. Thus the high incidence of hearing loss, mental retardation, and

central nervous system involvement beyond the motor system are well documented, providing numerous causal bases for multiple coexisting language processing breakdowns.

The few studies of language of children with severe motoric involvement are equivocal and do not settle the issue of whether these children have language disorders beyond what can be attributed to mental retardation or hearing impairments. For example, Love (1964), in a study of the oral language behavior of 27 older (10- to 15-year-old) cerebral palsied children, concludes that his study does not provide evidence for a disorder of comprehension and formulation of oral symbols. An examination of Love's (1964) data reveals that these children did not perform inferiorly on receptive vocabulary using the *Peabody Picture Vocabulary Test* (Dunn, 1959) or a vocabulary definition task, but were significantly inferior on the expressive vocabulary naming task. Love (1964), however, concludes the following:

> The cerebral palsied subjects showed no greater discrepancy between their receptive and expressive vocabularies than did their controls, suggesting the absence of a clinical naming disorder.[*]

To accept Love's (1964) conclusion, one must accept that an expressive vocabulary deficit is established in reference to the level of vocabulary comprehension, not to control subjects matched for IQ and chronologic age.

Myers (1965) reported results of the Illinois Test of Psycholinguistic Abilities (Kirk and McCarthy, 1961) with 28 spastic, 24 athetoid, and 32 normal children, controlling for age and IQ. Findings revealed significant differences favoring the spastic group in the automatic sequential subtests, and the athetoid group on the representational subtests. The

---

[*]From Love, R.J., Oral language behavior of older cerebral palsied children. *Journal of Speech and Hearing Research,* **7,** 357 (1964).

normal children scored uniformly higher than either of the two groups with cerebral palsy.

The relationship between significant motor speech disorders and language disorders awaits further investigative description. Still to be disentangled are a number of questions, among them: Do these children have language disorders beyond what can be attributed to retardation and/or hearing disorders? (Love [1964] suggests no; Myers [1965] suggests yes.) Do these children use the same early words as children free to explore their environment? What functions do their early communicative attempts entail? What relationships are expressed in two- and three-word utterances? If motor restrictions limit output, is semantic information retained at the expense of syntactic information? Although these questions offer provocative natural experiments testing theories of language acquisition, such studies have not yet been reported.

Relationship between speech mechanism structural disorders and language disorders

To exemplify structural disorders of the peripheral speech mechanism and concomitant language disorders, we have chosen two exemplary types of children, those with cleft lip and palate affecting the speech production process and those with tracheotomies for prolonged periods during early language development. As with the other disorders affecting speech production, these structural disorders rarely occur as isolated phenomena, but usually are accompanied by other circumstances that may contribute to any evident language deficits. Therefore, even though language deficits may be described in these groups of children, establishing a cause-effect relationship between the structural disorder and the deficient language usually is not possible, since other variables interact and may be responsible.

Cleft lip and palate and language disorders. The study of language disorders in children with cleft lip and palate received its impetus from the research of Spriestersbach, Darley, and Morris (1958) and was extended by Morris in 1962. Since that time many studies have appeared using a variety of language measures and research methodologies (Brennan and Cullinan, 1974; Nation, 1970a,b; Philips and Harrison, 1969; Smith and McWilliams, 1968; and others).

Children with cleft palate tend to be reduced across the language measures studied. Although these differences become less pronounced as the children reach ages 5 and 6, Pannbacker (1975) concluded that adult speakers with cleft lip and palate used shorter responses than did the normal control subjects.

The question of primary interest here is why these children should have language disorders, since their major difficulty is a structural defect of the speech mechanism creating resonation and articulation disruptions. Do these speech production disruptions create the language disorder?

Most of the available information indicates that this is not the case. When the heterogeneity of the population with cleft lip and palate is considered and the variables inherent in this population are studied, it appears that other variables are responsible for the onset and development of the language disorder.

From his data, Nation (1970a,b) hypothesized that the determinants most responsible for the vocabulary reduction in his preschool subjects were hearing loss and length of hospitilization. The relationship of hearing loss, including mild chronic conductive hearing losses, to language development is becoming clearer and was discussed in Chapter 5 when we considered the Speech to Language Processing Stage. The information on otitis media and language development is relevant to the study of language disorders in children with cleft lip and palate.

However, we cannot rule out the relationship between the difficulties in articulation and resonation and the developing language system of the child with cleft lip and palate. In children with cleft lip and palate who have chronic conductive hearing losses, their reduced hearing may prevent them from discriminating and fully utilizing their own speech productions for further language processing. In this hypothesis, hearing loss is again implicated as the more direct basis for the language disorder rather than the articulation-resonation disorder.

Another hypothesis related to feedback systems was suggested by Philips and Harrison (1969), who speculated that the language disorder present could be caused by the rejection of the children's speech production by parents, who do not in turn provide adequate feedback and stimulation.

Thus children with cleft lip and palate provide a variety of variables to study in determining the cause-effect relationships for the language disorders they exhibit. We need to discover when the onset of these disorders occurs if we are to understand the relationship of speech production processes to language processing.

Prolonged tracheotomies and language disorders. The presence of multiple causal factors contributing to any presented language disorder probably is nowhere more apparent than in children who have required tracheotomies, usually for life-threatening medical problems. Frequently, these children have sustained neurologic impairment, have required prolonged hospitalizations, have multiple handicaps including significant

mental retardation, and are restricted in movement for prolonged periods, all factors that may negatively influence language. Disordered language in this group would be expected to result from neurologically based higher processing breakdowns secondary to any neurologic complications. However, clinically we have seen several children who have had tracheotomies for prolonged periods who seem to be developing well in other cognitive areas and in language comprehension but who have notable language formulation deficits. Typically these children have had laryngeal or tracheal atresia or stenosis (Baker and Savetsky, 1966; Cohen, 1971; Holinger, Johnson, and Schiller, 1954).

Although there have been reports of the use of an artificial larynx with patients with temporary tracheotomies (Summers, 1973), we know of no studies describing the language development and disorders of children with tracheotomies over prolonged periods of time. In a hospital-based practice, however, we have seen perhaps six children who because of tracheal or laryngeal stenosis have required tracheotomies for periods ranging from several months to over 8 years. We have observed that as infants these children frequently fail to babble, seemingly because of the lack of auditory feedback. Provided with mirrors in their cribs, however, often they will resume babbling, again gaining reinforcement from visual feedback. Typically such children are significantly delayed in the onset of speech and have some language limitations later in development, although certainly much of this delay can be attributed to the medical problems and to the prolonged hospitalization involved.

In the preceding discussion a number of variables common to each of these speech production disorders emerge. First, relatively little research has been reported that describes the language abilities in most of these children. Second, often children with speech production disorders have multiple causal variables involving hearing and the central nervous system. Thus frequently it is not possible to confine breakdowns to the process of speech production, and therefore it is often difficult or impossible to study a "pure" speech production breakdown and to hypothesize a "backup" effect on language abilities and development. For example, while children with cleft palate present speech production disorders, so also do they typically present sensation restrictions. Any described language deficit, therefore, cannot be attributed solely to the speech production breakdown but also must take into account the sensation limitations.

Finally, although the relationship between speech production breakdowns and language disorders may be a neglected area of investigation, study in this area holds the key for testing theories of the role of motor behavior in the development of language and arriving at a better understanding of the interdependencies that may be present.

Although hypothesizing a backup effect in which the speech production disruption negatively influences language development is tempting, certainly the relationship between variables in such children is complex and requires further investigation. In any event, for the present we cannot simply dismiss the process of speech production as a one-way executor of higher-planned language. Rather, the interdependence and two-way interaction of the higher language processes and the process of speech production must be considered. Certainly a basic need is a more extensive description of the language abilities and development of children presenting speech production disorders. It becomes an intriguing cause-effect relationship study where issues of multiple causation, chains of cause-effect relationships, and other aspects of causation enter into the analysis and interpretation.

chapter 8

Assessment of child language disorders

As the material presented in the previous chapters has suggested, child language disorders come in many faces and facets. There is no single, homogeneous population of children with language disorders. Behavior differs, performance differs, development differs, age differs, processing differs, causation differs, and so forth. In addition, children with language disorders may have other concomitant intrinsic and extrinsic developmental problems. Confronted with this vast array of differences, how does the speech-language pathologist diagnose, assess, manage, and treat these children?

ASSESSMENT: ONE PART OF DIAGNOSIS

A fundamental step in the diagnostic process is to differentiate through measurement each client's speech and language disorder. Assessment of child language disorders therefore is viewed here as the selection and use of appropriate measurement tools for determining the nature and severity of each child's language disorder. This assessment task is crucial to the understanding of child language disorders.

The speech-language pathologist must be able to measure a wide range of behaviors,

both verbal and nonverbal, in response to the type of stimulation he provides to the child. He must use a variety of assessment tools, procedures, and tests that detail language behavior and processes. These assessment procedures assist him in quantifying and comparing the symptoms of the disorder with normative data and with patterns of language performance seen in these children.

In essence the speech-language pathologist must become a measurement expert. He must know what each tool will do, how well each performs, and whether or not a specific tool is available. He must know what his observations tell him about underlying processes; he must know when he can infer safely and when the inferences are less secure. He becomes a calibrated measuring device, using many forms and types of measurements for assessing the variety of children with language disorders.

Many tests, tools, and procedures are now available for assessing child language disorders. From the time when no commercial tools were available and speech-language pathologists relied upon their own tool-making skill, we have arrived at a point of great proliferation and availability of commercial tools, clinically designed measurement protocols, and research instruments. Some of these tools are highly standardized; others simply are nicely packaged.

There also are a range of resources available to study and learn about tests and test procedures, including textbooks about child language disorders (Eisenson, 1972; Irwin and Marge, 1972; Muma, 1978; Wiig and Semel, 1976, 1980), books discussing the diagnostic process (Darley, 1964; Darley and Spriestersbach, 1978; Emerick and Hatten, 1979; Hutchinson, Hanson, and Mecham, 1979; Nation and Aram, 1977), books that evaluate the tests available (Darley, 1979), books that present tools that have been used in research (Johnson, 1976; Johnson and Bommarito, 1971), as well as research articles where tools that have been used are described (Aten, 1974; Aten and Davis, 1968; Weiner, 1972).

Issues surrounding testing have been discussed extensively in our profession (Nation and Aram, 1977), particularly topics such as reliability, validity, sampling, standardization, formal and informal procedures, and clinical adequacy of tools. Darley's (1979) contributors present their evaluations of commercial tools focusing on many of these issues.

It is not our intent in this chapter to address the many issues about testing or the many articles addressing the evaluation of specific assessment instruments. The fundamental purpose of Chapter 8 is to provide readers with a resource by which they can locate, select, and review assessment tools based on the material and working definitions detailed in this book. We will provide catalogs of assessment tools organized around the three processing segments of the CLPM. We will follow the presentation of this resource material by illustrating the relationship of assessment to the comprehensive diagnostic process, and then we will provide the student with a series of study questions by which he can apply his knowledge of child language disorders to the selection of assessment tools.

CLPM PROVIDES ORGANIZATIONAL BASIS FOR CATALOGING ASSESSMENT TOOLS

As presented in Chapter 3, the CLPM is composed of one major processing unit and two observational units. These three units provide the basis for organizing what we want to measure, for observing and measuring, and for relating our measurements of responses to underlying language processes.

The two observational units allow for inferences to be made about underlying processing disruptions. The design of the CLPM allows the speech-language pathologist to delimit responses that reveal information primarily about language input processing from responses that reveal information primarily about language output processing. Careful use of the CLPM allows for differentiation among types of language disorders.

We will present three catalogs of assessment tools corresponding to the processing segments of the CLPM: (1) speech to language, (2) language to thought to language, and (3) language to speech. Each catalog will include the name, author, and reference for the tool; information about the nature of the stimuli; the processing stages being tapped; and the behaviors being observed within the two observational units.

The tools catalogued are not to be considered an endorsement on our part of the quality or usefulness of the particular tool. They are included to provide the reader with a wide range of potential selections for assessment. Since we are still some way from understanding child language disorders and their causes, we contend that students should be exposed to a wide variety of potential assessment tools that have been derived from different theoretical and practical considerations. To provide a preselected set of tools in our view would bias the student. A major part of our professional learning is spent in evaluating tools. What would be an appropriate selection for one child may be unfortunate for another. The literature about each tool should be reviewed to determine its appropriateness for assessment. The evaluations and criteria used by the contributors to Darley's (1979) book can serve as models by which tools may be evaluated.

Another major point must be made about the three catalogs. Many tools have been constructed to *test for* certain behaviors, processes, skills, and so forth. However, we are aware that these tools, although developed for one purpose, may be used for assessing other types of information. Our position on cataloging has been to place the tool in the processing segment of *best fit,* particularly as determined by the author of the tool. Those who use these catalogs may well revise the catalog by multiple placement of tools based on their interpretation of what skill may be tapped by the tool. For example, while we have placed Wepman's Auditory Discrimination Test (1958) in the speech to language processing segment as a test for auditory discrimination, some may see it as a tool for tapping metalinguistic skills because of the judgments required of the child and would therefore also place it within the language to thought to language processing segment.

SPEECH TO LANGUAGE PROCESSING SEGMENT

In Chapter 3 the Speech to Language Processing Segment was introduced, and in Chapter 5 it was discussed in detail. Two processing stages were identified in this segment: (1) sensation and (2) perception. As we said earlier, this segment primarily is involved in processing auditory information prior to the time when comprehension of the stimulus takes place. We also included the prelinguistic processing of phonetic data in this segment.

When assessing the Speech to Language Processing Segment, we are interested in tests, tools, and procedures that reveal how the child responds to a variety of auditory stimuli. We ask basic questions such as the following: Can the child hear? How loud must a stimulus be before he indicates that he hears the sounds? Can he distinguish among sounds that differ by minor amounts as well as by more distinct differences? Can the child attend to sounds? Can the child retain a sequence of sounds and report the nature of that sequence correctly? Can the child respond appropriately when the sounds are presented at a fast rate?

Audiologic assessment

The audiologist's professional concern is the measurement and treatment of hearing and its disorders. Since audiologic testing procedures comprise an entire field of study, and readers of the present text are expected to have obtained course work in this area, no attempt will be made here to detail this information beyond a few summary statements and references for further study.

Early in the history of the audiology profession, assessment focused on the severity and nature of any loss or decrement in sensation and discrimination. Assessment procedures primarily consisted of attempts to specify pure tone and speech reception or detection thresholds and speech discrimination abilities. A further goal was specification of the hearing loss as conductive or sensorineural.

As the profession advanced, increased attention was devoted to (1) more objective specification of middle ear functions; (2) the functioning of the auditory system beyond determination of levels of sensation and discrimination, with specification of site of auditory lesions; and (3) the functioning of higher or more "central auditory" abilities. Site of lesion testing and central auditory testing have led the audiologist "up the brainstem to the cortex," while parallel interests of speech-

TABLE 8-1. *Catalog of audiologic assessment tools organized by site of lesion**

Procedure	Conductive	Cochlear	Eighth nerve	Brainstem	Cortical	Functional
Behavioral response						
Pure-tone air and bone conduction thresholds	X	X	X	X	X	X
Spondee thresholds	X	X	X	X	X	X
Speech discrimination in quiet	X	X	X	X	X	X
Alternate Binaural Loudness Balance (ABLB)		(recruitment)	(decruitment)			
Monaural Loudness Balance (MLB)		X	X			
Short Increment Sensitivity Index (SISI)		X	X (high level)			
Tone decay						
Bekesy (conventional)	Type I	Type II	Type III, IV			Type V
Critical-Off Time (COT)			X			X
Lengthened-Off Time (LOT)						X
Bekesy Comfortable Loudness (BCL)			X			
Bekesy Ascending-Descending Gap Evaluation (BADGE)						
Forward-backward tracings						
Brief-tone audiometry		X	X			
Aural Overload Test		X	X			
Frequency DLs		X				
Performance-Intensity Function (PI-PB)			X			
Synthetic Sentence Identification with Ipsilateral Competing Message (SSI-ICM)			X	X		
Synthetic Sentence Identification with Contralateral Competing Message (SSI-CCM)					X	
Speech-in noise				X	X	
Binaural fusion				X		
Rapidly alternating sentences				X		
Masking Level Differences (MLDs)				X		
Mid-plane balancing						

Staggered Spondaic Word Test (SSW)

Competing Environmental Sounds (CES)

Time Altered Speech (compression and expansion)

Rush Hughes Speech Discrimination Test

NU No. 6 Competing Message Test

Auditory pitch pattern perception

Dichotic digits, syllables, etc.

Spondee threshold and pure-tone discrepancy

Stenger Test

Shadow Curve

Delayed Auditory Feedback (DAF)

Doerfler-Steward Test

Lombard Test

Swinging (Shifting) Story Test

Electrophysiologic response

Immittance measurements

Tympanometry

Acoustic reflex thresholds

Static compliance

Stapedial reflex decay

Acoustic reflex latency test

Eustachian tube function tests (Pressure-swallow testing, Valsalva, Toynbee, etc.)

Auditory evoked response potentials

Electrocochleography (ECoG)

Brainstem Auditory Evoked Potentials (BAEP)

Cortical Auditory Evoked Potentials

Electrodermal audiometry

*Prepared by Craig Newman, Communication Sciences, Case Western Reserve University, Cleveland, Ohio language pathologists have led them "down from the cortex" to consider prelinguistic auditory operations or what we have referred to as speech to language processing. Thus, there has come to be considerable overlap in what is examined when speech-language pathologists examine auditory processing or speech perception and when the audiologist measures central auditory functions.

Numerous audiologic assessment tools are employed and are categorized in a number of ways. One broad distinction has been between techniques that rely on behavioral responses and those where the response is electrophysiologic. Most forms of audiologic assessment fall into the former category, including pure-tone air and bone conduction thresholds, speech reception thresholds, short increment sensitivity index testing (SISI), and the central auditory test batteries. Electrophysiologic assessments achieve greater objectivity and are often employed in young or uncooperative patients. Such measures include evoked response audiometry, electro-cochleography, and tympanometry among others.

Audiologic assessment procedures also are categorized in terms of the population (often determined by age) for which they are best appropriate. Thus a series of hearing tools are available for use with neonates, including the Crib-o-gram (Simmons and Russ, 1974) and the High Risk Register (Downs and Silver, 1972). Similarly, visual response audiometry (VRA), in which the child is conditioned to look at the visual reinforcer when he hears the sounds, and tangible reinforcement operant conditioning (TROCA) are typically employed with infants and young children.

Many retrocochlear assessment procedures (with the notable exception of evoked response audiometry) require reliable behavioral responses by the child and thus are often not usable with preschool children. Similarly, the current central auditory test batteries are

difficult to use with children below 5 to 6 years of age. Furthermore, children with significant psychologic or cognitive impairments, whatever their age, cannot fully comply with behavioral testing. Thus a profoundly retarded 8-year-old, functioning under a 2-year-old level, may well have to be tested with visual reinforcement audiometry or through electrophysiologic measurement. Similarly, autistic children may not accept earphones, comply with conditioning techniques, or provide reliable responses. Thus electrophysiologic measurement, most likely evoked response audiometry, may be the necessary assessment tool.

Audiologic assessment procedures are detailed in numerous audiology texts. For further study, the reader is referred to Katz (1978), Keith (1977), Martin (1978), Northern and Downs (1978), and Rose (1971). In addition, Brooks (1979) provides an extensive review of information related to design factors in the identification and assessment of hearing loss. He presents literature on the success and failure of techniques for use with young children and infants.

Probably one of the primary means of categorizing audiometric assessment procedures is in terms of site of lesion under examination. Table 8-1 provides one such summary of auditory tests grouped in this manner, separated by tests requiring (1) a behavioral response and (2) an electrophysiologic response.

Assessment of auditory operations

Many tools and procedures have been devised to answer questions about auditory perceptual processing and its relationship to child language disorders. These tools have generally been defined operationally in terms of the task expected of the child; the stimulus is specified in a precise way as is the response modality and type. Then if failure occurs on the task, the inference is made that the underlying auditory process (operation) is disrupted.

In Chapter 5 we summarized a vast amount of information about auditory perceptual processing and child language disorders. We emphasized that the findings of the studies were equivocal in terms of establishing a relationship, particularly a causal relationship, between auditory processing (perceptual) dysfunctions and child language disorders. We pointed out the difficulties in interpreting the data available about the auditory operations that we delineated as part of speech to language processing and therefore ended that chapter with a set of precautions to be kept in mind when assessing this relationship. Rapin and Wilson (1978) are in agreement with this cautious position. They, too, feel that the information on auditory perception in child language disorders is too sparse to be useful in clinical diagnosis.

We therefore stress taking a conservative approach when interpreting the relationship of auditory processing measures to child language disorders. However, the state of the art between auditory perceptual processing and language, both normal and disordered, should not be discouraging to us. Rather it should challenge us to discover more before proceeding with treatment based on undocumented assumptions about the relationship.

With these precautions in mind, we present Table 8-2 as a catalog of some of the assessment tools used to measure the auditory operations that were enumerated and discussed in Chapter 5. Because of the vast number of standardized, experimental, and clinical tools available, it is not possible to present an exhaustive listing of every measure of these auditory operations. Rather we have attempted to include what we consider to be a representative group of such tools, most of which are commercially available. This listing therefore is intended as a reference rather than an exhaustive catalog.

In Table 8-2 the name and source of each tool is listed on the left. The stimulus is specified in terms of providing visual (V) or auditory (A) input, further specifying auditory input as single words, digits, speech sounds, or connected speech. The primary auditory operation(s) under test are then indicated by an X. Typically, auditory tasks require more than one auditory operation for completion. In the Boston University Discrimination Test (Pronovost, 1953), for example, a child must attend to the stimulus at the rate presented in addition to discriminating the word presented. However, we have categorized this test as one of discrimination, since this is the primary operation that it addresses.

The response modality is indicated as nonverbal or verbal. We have indicated whether or not we are primarily observing the use of the child's language directly, in which case we have indicated a 2 related to observational unit two in the CLPM. If we are primarily observing the child's response to language presented to him, we have indicated a 1 referring to observational unit one (refer to Chapter 3 for discussion of the observational units). Finally, on the far right of Table 8-2 we have indicated the age range for which the tool was developed, usually the age range for which normative data are available.

Summarizing tools in this manner allows students and clinicians to group tools assessing a particular operation, to gain broad information as to the stimulus and response requirements of the tool, and to judge the age range for which the tool is appropriate.

LANGUAGE TO THOUGHT TO LANGUAGE SEGMENT

The Language to Thought to Language processing segment is concerned with how the child derives linguistic data from the auditory stimulus for comprehension, how he re-

Text continued on p. 186.

TABLE 8-2. *Tools for assessing auditory operations*

Test and reference	Stimulus		Attention	Rate
	Modality	Nature of auditory stimulus		
Auditory Discrimination Test Wepman, J., *Auditory Discrimination Test*. Chicago: Language Research Associates (1958).	A	Word Pairs		
Auditory Memory For Speech Sounds Metraux, R.W., Auditory memory span for speech sounds of speech defective children compared with normal children. *Journal of Speech Disorders*, **6,** 33-36 (1942). Metraux, R.W., Auditory memory span for speech sounds: Norms for children. *Journal of Speech Disorders*, **9,** 31-38 (1944).	A	Series of vowels, diphthongs and consonants		
Auditory Memory Span Test Wepman, J.M., and Morency, A., *Auditory Memory Span Test*. Chicago: Language Research Associates (1973).	A	Word sequences 2-6 words in length		
Auditory Pointing Test Fudala, J.B., Kunze, L.H., and Ross, J.D., *Auditory Pointing Test*. San Rafael, Cal.: Academic Therapy Publications (1974).	V and A	Single syllable words 2-10 words in length		
Auditory Sequential Memory Test Wepman, J.M., and Morency, A., *The Auditory Sequential Memory Test*. Chicago: Language Research Associates (1973).	A	Digits		
Boston University Discrimination Test Pronovost, W., *Boston University Speech Discrimination Test*. Cedar Falls, Iowa: Go-Mo Products (1953).	V and A	Single words		
Denver Auditory Phoneme Sequencing Test Aten, J., *The Denver Auditory Phoneme Sequencing Test*. Houston: College Hill Press (1979).	V and A	Words, sequence of words		
Detroit Test Of Learning Aptitude Baker, H.J., and Leland, B., *Detroit Tests*. Indianapolis: The Bobbs-Merrill Co. (1959). 1. Auditory Attention Span for Unrelated Words 2. Auditory Attention Span for Related Words 3. Oral Commissions 4. Oral Directions	 A A A A	 Words Sentences 6-27 syllables Commands Commands		

Auditory operations			Response		
Discrimination	Memory	Sequencing	Modality	Observational unit	Age range
X			Verbal: same-different	1	5-0 to 8-0 4-6 to 12-5
	X		Verbal-repeat sounds	2	4-6 to 12-5
	X		Verbal repetition	2	5-0 to 8-0
	X		Pointing	1	5-0 to 10-11
	X	X	Verbal repetition	2	5-0 to 8-0
X			Pointing	1	K to first grade
	X	X	Pointing	1	5-0 to 13-0
	X		Verbal	2	3-0 to 19-0
	X		Verbal	2	3-0 to 19-0
	X		Performance	1	3-0 to 8-3
	X		Performance	1	6-3 to 19-0

Continued.

TABLE 8-2. *Tools for assessing auditory operations—cont'd*

Test and reference	Stimulus		Attention	Rate
	Modality	Nature of auditory stimulus		
Flowers-Costello Tests Of Central Auditory Abilities Flowers, A., Costello, M., and Small, V., *Flowers-Costello Test of Central Auditory Abilities*. Dearborn, Mich.: Perceptual Learning Systems (1970).				
1. Low Pass Filter Speech Test	V and A	Sentences	X	
2. Competing Message Test	V and A	Sentences	X	
Goldman-Fristoe-Woodcock Auditory Skills Test Battery Goldman, R., Fristoe, M., and Woodcock, R., *Goldman-Fristoe-Woodcock Auditory Skills Test Battery*. Circle Pines, Minn.: American Guidance Service (1974).				
1. Auditory Selective Attention Subtest	V and A	Words	X	
2. Diagnostic Auditory Discrimination Subtest	V and A	Words		
3. Auditory Memory Subtest	V and A	Words		
4. Sound Symbol Subtest	V and A	Nonsense syllables, isolated sounds		
Goldman Fristoe-Woodcock Test Of Auditory Discrimination Goldman, R., Fristoe, M., and Woodcock, R., *Goldman-Fristoe-Woodcock Test of Auditory Discrimination*. Circle Pines, Minn.: American Guidance Service Inc. (1970).	V and A	Words		
Illinois Test Of Psycholinguistic Abilities Kirk, S.A., McCarthy, J.J., and Kirk, W.D., *The Illinois Test of Psycholinguistic Abilities*. Champaign, Ill.: University of Illinois Press (1968). Auditory Sequential Memory	A	Digits		
Lindamood Auditory Conceptualization Test Lindamood, C.H., and Lindamood, P.C., *Lindamood Auditory Conceptualization Test*. Boston: Teaching Resources Corp. (1969).	V and A	Phonemes, nonsense syllables		
Rosewell-Chall Auditory Blending Test Roswell, F.G., and Chall, J.S., *Roswell-Chall Auditory Blending Test*. Planetarium Station, N.Y.: Essay Press (1963).	A	Isolated phonemes		

Auditory operations			Response		Age range
Discrimination	Memory	Sequencing	Modality	Observational unit	
			Pointing	1	K to sixth grade
			Pointing	1	K to sixth grade
			Pointing	1	3-0 to 80+
X			Pointing	1	3-0 to 80+
	X	X	Verbal, pointing, arranging pictures	1 2	3-0 to 80+
X		X	Pointing, verbal, writing	1 2	3-0 to 80+
X			Pointing	1	3-8 to 70+
	X		Verbal	2	2-0 to 10-3
		X	Arrange blocks	1	K to twelfth grade
	X		Verbal: blending phonemes	2	1st to fourth grade

Continued.

TABLE 8-2. *Tools for assessing auditory operations—cont'd*

Test and reference	Stimulus		Attention	Rate
	Modality	Nature of auditory stimulus		
Screening Test For Auditory Perception Kimmell, G.M., and Wahl, J., *Screening Test for Auditory Perception.* San Rafael, Cal.: Academic Therapy Publications (1969).	A	Words, rhythmic taps		
Short Term Auditory Retrieval And Storage Test Flowers, A., *Short Term Auditory Retrieval and Storage Test.* Dearborn, Michigan: Perceptual Learning Systems (1972).	V and A	Word pairs Word sequences		
Sound Discrimination Irwin, O.C., *Communication Variables of Cerebral Palsied and Mentally Retarded Children.* Springfield: C.C. Thomas (1972).	A	Word pairs		
Templin Sound Discrimination Test Templin, M., *Certain Language Skills in Children.* Minneapolis: University of Minnesota Press (1957). 1. Nonsense Syllables 2. Picture Sound	 A V and A	 Nonmeaningful CV syllables Words		
Test Of Listening Accuracy In Children Mecham, M.J., Jex, J.L., and Jones, J.D., *Test of Listening Accuracy in Children.* Provo, Utah: Brigham Young University Press (1969).	V and A	Words		
Washington Speech Sound Discrimination Test Prather, E.M., Miner, A., Addicott, M.A., and Sunderland, L., *Washington Speech Sound Discrimination Test.* Danville, Iowa: Interstate Printers and Publishers Inc. (1971).	V and A	Words		
Word Intelligibility By Picture Identification Ross, M., and Lerman, J., *Word Intelligibility by Picture Identification.* Pittsburgh: Stanwix House, Inc. (1971).	V and A	Words		

Auditory operations			Response		
Discrimination	Memory	Sequencing	Modality	Observational unit	Age range
X	X		Mark score sheet	1	8-0 to 12-0
	X		Mark in test booklet		1st to sixth grade
X			Verbal: same/different	1	6-0 to 16-0
X			Verbal: same/different	1	6-0 to 8-0
X			Pointing	1	3-0 to 5-0
X			Mark score sheet	1	5-0 to 9-0
X			Pointing	1	3-5 to 5-5
X			Pointing	1	4-7 to 13-9

lates this linguistic information to other cognitive, sensory, and perceptual data for language integration, and how he creates from his store of language and cognitive information messages to convey to listeners.

Assessment of this segment of the CLPM addresses the tools, procedures, and tests that tap into one or more aspects of comprehension, integration, repetition, and formulation at one or more levels of language. Thus the domain of this segment is directly concerned with assessing language as patterns of performance, that is, relating the language processes within this segment to levels of language behavior. The responses asked for and measured within the two observational units of the CLPM can be either nonverbal or verbal responses that reveal the child's language and cognitive knowledge.

A wide range of tools has been developed to gather information about the child's language and cognitive ability. As with the tools measuring the auditory operations, the number of instruments available is ever expanding and cannot be exhaustively surveyed in any one listing. Again, we have chosen to concentrate on commercially available tools for the most part, including tests we perceive as being widely used in the profession.

Tool selection considerations

While attempts to describe semantics have delineated various aspects of semantics (semantic features, semantic fields, semantic relations, the lexicon), most formal and informal assessment tools appropriate for child populations have been directed toward the lexicon and toward semantic relations. Of the standardized procedures for semantic comprehension, the Peabody Picture Vocabulary Test (PPVT) and the Full Range Picture Vocabulary Scale cover the broadest age range; however, they are restricted to comprehension of noun and verb forms. The Test for Auditory Comprehension of Language, the vocabulary subtest of the Assessment of Children's Language Comprehension (ACLC), and the Boehm Test of Basic Concepts examine a broader range of semantic concepts but are more restricted in the age groups for which they are applicable. In addition to these standardized procedures, numerous nonstandard procedures for assessing semantics have been reported in the literature, such as the Basic Concept Inventory. If standardized tests are employed for measuring semantic comprehension, selection of several measures would seem to be indicated to accommodate age and ability range.

Standardized semantic formulation tools are few in number, limited in age range, and limited in semantic concepts tapped. Beyond the vocabulary naming or definition items on standardized intelligence tests, there appears to be no extensively developed or standardized measures of expressive semantics. Typically measures of semantic formulation have been developed as part of research protocols with particular groups of language impaired children; for example, Nation's (1972) Vocabulary Usage Test, an expressive adaptation of the PPVT, was first developed for use with children who have cleft palate and has been standardized only on a small group of normal children. Similarly the Environmental Language Inventory (ELI) was initially developed for use with retarded children but subsequently has been adapted for use with diverse groups of children. Other expressive lexical measures include the type/token ratio (Johnson, Darley, and Spriestersbach, 1963), the number of in class words per unit of time (for example, number of animal names offered in 90 seconds), and verbal analogy and opposite tests (such as those included in the Detroit Test of Learning Abilities), which provide measures of semantic relatedness. Probably the most widely used method of describing semantic formulation is to analyze the semantic relations in the spontaneous speech samle of children under study. In view of the very few standardized tools available to measure semantic formulation, nonstandardized procedures may have to be developed for assessing the diverse types of language disordered children.

In contrast to the dearth of standardized tools available for measuring semantics, several appropriate options are available for the study of syntax; these usually include measures of word order and inflectional markers. For syntactic comprehension the Assessment of Children's Language Comprehension, The Miller-Yoder Test of Grammatical Comprehension, and the Northwestern Syntax Screening Test are probably the most frequently used, the former two being appropriate for lower functioning children and the latter (NSST) requiring higher performance and providing norms up to 8 years of age. The Token Test for Children, although providing very valuable information regarding ability to comprehend stimuli of increasing length and grammatical complexity, is not standardized for children below 4 years of age and requires knowledge of color and shape.

The chief standardized tools available for measuring syntactic formulation include the expressive part of the Northwestern Syntax Screening Test and the Grammatic Closure subtest of the Illinois Test of Psycholinguistic Abilities. A number of immediate repetition tasks have been developed to elicit syntactic information, but none provides standardization information (for example, Carrow Elicited Language Inventory; Aram's Developmental Sentences). Furthermore the validity of using sentence repetition tasks to measure expressive syntax (including the NSST) has been questioned, particularly without comparison to a spontaneously generated speech sample. Except for various methods of analyzing spontaneous speech samples, there are few tools available for measuring expressive syntax for children who are not yet using complete sentences. Aram and Nation (1975) used an expressive adaptation of the ACLC with younger/lower functioning language disordered children. While standardized tools are available for the older/more able children, tools may have to be developed for assessing younger/lower functioning children.

It is clear that much research has been done that describes the communicative performance of normal children in various contexts, an area that has frequently been termed communicative competence or pragmatics and that we view as a function of the integration processing stage. Although considerable literature has appeared in this area, assessment approaches continue to be in the experimental stages of development, and few provide any standardized information.

Because of the diverse approaches taken in the literature to the study of communicative performance and because of the lack of standardized tools available, speech pathologists will need to give considerable attention to the selection of assessment procedures in this area. Prutting (1979) and Miller (1978) provide an important starting point. They have summarized much of the literature and have applied this information to language disordered children. Prutting (1979) has focused on developmental stages of pragmatic acquisition, whereas Miller (1978) has developed a protocol for systematically observing the communicative interactions of language disordered children.

Organization of the assessment catalog

Table 8-3 summarizes representative tools available for assessing language and cognitive knowledge and performance within the language to thought to language processing segment of the CLPM. The table is organized in the following way:

1. The first section, *test and reference,* provides the name of the test and its primary

Text continued on p. 204.

TABLE 8-3. *Tools for assessing language and cognitive knowledge and performance*

Test and reference	Stimulus		Language processing stages			
	Modality	Nature of auditory stimulus	Compre-hension	Integra-tion	Formu-lation	Repeti-tion
Assessment Of Children's Language Comprehension Foster, R., Giddan, J.J., and Stark, J., *Manual for the Assessment of Children's Language Comprehension.* Palo Alto, Calif.: Consulting Psychologists Press (1973).	V and A	Words and 1-4 element phrases	X			
Assessment In Infancy: Ordinal Scales Of Psychological Development Uzgiris, I.C., and Hunt, J., *Assessment in Infancy: Ordinal Scales of Psychological Development.* Urbana, Ill.: University of Illinois Press (1975).	V and A	Nonmeaningful vocalizations, words		X		
Bankson Language Screening Test Bankson, N.W., *Bankson Language Screening Test.* Baltimore: University Park Press (1977).	V and A	Words, sentences	X		X	
Basic Concept Inventory Englemann, S., *The Basic Concept Inventory.* Chicago: Follett Educational Corporation (1967).	V and A	Words, sentences, nonverbal patterns and digits	X			
Bayley Scales Of Infant Development Bayley, N., *Bayley Scales of Infant Development.* N.Y.: Psychological Corporation of America (1969). Aram, D.M., and Nation, J.E., Intelligence tests for children: A language analysis. *Ohio Journal of Speech and Hearing,* **6,** 22-43 (1971).	V and A	Words, phrases and commands		X		
Berry-Talbott Tests Of Language: I. Comprehension Of Grammar Berry, M., *Berry-Talbott Tests of Language: I. Comprehension of Grammar.* Rockford, Ill.: 4322 Pinecrest Road (1966).	V and A	Nonsense words in sentence completion task			X	
Boehm Test Of Basic Concepts Boehm, A.E., *Boehm Test of Basic Concepts.* N.Y.: Psych. Corp. (1971).	V and A	Words, sentences	X			

Language level			Intelligence, cognitive, developmental	Multi-dimen-sional	Response		Age range
Pragmatic	Semantic	Syntactic			Modality	Observa-tional unit	
	X	X			Pointing	1	3-0 to 6-11
			X		Spontaneous vocalizations, sound and word imitation, performance	1 2	0 to 2-0
				X	Verbal, pointing	1 2	4-1 to 8-0
			X	X	Verbal and nonverbal performance	1 2	3-0 to 10-0
			X		Vocal/verbal performance	1 2	0.2 to 2-6
		X			Verbal: nonsense words	2	5-0 to 8-0
X			X		Marks test booklet	1	K to second grade

Continued.

TABLE 8-3. *Tools for assessing language and cognitive knowledge and performance—cont'd*

Test and reference	Stimulus		Language processing stages			
	Modality	Nature of auditory stimulus	Compre-hension	Integra-tion	Formu-lation	Repeti-tion
Carrow Elicited Language Inventory Carrow-Woolfolk, E., *Carrow Elicited Language Inventory.* Austin, Tex.: Learning Concepts (1974).	A	Sentences				
Cattell Infant Intelligence Scale Cattell, P., *The Measurement of Intelligence of Infants and Young Children.* N.Y.: The Psychological Corporation (1947). Aram, D.M., and Nation, J.E., Intelligence tests for children: A language analysis. *Ohio Journal of Speech and Hearing,* **6,** 22-43 (1971).	V and A	Words, sentences		X		
Chicago Non Verbal Examination Brown, A.W., and Stein, S., *Chicago Non Verbal Examination.* N.Y.: The Psychological Corp. (1936).	A			X		
Clinical Evaluation Of Language Function Semel, E.M., and Wiig, E.H., *Clinical Evaluation of Language Functions: Examiner's Manual.* Columbus, Ohio: Charles E. Merrill Pub. Co. (1980).	V and A	Words, commands, sentence completion				
Columbia Mental Maturity Scale Burgemeister, B., Blum, L., and Lorge, I., *Columbia Mental Maturity Scale.* N.Y.: Harcourt Brace Jovanovich, Inc. (1953).	V			X		
Communicative Evaluation Chart From Infancy To Five Years Anderson, M., Miles, M., and Matheny, P., *Communicative Evaluation Chart from Infancy to Five Years.* Cambridge, Mass.: Educators Publishing Service, Inc. (1963).	V and A	Parent informant	X		X	
Del Rio Language Screening Test English/Spanish Toronto, A.S., Leverman, D., Hanna, C., Rosensweig, P., and Maldonado, A., *Del Rio Language Screening Test English/Spanish.* National Education Laboratory Pub. (1975).	V and A	Words, sentences, commands, stories	X			X

| Language level | | | Intelligence, cognitive, developmental | Multi-dimensional | Response | | Age range |
Pragmatic	Semantic	Syntactic			Modality	Observational unit	
		X			Verbal: imitation of sentences	2	3-0 to 7-11
			X		Verbal and performance	1 2	0-3 to 2-6
			X		Performance	1	6-0 to 14+
				X	Verbal and performance	1 2	K to tenth grade
			X		Pointing	1	3-6 to 9-11
				X	Verbal and performance	1 2	0-3 to 5-0
				X	Verbal and performance	1 2	3-0 to 6-11

Continued.

TABLE 8-3. *Tools for assessing language and cognitive knowledge and performance—cont'd*

Test and reference	Stimulus		Language processing stages			
	Modality	Nature of auditory stimulus	Compre-hension	Integra-tion	Formu-lation	Repeti-tion
Denver Developmental Screening Test Frankenburg, W.K., and Dodd, J.B., *Denver Developmental Screening Test.* Denver: University of Colorado Medical Center (1967). Frankenburg, W., Dodds, J., and Fandal, A., *Denver Developmental Screening Test.* Denver: University of Colorado Medical Center (1970).	V and A	Sentences, commands, questions, sentence completion		X		
Detroit Tests Of Learning Aptitude Baker, J.H., and Leland, B., *Detroit Tests of Learning Aptitude.* Indianapolis: The Bobbs-Merrill Co. (1959). 1. Verbal Absurdities 2. Verbal Opposites 3. Social Adjustment 4. Orientation 5. Likenesses and Differences	A A A A A	Connected speech Words Connected speech Questions, commands Words		X X X X X		
Developmental Potential Of Pre-school Children Haeussermann, E., *Developmental Potential of Preschool Children.* N.Y.: Grune & Stratton, Inc. (1958).	V and A	Words, commands, con-nected speech	X	X		
Developmental Sentences Aram, D.M., *Developmental Sentences.* Cleveland: Cleveland Hearing and Speech Center (1969).	A	Sentences				X
Developmental Sentence Scoring And Developmental Sentence Types Lee, L.L., *Developmental Sentence Analysis.* Evanston: Northwestern University Press (1974).	V and A	Variable			X	
Environmental Language Inventory MacDonald, J.D., and Nickols, *Environmental Language Inventory.* Columbus, Ohio: Charles E. Merrill (1978).	V and A	Phrases			X	

Language level			Intelligence, cognitive, developmental	Multi-dimensional	Response		Age range
Pragmatic	Semantic	Syntactic			Modality	Observational unit	
			X		Verbal and performance	2	0 to 6-0
			X	X			
1. X						2	5-3 to 16-6
	2. X					2	5-3 to 19-0
3. X						2	3-6 to 13-6
	4. X					2	3-0 to 13-6
	5. X					2	6-9 to 19-0
			X		Verbal and performance	1 2	2-0 to 6-6
		X			Verbal: sentence imitation	2	3-0 to 7-0
		X			Spontaneous language	2	DSS: 2-0 to 6-11 DST: no age range specified 2-0 to 2-11 (normals)
	X	X			Verbal	2	

Continued.

TABLE 8-3. *Tools for assessing language and cognitive knowledge and performance—cont'd*

Test and reference	Stimulus		Language processing stages			
	Modality	Nature of auditory stimulus	Compre-hension	Integra-tion	Formu-lation	Repeti-tion
Environmental Prelanguage Battery Horstmeier, D., and MacDonald, J.D., *Environmental Prelanguage Battery.* Columbus, Ohio: Charles E. Merrill (1978).						
1. Nonverbal	V and A	Words, commands, and phrases		X		
2. Verbal	V and A	Words commands, and phrases			X	X
Full-Range Picture Vocabulary Test Ammons, R.B., and Ammons, H.S., *Full-Range Picture Vocabulary Test.* Missoula, Mont.: Psychological Test Specialists (1948).	V and A	Words	X			
Goodenough-Harris Drawing Test Goodenough, R.L., and Harris, D.B., *Goodenough-Harris Drawing Test.* N.Y.: Harcourt Brace Jovanovich, Inc. (1963). Harris, D., *Children's Drawing as Measures of Intellectual Maturity.* N.Y.: Harcourt Brace Jovanovich, Inc. (1963).				X		
Houston Test For Language Development Crabtree, M., *Houston Test for Language Development.* Houston: Houston Test Co. (1963).	V and A	Sounds, commands, words	X		X	
Illinois Test Of Psycholinguistic Abilities Kirk, S.A., McCarthy, J., and Kirk, W.D., *Illinois Test of Psycholinguistic Abilities.* (Rev. ed.) Urbana, Ill.: University of Illinois Press (1968).						
1. Auditory Reception	A	Sentences	X			
2. Auditory Association	A	Sentence completion		X		
3. Verbal Expression	A	Words			X	
4. Grammatic Closure	V and A	Sentence completion			X	
5. Manual Expression	V				X	
Language Facility Test Dailey, J.T., *The Language Facility Test.* Alexandria, Va.: Allington Corporation (1977).	V and A	Prompts to tell story			X	

Language level			Intelligence, cognitive, developmental	Multi-dimensional	Response		Age range
agmatic	Semantic	Syntactic			Modality	Observational unit	
			X	X			
X					Vocal behavior	1 2	0-12 to 2-6
	X	X			Verbal	2	0-12 to 2-6
	X				Pointing	1	2-0 to adult
			X		Drawing	2	K to ninth grade
				X	Vocal, verbal and performance	1 2	0-6 to 3-0
				X			
	1. X				Yes/no	1	2-1 to 10-2
	2. X				Words	2	2-4 to 10-11
	3. X				Words	2	2-0 to 10-11
		4. X			Words	2	2-2 to 10-4
					Gestures	2	2-0 to 10-4
				X	Verbal: story	2	3-0 to 20-0

Continued.

TABLE 8-3. *Tools for assessing language and cognitive knowledge and performance —cont'd*

Test and reference	Stimulus		Language processing stages			
	Modality	Nature of auditory stimulus	Compre-hension	Integra-tion	Formu-lation	Repeti-tion
Language Sampling, Analysis And Training Tyack, D., and Gottsleben, R., *Language Sampling, Analysis and Training*. Palo Alto, Cal.: Consulting Psychologists Press (1974).	V and A	Variable			X	
Leiter International Performance Scale Leiter, R.G., *Leiter International Performance Scale*. Washington, D.C.: The Psychological Service Center Press (1948).	V			X		
Arthur, G., *Arthur Adaptation of the Leiter International Performance Scale*. Washington, D.C.: The Psychological Service Center Press (1952).	V			X		
McCarthy Scales Of Children's Abilities McCarthy, D., *McCarthy Scales of Children's Abilities*. N.Y.: Psychological Corp. (1970).	V and A	Words, word definitions, word associations, digits		X		
Memory For Sentences Spencer, E.M., *Memory for Sentences*. Unpublished dissertation, Evanston, Ill.: Northwestern University Press (1958).	A	Sentences				X
Merrill-Palmer Scale Of Mental Tests Stutsman, R., *Mental Measurement of Pre-school Children*. Yonkers-on Hudson, N.Y.: World Book Co. (1931). Aram, D.M., and Nation, J.E., Intelligence tests for children: A language analysis. *Ohio Journal of Speech and Hearing*, **6,** 22-43 (1971)	V and A	Words, connected speech, action-agent		X		

Language level			Intelligence, cognitive, developmental	Multidimensional	Response		Age range
Pragmatic	Semantic	Syntactic			Modality	Observational unit	
				X	Spontaneous language sample	2	2-0 to 6-0
			X		Block arrangement	1	2-0 to adult
			X		Block arrangement	1	3-0 to 8-0
			X		Verbal, performance	1 2	2-6 to 8-6
		X			Verbal: sentence imitation	2	4-0 to 9-6
			X		Verbal and performance	1 2	1-6 to 5-11

Continued.

TABLE 8-3. *Tools for assessing language and cognitive knowledge and performance —cont'd*

Test and reference	Stimulus		Language processing stages			
	Modality	Nature of auditory stimulus	Compre-hension	Integra-tion.	Formu-lation	Repeti tion
Michigan Picture Language Inventory Lerea, L., *Michigan Picture Language Inventory*. Ann Arbor, Mich.: University of Michigan Press (1958). Wolski, W., *The Michigan Picture Language Inventory*. Ann Arbor, Mich.: University of Michigan Press (1962).	V and A	Words	X		X	
Miller-Yoder Test Of Grammatical Comprehension Miller, J.F., and Yoder, D.E., *The Miller-Yoder Test of Grammatical Comprehension: Experimental Edition*. Madison, Wisc.: Department of Communicative Disorders, University of Wisconsin (1972).	V and A	Sentences	X			
Northwestern Syntax Screening Test Lee, L.L., *Northwestern Syntax Screening Test*. Evanston, Ill.: Northwestern University Press (1969).	V and A	Sentences	X		X	
Oral Language Sentence Imitation Test And Oral Language Sentence Diagnostic Inventory Zachman, L., Hulsingh, R., Jorgensen, C., and Barrett, M., *Oral Language Sentence Imitation Test and Oral Language Sentence Diagnostic Inventory*. Moline, Ill.: Lingui Systems, Inc. (1976).	A A	Phonemes Sentences				X X
Parsons Language Sample Spradlin, J.E., Assessment of speech language of retarded children. The Parsons language sample. *Journal of Speech and Hearing Disorders*, Monograph Suppl. **10,** 8-31 (1963).	V and A	Questions, digits, words, sentences, commands	X		X	X
Peabody Picture Vocabulary Test Dunn, L.M., *Expanded Manual for the Peabody Picture Vocabulary Test*. Circle Pines, Minn.: American Guidance Service, Inc. (1965).	V and A	Words	X			

| Language level | | | Intelligence, cognitive, de-velopmental | Multi-dimen-sional | Response | | Age range |
Pragmatic	Semantic	Syntactic			Modality	Observa-tional unit	
	X	X			Verbal: words and pointing	1 2	4-0 to 6-0
		X			Pointing	1	3-0 to 6-0
		X			Pointing, sentence	1 2	3-0 to 7-11
		X X			Verbal: imitation Verbal: imitation	2 2	none given
				X	Verbal and perfor-mance	1 2	7-11 to 15-8 (mentally retarded subjects)
	X				Pointing	1	2-6 to 18-0

Continued.

TABLE 8-3. *Tools for assessing language and cognitive knowledge and performance—cont'd*

Test and reference	Stimulus		Language processing stages			
	Modality	Nature of auditory stimulus	Compre-hension	Integra-tion	Formu-lation	Repeti-tion
Pictorial Test Of Intelligence French, J.L., *Pictorial Test of Intelligence*. Boston: Houghton-Mifflin Co. (1960). Aram, D.M., and Nation, J.E., Intelligence tests for children: A language analysis. *Ohio Journal of Speech and Hearing*, **6**, 22-43 (1971).	V and A	Words, commands, connected speech		X		
Picture Articulation And Language Screening Test Rodgers, W.C., *Picture Articulation and Language Screening Test*. Salt Lake: Word Making Productions (1976).	V and A	Question	X		X	
Picture Story Language Test Myklebust, H., *Development and Disorders of Written Language: Picture Story Language Test,* Vol. I, N.Y.: Grune & Stratton, Inc. (1965).	V				X	
Porch Index Of Communicative Ability In Children Porch, B.E., *Porch Index of Communicative Ability in Children*. Palo Alto, Cal.: Consulting Psychologist Press (1974).	V and A	Connected speech	X		X	
Preschool Language Assessment Instrument Blank, M., Rose, S., and Berlin, L., *Preschool Language Assessment Instrument*. N.Y.: Grune & Stratton (1978).	V and A	Connected speech, sentences, commands, sentence completion		X		
Preschool Language Scale Zimmerman, I., Steiner, V., and Evatt, R., *Preschool Language Mantal*. Columbus, OH: Charles E. Merrill Publishing Co. (1969).	V and A	Words, commands, questions, digits, action-agent	X		X	
Receptive-Expressive Emergent Language Scale (Reel) Bzoch, K., and League, R., *Assessing Language Skills in Infancy*. Gainesville, Fla.: Tree of Life Press (1971).	Parent informant					

Language level			Intelligence, cognitive, developmental	Multi-dimensional	Response		Age range
Pragmatic	Semantic	Syntactic			Modality	Observational unit	
			X		Verbal and performance	1 2	3-0 to 8-0
				X	Verbal, pointing	1 2	None given (preschool)
				X	Written language	2	7-0 to 17-0
				X	Verbal, reading, performance	1 2	Preschool to 12-0
				X	Verbal and performance	1 2	3-0 to 6-0
				X	Verbal and performance	1 2	1-6 to 7-0
				X	Parent informant		0-0 to 3-0

Continued.

TABLE 8-3. *Tools for assessing language and cognitive knowledge and performance—cont'd*

	Stimulus		Language processing stages			
Test and reference	**Modality**	**Nature of auditory stimulus**	**Compre-hension**	**Integra-tion**	**Formu-lation**	**Repeti-tion**
Reynell Developmental Language Scales Reynell, J., *Reynell Developmental Language Scales: Manual.* (Experimental Edition) Buckinghamshire, England: National Foundation for Educational Research in England and Wales (1969).	V and A	Connected speech, naming	X		X	
Sequenced Inventory Of Communication Development Hendrick, D.L., Prather, E.M., and Tobin, A.R., *Sequenced Inventory of Communication Development.* Seattle: University of Washington Press (1975).	V and A	Nonverbal sounds, words, commands, CV, digits, sentences	X		X	
Stanford-Binet Intelligence Scale Terman, L.M., and Merrill, M.A., *Stanford-Binet Intelligence Scale: Manual for the Third Revision,* Form L-M. Boston: Houghton Mifflin Co. (1960). Aram, D.M., and Nation, J.E., Intelligence tests for children: A language analysis. *Ohio Journal of Speech and Hearing,* **6,** 22-43 (1971).	V and A	Connected speech, sentences		X		
Test Of Auditory Comprehension Of Language Carrow-Woolfork, E., *Test for Auditory Comprehension of Language.* Austin, Tex.: Learning Concepts (1973).	V and A	Words, sentences	X			
Test Of Language Development Scale Newcomer, P., and Hammill, D., *Test of Language Development.* Austin, Tex.: Empiric Press (1977).	V and A	Words, sentences, sentence completion	X		X	

| Language level | | | Intelligence, cognitive, developmental | Multi-dimensional | Response | | Age range |
Pragmatic	Semantic	Syntactic			Modality	Observational unit	
				X	Verbal and performance	1 2	0-6 to 6-0
				X	Vocal, verbal and performance	1 2	0-4 to 4-0
			X		Verbal and performance	1 2	2-0 to adults
	X	X			Pointing	1	3-0 to 6-11
				X	Verbal, pointing	1 2	4-0 to 8-11

Continued.

TABLE 8-3. *Tools for assessing language and cognitive knowledge and performance —cont'd*

| Test and reference | Stimulus | | Language processing stages | | | |
	Modality	Nature of auditory stimulus	Compre-hension	Integra-tion.	Formu-lation	Repeti-tion
Tina Bangs Language Scale Bangs, T.E., Evaluating children with language delay. *Journal of Speech and Hearing Disorders,* **26,** 6-18 (1961). Bangs, T.E., *Language and Learning Disorders of the Pre-academic Child.* N.Y.: Appleton-Century-Crofts (1968).	V and A	Words, commands, analogies, sentence completion, sentences	X		X	
Token Test For Children DiSimoni, F., *Token Test for Children.* Boston: Teaching Resources Cor. (1978).	V and A	Commands varying in length and complexity	X			
Utah Test Of Language Development Mecham, M., Jex, J., and Jones, J., *Utah Test of Language Development.* Salt Lake City: Communication Research Associates (1967).	V and A	Connected speech			X	
Vane Evaluation Of Language Scale Vane, L., *Vane Evaluation of Language Scale.* Brandon, Vermont: Clinical Psychology Pub. Co. (1975).	V and A	Commands, sentences	X		X	
Verbal Language Development Scale Mecham, M., *Verbal Language Development Scale.* Circle Pines, Minn.: American Guidance Service, Inc. (1958).	Parent informant		X		X	

reference. At times other relevant references are included.

2. The second section, *stimulus,* includes the stimulus modalities employed in the test and the nature of the auditory stimulation presented.

3. The third section, *language processing stages,* specifies with an X the principal stage(s) tapped by the tool. If multiple processing stages are incorporated into the tool, no X will be placed in this section. Instead the tool will be listed as a multidimensional tool.

We have included certain developmental and intelligence measures under the processing stage of integration because many of these tools tap the child's cognitive development.

4. The fourth section, *language level,* specifies with an X the primary language level(s) under test. If more than two language levels are assessed by the tool, no X will appear in this section. Instead the tool will be listed as a multidimensional tool. As we suggested in Chapter 6, the processing stages of comprehension and formulation are the stages pri-

| Language level | | | Intelligence, cognitive, developmental | Multi-dimen-sional | Response | | Age range |
Pragmatic	Semantic	Syntactic			Modality	Observa-tional unit	
				X	Verbal and performance	1 2	2-0 to 6-0
	X				Performance	1	3-0 to 12-5
				X	Verbal and performance		1-6 to 14-5
				X	Verbal and performance	1 2	2-6 to 6-6
				X	Parent informant		0-0 to 16-0

Continued.

narily responsible for syntactic and semantic processing. Gaining significance from semantic information, however, also has been attributed to the process of integration, since semantic information is understood in reference to past experience, other sensory information, and the child's level of cognitive ability. We have also attributed to the process of integration pragmatics, including the functions of communication and modifications of the language code to meet contextual constraints.

5. The fifth section simply indicates with an X if the tool is considered primarily a cognitive, developmental, or intelligence measure, although it may assess language performance and behavior as well.

6. The sixth section indicates with an X if the tool is multidimensional, that is, if it assesses multiple language processing stages and language levels. Some test batteries assess multiple aspects of language development, for example the Sequenced Inventory of Communication Development (Hendrick,

TABLE 8-3. *Tools for assessing language and cognitive knowledge and performance—cont'd*

Test and reference	Stimulus		Language processing stages			
	Modality	Nature of auditory stimulus	Compre-hension	Integra-tion.	Formu-lation	Repeti-tion
Vocabulary Comprehension Scale Bangs, T.E., *Vocabulary Comprehension Scale*. Boston: Teaching Resources Corporation (1975).	V and A	Connected speech	X			
Vocabulary Usage Test Nation, J.E., A vocabulary usage test. *Journal of Psycholinguistic Research,* **1,** 221-231 (1972).	V and A	Sentence completion			X	
Weschler Intelligence Scale For Children Weschler, D., *Manual for the Weschler Intelligence Scale for Children*. N.Y.: The Psychological Corporation (1949). Aram, D.M., and Nation, J.E., Intelligence tests for children: A language analysis. *Ohio Journal of Speech and Hearing,* **6,** 22-43 (1971).	V and A	Questions, commands, sentence completion, similarities, digits, define words		X		
Weschler Preschool And Primary Scale Of Intelligence Weschler, D., *Weschler Preschool and Primary Scale of Intelligence*. N.Y.: The Psychological Corporation (1963). Aram, D.M., and Nation, J.E., Intelligence tests for children: A language analysis. *Ohio Journal of Speech and Hearing,* **6,** 22-43 (1971).	V and A	Questions, commands, sentences, sentence completion, similarities, define words		X		

Prather and Tobin, 1975) or the Houston Test for Language Development (Crabtree, 1963). Other provide brief screening of diverse language abilities, for example the Bankson Language Screening Test (Bankson, 1977). Still others have been developed to measure multiple aspects of language in specified groups of children, for example the Parson's Language Sample (Spradlin, 1963) for use with mentally retarded children. Tests that measure multidimensional aspects of children's language ability are incorporated in Table 8-3, including tests that are administered to the child by an examiner and those which are based on information about the child's language obtained from parent informants.

7. The seventh section, *response,* includes the verbal and nonverbal response modality and the observational unit from the CLPM

| Language level | | | Intelligence, cognitive, developmental | Multi-dimen-sional | Response | | Age range |
ragmatic	Semantic	Syntactic			Modality	Observa-tional unit	
	X				Performance	1	2-0 to 5-6
	X				Verbal	2	2-10 to 5-3
			X		Verbal and performance		5-0 to 15-0
			X		Verbal and performance		4-0 to 6-6

at is primarily employed for making the observation.

8. The eighth section states the age range r which the tool is applicable.

ANGUAGE TO SPEECH ROCESSING SEGMENT

The Language to Speech Processing Segent of the CLPM concerns the transduction of the message into the sequence of movements that will ultimately be produced as speech. This segment includes two processing stages: (1) speech programming and (2) speech production.

Speech programming disruptions have been seen to give rise to some types of phonologic disorders as well as to developmental verbal apraxia. These disorders were discussed in Chapter 7. We have viewed speech production as postlinguistic processing; if disrupted, it results in speech disorders, not language disorders, except in possible indirect interactions as suggested in Chapter 7.

Speech programming tools

The tools typically used to assess speech programming have taken samples of the speech sound system in spontaneous speech and in single word productions. These tools have generally aimed to inventory phonetic-phonemic-phonologic systems and more recently have included analysis of phonologic processes. Most of the commercially available tools have been described as articulation tests.

Although assessment of the speech sound system has traditionally relied on use of the standardized articulation tests, researchers in child phonology generally agree that these tests do not provide a representative sample of a child's phonologic abilities. Shortcomings of traditional articulation tests are (1) they do not conform either to the typical syllabic shape of words or to the relative frequencies of phonemes in children's natural speech, (2) they do not provide for analysis of error patterns, and (3) they do not relate the number of different sounds in error to consistency of error to determine a severity index. Phonologic assessment tools are appearing that meet some of these criticisms; however, they often require collection of spontaneous speech samples. It seems that a modification of current tests or some compromise between traditional articulation testing and the analysis of lengthy spontaneous speech samples needs to be made. Winitz (1969) has suggested that procedures for sampling a child's speech sound system should include a constant set of stimulus words that elicit sounds in several contexts and comparisons between spontaneous and imitated productions. Whether the outcome of this test is a measure of correctness (for example, in what percentage of instances a sound was correctly produced) or an analysis of the error pattern, it seems clear that the test of production should in some way be related to phonologic perception measures.

Table 8-4, organized similarly to Table 8-2 and Table 8-3, summarizes most of these commercially available tools.

Speech production assessment

While some language disordered children may present disruptions of the process of speech production, except for indirect interactions, we do not see these speech disruptions giving rise to language disorders. As we have stated, disruptions of this final processing stage produce speech disorders, not language disorders. Here diagnosticians have examined the structural and functional (motoric) intactness of the speech mechanism, including breathing for speech, phonation, resonation, articulation, and prosodation subprocesses. Nation and Aram (1977) discuss each of these subprocesses inherent in the speech production processing stage.

A principal approach to assessment of speech production, apart from such tools as articulation tests, has been through the speech mechanism examination. Structural assessments include examination of the speech mechanism at rest through both direct and indirect observation. Therefore the structural intactness of the lips, teeth, and tongue can be observed directly; the palatal and nasal structural adequacy can be only partially observed from unaided inspection, while the vocal folds require instrumental aids for even indirect observation.

Functioning of the peripheral speech mechanism is assessed through both speech and nonspeech activities. For example, while tongue movement is observed during speaking, a series of nonspeech activities is generally incorporated to assess the range and rate of tongue movement. Such nonspeech activities include tongue elevation to the upper lip and/or alveolar ridge, protrusion,

Test and reference	Stimulus		Response		Age range
	Modality	Nature of auditory stimulus	Linguistic unit	Observational unit	
Arizona Articulation Proficiency Scale Fudala, J.B., *Arizona Articulation Proficiency Scale.* Los Angeles: Western Psychological Services (1970).	V and A	Questions, sentences	Words, read sentences	2	3-0 to 11-0
Articulation Testing For Use With Children With Cerebral Palsy Irwin, O.C., A manual of articulation testing with children with cerebral palsy. *Cerebral Palsy Review,* **22,** 1-24. (1961).	A	Words	Words	2	3-0 to 16-0
Austin Spanish Articulation Test Carrow, E., *Austin Spanish Articulation Test.* Boston: Teaching Resources Corp. (1974).	V and A	Sentence completion	Words	2	4-0 to 7-0
Bzoch Error Pattern Diagnostic Articulation Test Bzoch, K.R., Introduction to section C: Measurement of parameters of cleft palate speech. In W.C. Grabb, S.W. Rosenstein, and K.R. Bzoch, *Cleft Lip and Palate: Surgical, Dental, and Speech Aspects.* Boston: Little Brown & Co. (1971).	A	Words	Words	2	3-0 to 6-0
Compton-Hutton Phonological Assessment Comptom, A.J., and Hutton, J.S., *Comptom-Hutton Phonological Assessment.* San Francisco: Carousel House (1978).	V and A	Sentence completion	Words	2	3-0 to adult
The Assessment Of Phonological Processes Hodson, B.W., *The Assessment of Phonological Processes.* Danville, Ill.: The Interstate Printers & Publishers, Inc. (1980).	V and A	Questions	Words	2	Preschool
Deep Test Of Articulation McDonald, E.T., *A Deep Test of Articulation.* Pittsburgh: Stanwix House, Inc. (1964). 1. Picture Form 2. Sentence Form McDonald, E.T., *A Screening Deep Test of Articulation.* Pittsburgh: Stanwix House, Inc. (1968).	V V	Sentences to read	Words Sentences	2 2	5-0 to 8-0 5-0 to 8-0

Continued.

TABLE 8-4. *Tools for assessing the speech sound system —cont'd*

Test and reference	Stimulus		Response		Age range
	Modality	Nature of auditory stimulus	Linguistic unit	Observational unit	
Denver Articulation Screening Exam Drumwright, A.F., *Denver Articulation Screening Exam*. Denver: University of Colorado Medical Center (1971). Drumwright, A., Van Natta, P., Camp, B., Frankenburg, W., and Drexler, H., The Denver articulation screening exam. *Journal of Speech and Hearing Disorders*, **38**, 3-14 (1973).	V and A	Words	Words: repetition	2	2-5 to 6-0
Developmental Articulation Test Hejna, R., *Developmental Articulation Test*. Ann Arbor, Mich.: Speech Materials (1958).	V		Words	2	3-0 to 8-0
Fisher-Logemann Test Of Articulation Competence Fisher, H.B., and Logemann, J.A.: *Fisher-Logemann Test of Articulation Competence*. Boston: Houghton Mifflin Co. (1971). 1. Picture 2. Sentence	V V	Sentences	Words Sentences	2 2	3-0 to adult 3-0 to adult
Goldman-Fristoe Test Of Articulation Goldman, R., and Fristoe, M., *Goldman-Fristoe Test of Articulation*. Circle Pines, Minn.: American Guidance Service, Inc. (1969).	V A V and A	(1) Sounds in words (2) Stimulability-CV (3) Sounds in sentences	Single words Imitated CV Connected speech	2 2 2	6-0 to 16+ 6-0 to 16+ 6-0 to 16+
Iowa Pressure Articulation Test (see *Templin-Darley Tests of Articulation*) Morris, H.L., Spriestersbach, D.C., and Darley, F.L., An articulation test for assessing competency of velopharyngeal closure. *Journal of Speech and Hearing Research*, **4**, 48-55 (1961).	V and A V	(1) Sentence completion (2) Sentences	Words Read sentences	2	3-0 to 8-0 3-0 to 8-0
Laradon Articulation Scale Edmonston, W., *Laradon Articulation Scale*. Los Angeles: Western Psychological Services (1963).	V and A	Sentence completion	Words	2	3-0 to 8-6
Miami Imitative Ability Test Jacobs, R.J., Phillips, B.J., and Harrison, R., A stimu-	A	Consonants in CV combinations	Repetition of consonants in CV combi-	2	2-6 to 6-0

	V/A				Age
Analysis (NPA): A Procedure for Phonological Analysis of Continuous Speech Samples. N.Y.: John Wiley & Sons (1980).		sation			
P-B Articulation Test VanDemark, D.R., Swickard, S.L., A preschool articulation test to assess velopharyngeal competency. *Cleft Palate Journal*, **17**, 175–179 (1980).	V		2	Words with /p/ or /b/	2-6 to 4-2
Phonological Process Analysis Weiner, F.F., *Phonological Process Analysis.* Baltimore: University Park Press (1979).	V and A	Sentence completion, elicited imitation	2	Spontaneous words and work imitation	2-0 to 5-0
Photo Articulation Test Pendergast, K., Dickey, S.E., Selman, J.W., and Soder, A., *Photo Articulation Test.* Danville, Illinois: The Interstate Printers & Publishers Inc. (1969).	V		2	Single words, connected speech	3-0 to 12-0
Predictive Screening Test Of Articulation Van Riper, C., and Erickson, R., *Predictive Screening Tests of Articulation.* Kalamazoo, Mich.: Western Michigan University Press (1968).	A	Words, syllables and sentences	2	Words, syllable and sentence imitation	First grade level
Procedures For The Phonological Analysis Of Children's Language Ingram, D. *Procedures for the Phonological Analysis of Children's Language.* Baltimore: University Park Press (In Press).	V and A	Questions, conversation, repetition	2	Any verbal response	All ages
Riley Articulation And Language Test Riley, G., *Riley Articulation and Language Test*, Beverly Hills, Calif.: Western Psychological Services (1966).	A	Word, sentences	2	Word and sentence imitation	4-0 to 8-0
Screening Speech Articulation Test Mecham, M., Jex, J.L., and Jones, J.D., *Screening Speech Articulation Test.* Salt Lake City: Communication Research Associates (1970).	V		2	Words	3-0 to 8-6
Templin-Darley Tests Of Articulation Templin, M.C., and Darley, F.L., *Templin-Darley Test of Articulation.* (2nd ed.) Iowa City, Iowa: Bureau of Educational Research and Service, University of Iowa (1969). 1. Picture 2. Sentences	V and A V	Sentence completion Sentences to read	2 2	Words Sentences	3-0 to 8-0 3-0 to 8-0

lateralization, and depression. The examiner may also include tests of rapid alternating movements of the tongue such as lateralization to the left and right corners of the mouth, rapid repetitions of /tʌ/ or /kʌ/ or /pʌtəkə/, typically termed oral diadochokinetic movements. Finally the examiner often contrasts the function of the particular structure of the peripheral speech mechanism during vegetative versus speech activities. To assess vegetative activities of the tongue, for example, he may observe the child as he chews a cracker, as he drinks from a glass (observing movement of the tongue during swallowing), as he licks a sucker or licks peanut butter from his upper lip.

Several authors have written extensively about the purpose and techniques employed in assessment of the speech mechanism. For more specific discussions of these assessment procedures, refer to the following sources: Darley, Aronson, and Brown (1975); Darley and Spriestersbach (1978); Dworkin and Culatta (1980); Emerick and Hatten (1979); Johnson, Darley, and Spriestersbach (1963); Nation and Aram (1977); Westlake and Rutherford (1961).

Issues in assessment of speech programming and speech production

A central issue speech-language pathologists must address in assessing speech programming and speech production in language disordered children is whether the observed language disorder arises from a rule-based or from a motor-based breakdown. This is not an easy differentiation to make in any client but is particularly difficult with young children who present very little language on which to base a judgment. Until more speech develops, the speech-language pathologist may not be able to make this differentiation fully, although a number of observations contribute to making the distinction:

1. Observation of the speech mechanism during nonspeech activities. If such functioning is abnormal, this does not rule out the possibility of a language-based disorder, but it does indicate at least some degree of motor involvement.

2. Assessment of language comprehension ability in comparison to language formulation. If a wide discrepancy exists in favor of comprehension, the likelihood of a speech programming and/or speech production breakdown increases. If little discrepancy is present, the likelihood of these postlinguistic processing disruptions decreases but is not eliminated, since many severely impaired children have multiple processing limitations.

3. Observation of the diversity of vocalizations that a child presents. While this is far from a fail-safe clue, our experience has been that often children with little diversity in speech sound production present speech programming and/or speech production disorders whereas those with somewhat greater diversity typically present language-based disorders.

4. Observation of the child's responses to speech sound imitation. These responses provide valuable but not infallible evidence for differentiating language versus speech disorders. Children with speech production breakdowns will evidence problems of motor control in their attempts to imitate. Young children with speech programming breakdowns rarely can imitate many consonants and tend to produce undifferentiated schwa-like vowels in CV-imitation tasks. While children with severe formulation disruptions also may show these difficulties, children with language-based disorders typically are better imitators than children with postlinguistic breakdowns are.

5. Analysis of phonetic versus phonologic errors using what little speech is available. As suggested by Nation and Aram (1977), such an analysis provides persuasive evidence when sufficient speech is present.

COMMENTS ON ASSESSMENT
Issue of standardized and formal-informal assessment tools

An important point should be made at this time. We do not believe that assessment of child language disorders is done only from or even primarily from standardized assessment tools. This is an issue of some importance in the profession of speech-language pathology. Nation and Aram (1977) have expressed their concern over the growing movement of reliance on standardized psychometric measures, and they caution their readers that "testing is not diagnosis." Leonard, Prutting, Perozzi, and Berkley (1978) raise cautions along similar lines, and Muma (1979) has objected to the use of standardized measures that derive from psychometric models. He expresses his objections on two grounds: (1) the child's behavior is made to fit the psychometric model rather than the other way around, and (2) the psychometric model is primarily methodologic rather than clinically substantive and therefore does not fit with theories of clinical assessment.

Finally, Berry (1980) has come out strongly against the use of diagnostic and commercial tests. She states:

> Students and teachers may be disconcerted by the absence of diagnostic tests. They have been omitted from all discussions of evaluation in this book because formal assessment measures rarely tell us what we need to know about the true status of a child's language development. . . . Tests do not ferret out the problems the child has in comprehending or expressing his intentions and his dynamic interactions in oral communication with children in his environment. Instead commercial tests evaluate isolated segments of language: the literal meaning of words and sentences, the comprehension of lexical items, the understanding of grammatical "rules."*

---

*From Berry, M.F., *Teaching Linguistically Handicapped Children*. Englewood Cliffs, N.J.: Prentice-Hall, Inc., 7-8 (1980).

☐ **How does Berry (1980) believe that child language disorders should be evaluated if not through diagnostic tests?**

While standardized or commercial tests do have limitations, their use does provide several advantages to the clinician who knows what tests are appropriate to select and where, how, and when to use them. Issue has frequently been made of the reliability and validity of the samples obtained; for example, Prutting, Gallagher, and Mulac (1975) have questioned the reliability of the Northwestern Syntax Screening Test (Lee, 1969) as an indicator of spontaneous expressive syntax.

While we would agree that test results, frequently reported as scores, age equivalents, and percentiles, often do not provide substantive description and direction for therapy, such psychometric data are useful in many contexts. Test results are useful, for example, in determining whether or not the child performs similarly to other children of the same age and circumstances; in communicating the relative deficit or ability to other professionals; in comparing among skill areas; in quantitatively charting development; and in comparing or equating children for group placement or other situations in which child comparisons are necessary. We maintain that standardized testing is not the whole picture but that standardized tests and the normative data they provide are indispensable. Standardized or commercial tests should not be summarily dismissed. A speech-language pathologist from a conceptually rich background can select and appropriately use standardized or commercial tests as part of an overall assessment approach to child language disorders.

☐ **McLean and Snyder-McLean (1978) provide a thoughtful discussion of the use of standardized and nonstandardized assessment procedures. What major points do they raise about the advantages and disadvantages of each?**

Frequently assessment procedures have been dichotomized into formal and informal procedures. We want to make the point here that this dichotomy can lead to false impressions about the nature of assessment. Our position is simply that all assessment procedures can be formalized whether they stem from structured, standardized instruments or from observations of responses made by the child to a variety of stimuli. Formality stems from the diagnostician who structures the nature and purpose of any stimulation in relationship to the responses observed. If the diagnostician imposes a structure on his method of observation, then the observation becomes formal. Thus to us, all assessment procedures can be considered formal, even observation of those behaviors of the child that seem incidental to the task required. We believe this is a more appropriate position to take with students in training than posing a dichotomy, often arbitrary, that casts certain assessment procedures into a formal mode and others into an informal mode.

The spontaneous speech-language sample as an assessment tool

The spontaneous speech sample has become a staple of the speech-language pathologist's assessment repertoire. It has generated much research including investigations of the type of stimulation used, the material used for stimulation, the nature of the interaction between examiner and child, the number of responses needed, the number of times samples should be taken, the times at which the samples are taken, the place in which the samples are taken, the way to count the usable responses, what counts as a response, and ways to analyze and interpret the responses. It has been and continues to be one of the most frequently investigated assessment tools that we use.

A number of procedures have been devel-

oped to guide the analysis of spontaneous speech samples allowing for quantification and comparison with normative data. Chief among these procedures are the Developmental Sentence Types (DST) and Developmental Sentence Scoring (DSS) procedures (Lee, 1974), the Tyack and Gottsleben System (1974), the Engler, Hannah, and Longhurst approach (1973), the Crystal, Fletcher, and Garman (1976) analysis, and the Length-Complexity Index (Miner, 1969). Of these the DSS and the Crystal probably provide the most extensive analysis and normative base, but they are limited in the extensiveness of the grammatical forms analyzed.

Since the purpose of the present chapter is principally one of summarizing available assessment tools, we will not undertake a detailed discussion of the usefulness and procedures involved in the spontaneous speech sample. However, because of its importance in the overall assessment of language disordered children and its role in the issue of standardized versus nonstandardized tools, we want to underline its relevance in assessment.

It is our position that the information about a child's formulation of language obtained from any test instrument must be validated in respect to his spontaneous language. We maintain that the contrast between a child's response to testing procedures (especially when elicited imitation tasks are used) and his spontaneous language may be of important diagnostic significance. Can the child use the syntactic structures he produces in elicited imitation tasks in his spontaneous speech, or is he merely processing the information through repetition, bypassing formulation? On the other hand, can the child use structures in his spontaneous speech that he is not demonstrating on standardized syntax tests? We have raised these and other issues concerning the usefulness of a spontaneous speech sample in assessing child language disorders (Nation and Aram, 1977) as have many other writers (Bloom and Lahey, 1978; Lee, 1974).

Despite criticisms of standardized tests in terms of the reliability and validity of the measure obtained, many diagnosticians do not have the time available either to gather or analyze extended samples of spontaneous language. Furthermore, even spontaneous speech samples may be criticized in terms of the stimulus provided, the context (for example, clinic versus home), the persons present (clinician versus mother), and so forth. Thus anything short of an extensive language sample obtained in multiple contexts may be questioned in terms of its representativeness. Reality factors, including time, expense to the parents, waiting lists, and the child's non-familiarity with the examiner, impose limitations on what can and cannot be obtained in sessions of a fixed duration.

□ **Lee (1974), Bloom and Lahey (1978), Tyack and Gotts-leben (1974), and Crystal, Fletcher, and Garman (1976) have discussed elicitation and analysis of spontaneous speech samples. How does Lee (1974) suggest that the language sample be elicited? What difference does using the mother versus the clinician as the elicitor make (Olswang and Carpenter, 1978)? How do Lee's (1974), Tyack and Gottsleben's (1974), and Crystal, Fletcher, and Garman's (1974) systems of analysis of spontaneous speech samples differ?**

THE DIAGNOSTIC PROCESS

Chapter 8 thus far has concentrated on assessment as the measurement step in the comprehensive diagnostic process. At this point we want to develop briefly a framework for viewing assessment in relationship to this diagnostic process, a process that is designed to establish the nature and cause of a child's language disorder with the intent of providing a solution to that problem.

As a process, diagnosis has been ap-proached from a variety of professional orientations, and in particular the role of the speech-language pathologist in establishing cause-effect relationships has been questioned (Perkins, 1977; Rees, 1978). Nation and Aram (1977, 1982) have explicated the purposes of diagnosis and have developed a problem-solving orientation to this process based on the scientific method. This approach details a series of interacting steps, each including a set of tasks to be performed by the diagnostician in completing the process. This approach is applicable to all speech and language disorders including child language disorders. Fig. 8-1 and the accompanying outline prepared from Nation and Aram (1977, 1982) summarize the steps and tasks that make up the comprehensive diagnostic process:

1. Constituent analysis (case study)
   a. Categorize the constituents
   b. Evaluate the constituents
2. Clinical hypothesis
   a. Derive and evaluate the clinical hypotheses
   b. Formally state and order the hypotheses
3. Clinical design (measurement/assessment design)
   a. Determine the measurement plan
   b. Select measurement tools
   c. Develop testing strategy
4. Clinical testing (measurement/assessment)
   a. Prepare for testing and meet the client
   b. Carry out and adapt the testing strategy
   c. Close the testing session
5. Clinical analysis of measurement/assessment data
   a. Objectify the data
   b. Organize the data relative to the clinical hypotheses
6. Clinical interpretation
   a. Collate all available information
   b. Evaluate the significance of the information
   c. Formalize the diagnostic statement
   d. Evaluate the quality of the diagnosis
7. Conclusions
   a. Propose a management and treatment plan
   b. Hold an interpretive conference
   c. Prepare professional reports
   d. Complete all administrative and follow-up procedures

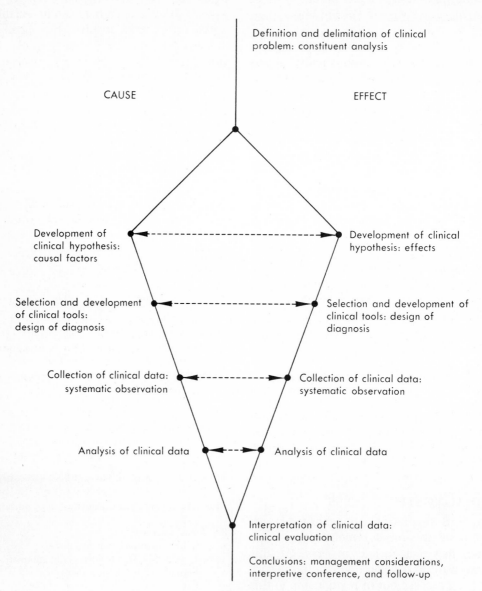

FIG. 8-1. Model of diagnostic process: a scientific framework. (From Nation, J.E., and Aram, D.M., *Diagnosis of Speech and Language Disorders*. St. Louis: The C.V. Mosby Co. [1977].)

From Fig. 8-1 and the outline, we can see that assessment is only one part of the diagnostic process; the emphasis is on the tools and procedures to be used to assess the cause-effect hypothesis that has been established from the case study. Information from the assessment allows the diagnostician to analyze these findings to determine what management and treatment plan should be put into effect.

The clinical hypothesis to be assessed in child language disorders

The diagnostic process calls for the derivation and evaluation of a clinical hypothesis for which assessment procedures are selected. In child language disorders the abstract clinical hypothesis is specified by our working definition. That definition is reiterated here for convenience.

Children with language disorders are those with disordered language behaviors related to language processing dysfunctions that appear as variable patterns of language performance and are shaped by the developmental context in which they occur.

The parts of this working definition were developed in detail in the preceding chapters of this book. In addition, we addressed causal factors for child language disorders, emphasizing an interactive developmental viewpoint. This information serves as the background for derivation of specific clinical hypotheses for each child. At this point the diagnostician can then select appropriate assessment tools designed for the specific clinical hypothesis, using the catalog of assessment tools provided in this chapter. It is important to reiterate here that in our approach assessment procedures are selected in relationship to each child's specific clinical hypothesis, including causation, language processing, language levels, ability of the child to respond to the nature of the tasks, and age of the child. We also evaluate the assessment tool in terms

of theoretical orientation, reliability, and validity. Therefore we do not subscribe to an assessment battery designed for categorical groups of suspected child language disorders.

Others have developed *assessment protocols* for use with child language disorders. Here we will include two for the reader to compare and contrast with the information presented in this book and Nation and Aram (1977, in press). The first by Miller (1978) is called a "developmental process approach." Miller's (1978) outline of the basic components of the assessment process and his overview of the format followed in assessment are presented in Table 8-5 and Fig. 8-2.

The second protocol for assessment has been developed by McLean and Snyder-McLean (1978) and follows their transactional model of child language disorders. Two figures are reproduced here. The first, Fig. 8-3, is a general format for assessment whereas the second, Fig. 8-4, individualizes the format by providing priorities based on the needs of the child as determined by the speech-language pathologist.

If we compare these two assessment protocols to the diagnostic process of Nation and Aram (1977, 1982), it becomes readily apparent that each author's use of assessment is closely allied to Nation and Aram's conceptualization of the diagnostic process. The major exception is that these authors do not specify what parts of their assessment protocols focus on causation and what parts focus on language behavior.

STUDY QUESTIONS

The following study questions are designed to familiarize the reader with the catalogs of tools presented in this chapter. Each study question will require the student to develop a clinical hypothesis based on the amplification of the working definition provided in this book. Once the hypothesis has been worked out, the student should explore the catalogs for selection of tools and then go to the tool references and other resources cited to

Text continued on p. 223.

TABLE 8-5. *Outline of the basic components of the assessment process* *

Why?	What?	How?

1. Identify potential problems
   a. Screening
     (1) Problem/no problem
     (2) Further evaluation
     (3) Referral to other professionals
2. Establish baseline functioning
   a. Determine developmental level
   b. Describe nature of behavioral difference
   c. Specify behavior needing remediation
3. Measure behavioral change within a teaching program
   a. Establish the nature of behavioral change resulting from program
     (1) Within context of teaching situation
     (2) Within natural environment
	1. Components of language system
	   a. Phonology
	     (1) Articulatory proficiency
	     (2) Phonological system
	   b. Syntax
	     (1) Sentence form/grammar
	     (2) Order relationships of constituents
	   c. Semantic
	     (1) Sentence function; meaning
	     (2) Case relationships
	     (3) Lexicon; concepts
	2. Processes
	   a. Comprehension
	     (1) Hearing acuity
	     (2) Auditory processing of linguistic units
	   b. Production
	     (1) Mechanism functioning
	     (2) Production of linguistic units
	   c. Pragmatics
	     (1) Communication functions
	     (1) Conversational competence
	   d. Cognitive development
		1. Procedures
		   a. Standardized tests
		   b. Nonstandardized tests
		   c. Developmental scales
		   d. Behavioral observation

*From Miller, J.F., Assessing children's language behavior: a developmental process approach. In R.L. Schiefelbusch, (Ed.), *Bases of Language Intervention*. Baltimore: University Park Press, 280 (1978).

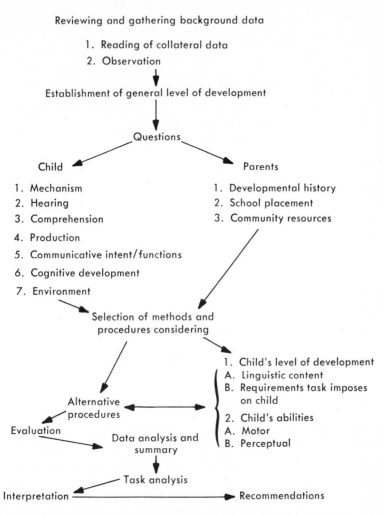

Reviewing and gathering background data

1. Reading of collateral data
2. Observation

Establishment of general level of development

Questions

Child

1. Mechanism
2. Hearing
3. Comprehension
4. Production
5. Communicative intent/functions
6. Cognitive development
7. Environment

Parents

1. Developmental history
2. School placement
3. Community resources

Selection of methods and
procedures considering

Alternative
procedures

Evaluation

Data analysis and
summary

1. Child's level of development
A. Linguistic content
B. Requirements task imposes
   on child
2. Child's abilities
A. Motor
B. Perceptual

Task analysis

Interpretation

Recommendations

FIG. 8-2. Overview of assessment format developed for establishing baseline functioning in interdisciplinary clinic. (From Miller, J.F., Assessing children's language behavior: a developmental process approach. In R.L. Schiefelbusch [Ed.], *Bases of Language Intervention*. Baltimore: University Park Press [1978].)

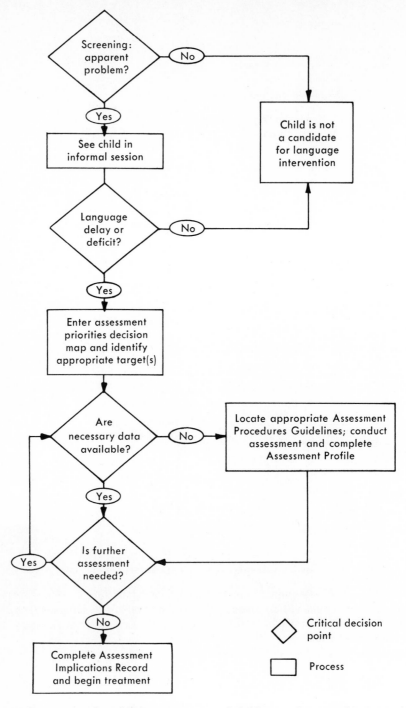

FIG. 8-3. Transactional model for assessment of children with severe language deficits. (From McLean, J.E., and Snyder-McLean, L.K., *A Transactional Approach to Early Language Training.* Columbus, Ohio: Charles E. Merrill Publishing Co. [1978].)

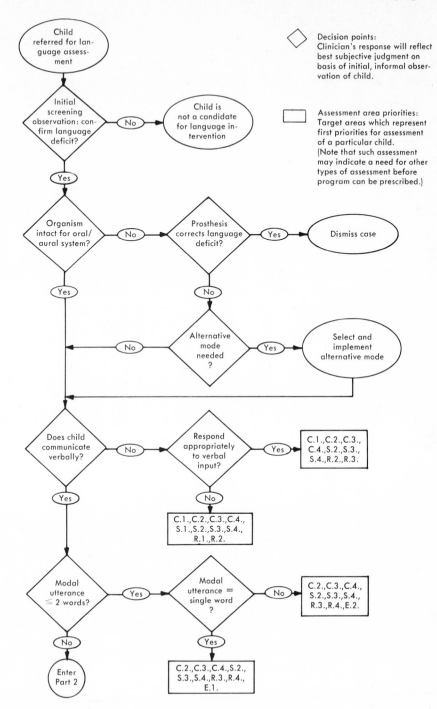

FIG. 8-4. Guidelines for determining assessment priorities. (From McLean, J.E., and Snyder-McLean, L.K., *A Transactional Approach to Early Language Training.* Columbus, Ohio: Charles E. Merrill Publishing Co. [1978].)   *Continued.*

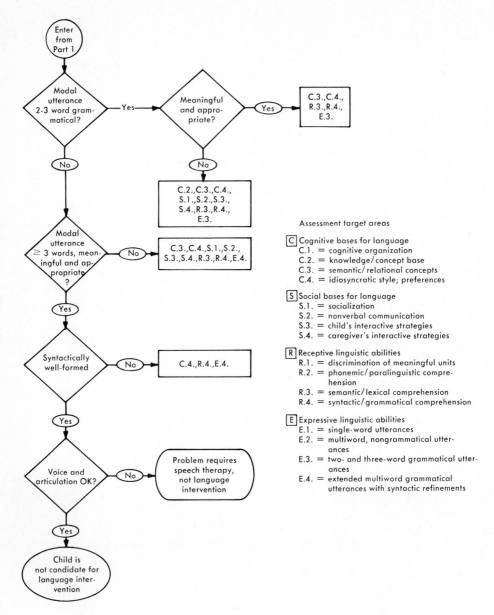

FIG. 8-4, cont'd. Guidelines for determining assessment priorities.

evaluate the appropriateness of each tool. These study questions then become a means of application of assessment procedures to child language disorders based on the CLPM.

1. If you were Eisenson (1972), what tools would you select for a child described as developmentally aphasic? Would you select the same tools if you followed the orientation provided in this book?

2. If you were required to establish a test battery for all children with language disorders between the ages of 3 and 5, what would you select for your battery? Could you justify this battery?

3. Aram and Nation (1971) have prepared a coding system of language performance that is tapped by a variety of intelligence tests. How do intelligence test items reveal differences between cognitive performance and language performance as revealed through the language processing stages of comprehension, integration, and formulation?

4. John, a 5-year-old boy, recently sustained significant trauma to the left cerebral hemisphere. What tools would you select to determine his current stage of language performance? Would these tools allow you to predict recovery of function?

5. What tools would you select to determine the language abilities of the following preschool children medically diagnosed as having (1) Treacher Collins syndrome, (2) fetal alcohol syndrome, (3) athetoid cerebral palsy, and (4) Down's syndrome?

6. How would you select tools to determine if a 4-year-old child who has been in four foster homes has any language delay related to environmental circumstances?

7. What tools would you select to follow the language progress of mentally retarded children to assist in determining if and when language treatment should be instituted?

8. A child referred has been described as echolalic. What tools could you select to determine if this child's behavior is truly echolalic or represents other language processing deficits?

9. Two children referred have been described as nonverbal. What tools will assist you in determining the basis for this lack of language usage?

10. Which language tools will assist in predicting if a preschool child will have learning disabilities when he enters school?

11. What set of tools will assist in differentiating children who have been described as apraxic from those thought to have developmental phonology problems?

12. How would you select tools to determine the pragmatic and semantic abilities of young hearing impaired children?

13. What tools would you select to obtain a comprehensive sample of a 3-year-old child's syntactic development, semantic development, and pragmatic development?

14. A 5-year-old child will not cooperate for standardized assessment of his language abilities. What alternate tools are available to you?

15. A 3-year-old does not seem to understand when he is spoken to. What tools would you select for evaluation of the presenting problem?

16. All incoming kindergarteners are to have speech and language abilities assessed. What tools might be useful for this purpose?

17. Stanley, introduced in Chapter 1, is an 8-year-old trainable mentally retarded child who uses only 25 different words, most of which are unintelligible to anyone other than family members. At least some of his limited language output may be attributed to disruptions of speech programming and/or speech production. Devise an assessment format for determining the relative contribution of these two final processing stages to the speech and language limitations that Stanley presents. Keep in mind the cognitive limitations that this child presents when devising specific tasks. Can an 8-year-old retarded child without a specific language problem do what you are requiring?

chapter 9

Management and treatment of child language disorders*

DIAGNOSIS IS THE BLUEPRINT FOR MANAGEMENT AND TREATMENT

Completion of the diagnostic process provides us with a description of a child's disordered language behavior, a delineation of suspected processing dysfunctions, an understanding of possible interacting causal factors, and information for prognostication. The diagnosis tells us what is wrong. Payoff to the client, however, comes when the diagnosis is translated into a management plan, an overall plan of action designed to change the child's language disorder. Diagnosis and management have a reciprocal relationship in that diagnostic findings assist the speech-language pathologist in making decisions about the best management and treatment plan for each child. Thus diagnosis is the blueprint for management and treatment.

Children with language disorders and their families require many professional services to meet the consequences of the disorder. The speech-language pathologist must take into account any number of professional, personal, and practical issues when formulating management and treatment plans for these children and their families. A series of decisions must be made which will be crucial in providing the best possible solution to the child and his family.

Chapter 9 centers around two fundamental purposes. First we will review approaches that have been developed for treating child language disorders, organizing this information within the Child Language Processing Model. In this way we intend to bring some convergence to the study of treatment of child language disorders. Second, we will discuss how treatment of child language disorders fits within the context of management plan decisions. This perspective on management and treatment also assists in bringing convergence from divergence in the study of child language disorders.

*At the onset we wish to clarify that our use of the term *treatment* subsumes the variety of terms used to discuss what is done to change child language disorders—terms such as therapy, intervention, instruction, and so forth. In this sense it holds no implications for a specific orientation or approach to working with child language disorders.

224

APPROACHES TO LANGUAGE TREATMENT

The speech-language pathologist must select a treatment approach designed to modify the child's difficulties in receiving, comprehending, integrating, formulating, and producing language. The speech-language pathologist's clinical experience comes into play in choosing the best possible approach for each child from among the variety of alternative approaches available. In each instance the approach chosen must be considered as an initial treatment decision, since modifications will undoubtedly take place as treatment progresses and more is learned about the child's ability to respond to the approach taken.

Therefore, the speech-language pathologist must be knowledgeable about the alternative approaches available that are useful at various ages, for the various levels of language, and for different patterns of performance across processes and behavior. However, the knowledge in child language development and disorders is voluminous and constantly changing; some information is outdated before it can be applied. Normal language development forms the basis for many of the treatment approaches that have been developed, yet it is still unclear how a child acquires language, and controversies exist as to whether this information can or should be applied in treatment of certain groups of children with language disorders (Bateman, 1974; Guess, Sailor and Baer, 1974; Miller and Yoder, 1974; Ruder and Smith, 1974).

What then are speech-language pathologists using to treat child language disorders? Are their selections idiosyncratic? Are there principles that govern the choices that are made? Are the choices made based on strong theoretical foundations? Are the choices made on models of intervention?

Addressing this issue, Nation (1982) has reviewed treatment principles and methods across a range of speech and language disorders. He concludes that it is difficult to determine from what theoretical basis the principles are derived and that often principles and methods are discussed as synonymous. He agrees with Perkins's (1977) statement that much of our treatment has derived from pragmatic, educated, trial and error approaches.

Muma has come out with the strongest statement we have read regarding the state of the art of treatment for children with language disorders. He states:

> Most of what is done in intervention is arbitrary, capricious, and authoritarian. We are very naive about what to do. There is good reason to be this way. We are only beginning to understand the nature and complexities of cognitive-linguistic-communicative systems. Theories of intervention are practically nonexistent. The positions at present are little more than authoritarianism. Although highly structured intervention programs are available, the probability is high that they may be of little relevance to individual needs.*

It appears that at this point in the development of our profession we have no clear, single orientation for treatment of child language disorders. However, there are treatment approaches available that have been guided by expert opinion, the opinion of those with extensive knowledge and experience derived from working with children with language disorders.

There are approaches designed for changing levels of language, approaches designed for subgroups of language disordered children—the retarded, the autistic, the aphasic, the deaf and hard of hearing, and so forth, approaches that have a processing orientation, and others.

---

*From Muma, J.R., *Language Handbook: Concepts, Assessment, Intervention.* Englewood Cliffs, N.J.: Prentice-Hall, Inc., 229 (1978).

Our historical heritage shaped the development of treatment approaches

In Chapter 2 we traced the historical heritage of child language disorders, taking the reader through the divergent perspectives that have shaped our current knowledge. This historical heritage presented the pioneering work of the three M's—McGinnis, Myklebust, and Morley—leading to the era of etiologic typologies. A major thrust occurred in changing our concepts of language and language disorders in the day of linguistic and psycholinguistic description, followed by the search for processing explanations. We concluded in Chapter 2 that most of these perspectives on child language disorders are still current and need to be brought together. The reader is encouraged to review Chapter 2 in parallel to this chapter.

A cursory review of treatment approaches to child language disorders quickly reveals that the approaches developed reflect the state of knowledge current at the time the approach was developed. Just as the description and theory of child language development and disorders have their heritage, so is there a heritage for the treatment approaches derived.

As was stated in Chapter 2, McGinnis (1963), Myklebust (1954), and Morley (1957, 1965, 1972) made major early contributions to the study of child language disorders and were presented as deserving a special place in our historical heritage. Their work led to the focus on etiologic classification, including treatment approaches. McGinnis and Myklebust remain as the primary examples of treatment approaches developed for childhood aphasia during the era of etiologic typologies, and in America controversy raged over whether the McGinnis approach or the Myklebust approach was best suited for these children. Each had his proponents.

The major focus in the day of psycholinguistic and linguistic description was on (1) detailed descriptions of levels of language behavior, (2) linguistic rules governing that behavior, and (3) identification and description of the stages and sequences of language development. Syntactic development provided the early impetus for study, but as the grammatical model of language became less explanatory, movement toward the semantic and pragmatic levels occurred. In the latter part of this period emphasis began to center on bridging the gap between language and communication, as language structure, cognition, pragmatics, and communicative interaction became related in more comprehensive schemas for understanding and treating child language disorders. During this period many of the approaches to language treatment emphasized the delay model, and programs were designed to facilitate the language disordered child's use of language *up* the stages of development, the emphasis being on increased use of language structures.

As part of our historical heritage we developed the *search for processing explanations;* this search encompassed two perspectives: (1) auditory processing explanations, and (2) multistage processing explanations. Unfortunately the outcome of much of this work as applied to treatment of child language disorders resulted in viewing the processes as *specific abilities* (Bloom and Lahey, 1978), and tasks were designed, much like those used in assessment, to treat the specific ability that had been assessed as deficient. The assumption made was that these abilities in some way underlie language behavior and if treated would generalize to what children knew about language and to their ability to use this information for communication.

In the following sections we will review the treatment approaches derived during these historical periods and integrate them within the CLPM. We will place the approaches into the processing segments of *best fit* based on our interpretation of the purposes and usefulness of the approaches. We will not describe the selected treatment approaches in detail nor discuss all that are available. Our intent is to exemplify treatment approaches within the CLPM as an orientation that brings convergence to the study of treatment of child language disorders.

SPEECH TO LANGUAGE PROCESSING
Deaf children

The teaching of language to the deaf and severely hearing impaired child is a specialized subject addressed in training programs for educators of the hearing impaired. Needless to say, these children require the specialized services of teachers of language, and these services are needed throughout their educational years. Lowell and Pollack (1974) and Graham (1976) provide summaries of remedial services to the deaf and hearing impaired and Ling (1976) and Ling and Ling (1978) can be consulted for more detailed treatment information.

Auditory processing orientations

One of the few auditory processing approaches to treatment of child language disorders was that of Eisenson (1972). Based on his underlying orientation that aphasic children have auditory perceptual problems, Eisenson (1972) developed a "speech sound (phonemic) processing" training program as part of his overall therapeutic approach to these children. Phonemic discrimination and sequencing form the basis of this program. Sequential activities are provided from first discriminating environmental, mechanical, and animate noises to more and more complex sequences of consonant-vowel combinations. Eisenson states that once the child is able to make the discriminations of the phonemic processing program, he should be ready for language production.

Myklebust (1954) and Johnson and Myklebust (1967) can also be included here because much of their approach for childhood aphasia stems from an auditory perceptual basis. Johnson and Myklebust (1967) have extended the concepts of receptive, expressive, and inner language presented by Myklebust (1954) to children described as having a psychoneurologic disability. For those children demonstrating generalized deficits in auditory learning, disorders of auditory language, and disorders of auditory expressive language, they present extensive educational procedures. Input stimulation is heavily stressed for these three groups of children with auditory impairment. The procedures require multimodality input of information, tying visual and tactile stimuli to the auditory in a simultaneous manner. The basis for this approach follows from the model that comprehension precedes expression and that the child must neurologically integrate perceptual information from various modalities if learning of language is to occur. Structured learning procedures are provided within natural situations.

More frequently approaches for treatment of auditory processing disruptions have been programs designed and kits sold for teaching children specific auditory tasks, a form of prescriptive treatment. The article by Falck (1973) is representative of this approach. She provides special-education personnel with a detailed outline of auditory processing units for teaching children with language disorders. For each auditory process that she identified she provides (1) its function, (2) signs of malfunction, and (3) programing possibilities.

In Chapter 5 we detailed the information on auditory perceptual processing and its relationship to language and communication, including representative research that has been done with language disordered children. In that chapter we raised a number of issues and precautions about the relationship of auditory processing to language. We suggest that the reader return to that information in his consideration of auditory processing treatment approaches.

Kleffner (1975) expresses similar feelings in this way: (1) invest your energies in direct treatment of the language disorder rather than in the auditory impairment; (2) although it is not difficult to discover failures on auditory tasks by language disordered children, do not attach too much importance to these failures because they tell us little about the language disorders; and (3) remain skeptical of the issue of auditory processing disruptions as causally related to language disorders.

Other approaches to treatment of child language disorders provide a focus on auditory processing, for example, treatment based on the Illinois Test of Psycholinguistic Abilities (ITPA), Wiig and Semel (1976, 1980), and Bangs (1968). However, we are reserving discussion of these multistage processing approaches until we consider the Language to Thought to Language Processing Segment.

LANGUAGE TO THOUGHT TO LANGUAGE PROCESSING

This processing segment encompasses the primary scope of child language disorders, and many of the treatment approaches developed fall within this segment. Treatment approaches that have been developed have derived from a number of historical perspectives: etiologic, linguistic-psycholinguistic, and processing. We will retain that primary organization here, pointing out how the different approaches focus on different processing stages within this segment, that is, comprehension, integration, and formulation.

Etiologic orientations

Childhood aphasia. Many of the early treatment approaches for child language disorders focused on the aphasic child. McGinnis (1963), one of the early leaders in this area, developed a teaching approach called the association method. We will discuss this later as we interpret this approach more in line with language to speech processing.

Diametrically opposed to McGinnis, the approach Myklebust (1954) took with childhood aphasia was highly unstructured. It was termed the "natural language approach" whereby the child was presented with auditory and other stimulation within as natural a situation as possible. The approach was highly representational and therefore tapped into the child's cognitive development extensively, or what Myklebust called "inner language." In his approach, treatment followed his concepts of child language development: inner language precedes receptive language which precedes expressive language.

Myklebust was heavily influenced by Piagetian thought in child development, which explains his highly symbolic representational approach to treatment of childhood aphasia. It is interesting to compare his approach to other current approaches to child language disorders that are based on communicative interaction and pragmatics. It is apparent that this natural language approach, often referred to as the cognitive approach to language learning, is having a resurgence, particularly in reference to the mentally retarded child. In essence, these approaches appear to focus on the processing stage of integration within the CLPM.

Direct language treatment is dependent upon placing the child in an appropriate group, and Ingram and Eisenson (1972) determine this primarily on mean words per utterance taken from a language sample. These group placements range from Group A (0 to 2 words—primary language level) to Group V (5 to 6 words). Again, they present sequential activities for each group centered on (1) basic constructions, (2) function words and affixes, (3) combinations of previously established formulations, and (4) question forms. Even though it has been discussed as representational behavior, we interpret this direct treatment approach as focusing on formulation of language, progressing from the one word stage to more and more complex syntactic structures.

Eisenson's (1972) primary approach to childhood aphasia was based on auditory processing as previously discussed. However, influenced by Ingram (1972), his approach was extended into what was termed representational behavior, particularly for the child who was nonverbal. Children go through a series of activities, defined as levels of representational behavior, that are preliminary to language training. The levels are:

Level 1: Object to object association

Level 2: Categorical matching

Level 3: Matching by associated function

The approach to "direct language training" presented in Eisenson was written by Ingram and Eisenson (1972) and is titled "Establishing and Developing Language in Congenitally Aphasic Children." The rationale behind the direct language training approach is based on stages or levels of language development in normal children. As they state: "Our program is based on helping the child to establish a 'grammar,' to learn with help and direct instruction how to produce utterances, or to make 'strings of words' that are akin to those of the speakers of his environment."*

Over the years Morley (1957, 1965, 1972) has maintained her views and classifications of child language disorders and has been in-

strumental in describing the relationships between etiologic categories and resultant language disorders. Her work is still influential among many American speech-language pathologists, and she was one of the early writers taking a processing orientation to childhood language disorders. However, in none of her three editions does Morley (1957, 1965, 1972) present information regarding her treatment approach for developmental aphasia, either the receptive or executive types. She states that:

1. The teaching of language to these children is based on neurologic maturation—language development cannot be taught until neurologic maturation is available.
2. Treatment is based on stimulation of the natural process of language development.
3. The first emphasis of treatment is on "input" based on the notion that comprehension precedes production.
4. The use of structured natural language by the parents is suggested as the primary mode of treatment.
5. Naming should be encouraged and developed through a number of procedures.
6. Treatment approaches should be designed to fit the individual needs of the child.

• • •

A number of articles have appeared that discuss treatment with other categorical groups of children, particularly the autistic and the mentally retarded. Many of these are discussions of specific therapy procedures and do not necessarily represent major treatment approaches. Many of these procedures stemmed from information that accrued during the day of psycholinguistic and linguistic description. A brief representative review of some of this material follows.

*From Ingram, D., and Eisenson, J., Therapeutic approaches III: Establishing and developing language in congenitally aphasic children. In J. Eisenson, *Aphasia in Children*. N.Y.: Harper and Row, Pub., 130 (1972).

Autistic children. The etiology of autism is still unclear; however, these children present major language to thought to language processing deficits, including comprehension, integration, and formulation of language.

With autistic or psychotic children, two basic treatment formats appear in the literature. The earliest and most assiduously applied has been some form of behavior modification. In a major review article on the conditioning of verbal behavior in these children, Hartung (1970) states that although there is much material, there is little that is systematic about the conditioning procedures that have been used, many of them idiosyncratic to the specific investigator reporting results. Hartung (1970) feels this information is often too limited to be of much use to others carrying out this treatment mode.

Schell, Stark, and Giddan (1967) and Stark, Giddan, and Meisel (1968) have provided extensive information about the development and use of verbal behavior in a single autistic child based on behavior modification procedures. Along similar lines, Goldstein and Lanyon (1971) have demonstrated how parents can be trained in "behavior change procedures" based on operant conditioning; these parents can then become teachers of their own children. Goldstein and Lanyon reported success with a 10-year-old autistic boy using modeling-reinforcement techniques.

The second basic treatment format has been the use of alternative forms of communication for these children. McLean and McLean (1974) have used wooden word symbols to achieve limited social transactions in two children that were nonverbal. Marshall and Hegrenes (1972) utilized a patterned language program using word cards that were then transferred to written communication. Concerning the child under observation, they concluded that patterned written language can be an effective secondary means of communication. Bonvillian and Nelson (1976) taught a mute 9-year-old autistic boy to communicate "extensively" through American Sign Language, including a full range of semantic relationships. Their results seem far more outstanding than those reported from other treatment approaches and may well be making a statement about the underlying processing basis for this condition.

Mentally retarded children. Language treatment for the mentally retarded has been a major thrust of speech-language pathology. Graham (1976) provided a summary account of language intervention approaches focused toward the mentally retarded child. She organized these approaches as (1) developmental approaches, (2) nondevelopmental approaches, (3) manual approaches, and (4) use of parents and peers in the intervention program.

As with cases of autism, a major treatment method that has been heavily used, particularly with the more severely retarded, is some form of behavior modification based on operant conditioning. Snyder, Lovitt, and Smith (1975) did a major review of 23 behavior analysis studies that had appeared since 1968. From this review they have made suggestions for improving behavior modification methodology for severely retarded children.

Behavior modification as a treatment approach in conjunction with the linguistic description emphasis led to the development of a number of treatment programs. Fristoe (1975, 1976) undertook a national survey of language treatment programs for mentally retarded children, many considered applicable to other developmentally delayed children. One hundred eighty-seven language programs were presented in the catalog developed by Fristoe (1975), 39 of which were in kit form and presented as an appendix (Fristoe, 1976) to the book edited by Lloyd (1976).

It is true that there are available any number of commercially packaged programs for child language disorders, many claiming to be successful with one or another group of children. However, many of these have not been tested or evaluated for effectiveness. As Berry (1980) states:

> Packaged programs are commercially available. Undoubtedly they assist the ill prepared "clinicians" to become "operational," but, as someone [Cazden, 1970] has commented, they have little if any lasting effects. Special language teachers [speech-language pathologists] will find them a feeble crutch producing a dependency that stifles the creative and halts challenging thought.*

Connell, Spradlin, and McReynolds (1977) also raise the question of the usefulness of many of the packaged programs for treatment of child language disorders. They believe that many of these programs are being distributed with little or no information about their clinical effectiveness, and they raise issues regarding the ethicality of their production and also of their use by speech-language pathologists.

Because of the intensive form that behavior modification takes for limited change, there have been personnel limitations. Several articles have dealt with the use of nonprofessionals as trainers of these children (Bidder, Bryant and Gray, 1975; Guess, Smith and Ensminger, 1971; Guralnick, 1972). Each of these has reported success in training college students, mothers, and psychiatric aides. It appears that others can be trained to work with severely retarded children operating at low language levels, providing behavior modification techniques to them to obtain changes in language usage.

Leonard (1975) and Jeffree, Wheldall, and Mittler (1973) used training programs with the retarded to facilitate use of two-word utterances. They developed language programs based on modeling and imitation with the added dimension of situational appropriateness, that is, language in context rather than the more imitative tasks used in many behavior modification programs.

It is interesting as an aside to note that in 1967, Peins used a client-centered communication therapy approach with a group of 10 institutionalized mentally retarded and delinquent adolescents that she described as deficient in all areas of oral communication.

A number of the treatment approaches we will take up in later sections of this chapter were also derived first for mentally retarded children and then later applied to other language disordered children. Many of them were derived from linguistic-psycholinguistic information, and they focused on obtaining language responses by working on what we would consider to be the processing stage of formulation. Based on the stage of language development achieved by the child, the treatment approaches were designed to increase linguistic performance according to stages of normal syntactic development.

Linguistic-psycholinguistic orientations

The treatment approaches that derived during the period of linguistic-psycholinguistic description centered heavily on the development of procedures for assisting the child through the stages and sequences of linguistic expression.

Syntactic emphasis. The heavy emphasis on syntax during this period led to a variety of approaches for treatment of syntactic development or programs designed to facilitate the use of some aspect of syntax, for example, wh- questions. The general order of these approaches often followed Lee's (1966, 1974) "developmental sentence types" or Brown's (1973) five stages of syntactic development. Basic syntactic relationships were taught, for

---

*From Berry, M.F., *Teaching Linguistically Handicapped Children*. Englewood Cliffs, N.J.: Prentice-Hall, Inc., 228 (1980).

example, subject + verb + object followed by morphologic markers and finally more complex transformations.

In 1975, Lee, Koenigsknecht, and Mulhern (1975) published *Interactive Language Development Teaching*, which was subtitled, *The Clinical Presentation of Grammatical Structure*. This approach was based on Lee's (1974) other work, *Developmental Sentence Analysis*, in which she detailed the developmental sequences of syntax. The approach attempts to model syntax approximating normal language usage as much as possible, building in spontaneous, nonimitative, and meaningful interchange between the clinician and the child.

The book presenting this method is detailed, providing lesson plans for the grammatical structures to be taught. It is important to note that Lee and others (1975) carefully state that this program has primarily been used with children of normal intelligence and hearing sensitivity. The following are guidelines presented for structuring the syntactic lessons:

1. Select a story topic that is within the child's experience.
2. Provide sufficient narrative to keep the child's attention.
3. Provide adequate build-up of semantic content for the target structures.
4. Introduce new structures as receptive tasks before eliciting them as targets.
5. Provide frequent review to stabilize structures previously introduced as target responses.
6. Clarify the concepts underlying the contentive vocabulary.
7. Include questions which elicit creative thinking.

They also list interchange techniques from most to least helpful for establishing the target syntactic structures: (1) complete model, (2) reduced model, (3) expansion requests, (4) repetition request, (5) repetition of error, (6) self-correction request, and (7) rephrased question.

Trantham and Pederson (1976) derived treatment implications for assisting language impaired children in abstracting and using grammatical rules. Their implications stemmed from their study of the language development of eight normal children.

The plan of their treatment program is to teach the grammatical rules in systematic steps in a well-structured program, providing suggestions for specific therapeutic procedures for teaching verbs, pronouns, negatives, interrogatives, and conjunctions. Included is drill for the missing structures, yet the authors caution that this is to be accomplished in ways designed to help the child generalize what is learned to more natural situations.

They do not advocate the use of telegraphic speech models as is sometimes done but rather insist that complete sentences be used by the clinician and the child. If the child is unable to use complete sentences, he is assisted in doing so. They make suggestions for the child with comprehension problems that prevent him from formulating appropriate syntactic structures. Throughout their program they take periodic language samples to compare the language impaired child to normal children on developmental sentence types (Lee, 1966, 1974) and mean sentence length.

Dever (1978) developed a program she calls *TALK: Teaching the American Language to Kids* that is designed to teach language disordered children English much in the same way it would be taught as a second language. The principles of the approach stem from applied English linguistics based on tagmemic theory. Dever's approach is based on the assumption that children with language disorders do not differ in the course of language development from normal children. Therefore her approach identifies and classifies where the child's current use of language is and then specifies sequentially where he needs to move. The three principles that guide her approach are:

1. Behavioral goals must be established that specify what the child should do when the program is completed.
2. The child's current language status must be specified behaviorally in relation to normal language development.
3. The procedures for getting the child from where he is to where he is going must be specified.

Given these principles, Dever (1978) however does not believe that teaching methodology is as important as the system that tagmemic grammar offers as a systematic approach to development of grammatical structure.

TALK is designed for children who have reached the basic use of intransitive and transitive clauses (Stage III 6 in Dever's system). Children having less grammatical structure she believes will have to be taught by different approaches. TALK has two basic components. First, there are formal lessons to teach grammatical patterns and, second, a more informal component for transfer of these patterns into situations so the child can learn where and how to use them.

The method includes the following procedural specifications: (1) pattern drill, (2) choral response, (3) individual responses, (4) the conversion principle (whereby the child is given a stimulus that must be restructured or converted in certain ways to offer a complete yet different response from the stimulus), (5) variant drills, (6) use of the group as a teaching tool, (7) rhythm, (8) the use of teacher aides as models, and (9) format and feedback of the tasks (task analysis whereby the teacher analyzes what to do to cause learning to take place and lets the child know if he is doing what he should be doing). Lesson plans

are provided as a framework for illustrating what is done with the TALK approach.

Bloom and Lahey (1978) have presented a comprehensive approach to the study of language development and language disorders. Their orientation is comprehensive in that it views language in three interacting developing dimensions (form, content, and use) and therefore goes beyond an emphasis on syntax. Even though more comprehensive in terms of their view of language and language disorders, their intervention approach focuses heavily on grammatical structure—that is, grammar as it relates to form, content, and use. Therefore, we are including it in this syntactic orientation section.

Bloom and Lahey consider their intervention program as a hypothesis whereby the knowledge available about normal language development is "exploited" for use with the language disordered child. In their plan for language learning they present underlying assumptions (principles) that govern intervention: (1) form, content, and use are interactive; (2) linguistic behaviors are emphasized regardless of the cause of the disorder; (3) normal language development provides the sequence for developing goals of intervention; and (4) goals are stated explicitly in terms of language production and only implicitly for language comprehension. This fourth assumption is drawn for interesting reasons. The authors state:

The reason for listing goals for production instead of or along with goals for comprehension is simply because more is known about the development of children's production of content/form/use interactions than is known about the development of children's comprehension of these interactions . . . A sequence of development related to comprehension cannot yet be even approximated.*

---

*From Bloom, L., and Lahey, M., *Language Development and Disorders*. New York: John WIley and Sons, 377 (1978).

Details of intervention goals are presented for form, content, and use starting with "precursory" goals focusing on sensory-motor activities and cognitive development. The remainder of their goals are sequenced in phases, the first three phases for early to later language learning and phases four through eight specified for later language learning. These eight phases are:

1. Single-word utterances
2. Emerging semantic-syntactic relations
3. Further semantic-syntactic development
4. Embedded relations and grammatical morphemes
5. Successive related utterances
6. Complex sentences
7. Syntactic connectives and modal verbs
8. Relative clauses

In 1974 The American Speech-Language and Hearing Association published a monograph under the editorship of McReynolds (1974) addressing the need to develop systematic procedures for training children's language. The focus of the articles included was on the linguistic structures that children learn thereby assisting clinicians in systematically developing treatment programs. The information centered on procedures for establishing baseline behaviors for the linguistic structures and adapting this information to clinical training programs where goals for behavioral change were set and measures taken to determine if the child generalized the material being taught. Suggestions were made for the development of a multiple baseline design treatment program incorporating information from the articles included within the monograph.

Others have used behavior modification procedures and techniques to change syntactic structures in certain groups of language disordered children. Gottsleben, Tyack, and Buschini (1974) reported on three children being seen in an institute for childhood aphasia. Programs were developed for each child based on a pretreatment analysis of his language. Posttreatment measures demonstrated that all three children used the target forms and constructions more frequently.

Mulac and Tomlinson (1977) and Hegde and Gierut (1979) used operant training techniques for teaching certain syntactic structures and found change in use of the structure under treatment. Generalization of treatment was a focus of both these studies. Mulac and Tomlinson (1977) found generalization to be 100% to untrained stimuli for the linguistic behaviors they treated, whereas Hedge and Gierut (1979) found that generalization outside the clinic only occurred in one of their experimental groups, those who received "an extended transfer program."

Leonard (1973) presented child-initiated and clinician-oriented procedures for applying rule learning in language disordered children. He discussed the use of expansion, modeling, and imitation as procedures as well as the use of behavioral methodology. Leonard (1974) used a modeling technique with eight language disordered children on two syntactic structures to determine the amount of generalization that took place. He found that generalization occurred on structures other than those taught and suggested that mastery of basic constructions is not essential to the development of more complex constructions. In another study, Wilcox and Leonard (1978) again used modeling to teach wh- questions in language disordered children and again found generalization beyond what was directly taught.

The example treatment approaches, procedures, and techniques considered in this section on syntactic orientations clearly focus on assisting the child to formulate grammatical responses according to normal acquisition of syntactic structures. We see most of these and similar approaches as concentrating on the formulation processing stage within the Language to Thought to Language Processing Segment.

Semantic emphasis. The day of linguistic and psycholinguistic description provided data about the development of semantic features and semantic relationships, which moved our understanding of semantic development beyond the simple counting of vocabulary items the child had acquired. These views of semantic development led to approaches to treatment that concentrated on meaning as much as or more than on vocabulary development per se. Studies such as those by Bloom (1970) and Leonard (1976) were instrumental in giving us better understanding of what occurs in early language acquisition, bridging the gap between early single-word development and the emergence of syntax. Grammars were written that corresponded to these early stages of development. And from this information several treatment approaches were derived for language disordered children at the semantic level of development.

The approach developed by Miller and Yoder (1974) stems from their work with mentally retarded children. However, it appears applicable to other children with delayed language development. They call their approach an "ontogenetic language teaching strategy" with the implication that treatment stems from knowledge about normal language development. From this basis they establish six criteria that guide their approach: (1) "exit behaviors" must be realistic; (2) normal psycholinguistic development guides the program; (3) paralinguistic variables that affect learning must be taken into account; (4) normal environmental interactions must be accounted for; (5) the child must be an active participant in the communicative experiences, both linguistic and nonlinguistic; and

(6) the language program must be systematic, and the language being taught must be specified.

The methodology for the approach is based on the criteria presented above and is set forth by Miller and Yoder (1974) as six operating principles, some overlapping the six criteria above. These operating principles specify stages of language development and the specific language structures to be taught, and they are based on the fundamental premise that language development stems from semantic concepts. Therefore the content of their teaching approach comes from their ordering of semantic functions in early language development. These functions are listed as:

1. Relational functions—single-word utterance level
2. Substantive functions
3. Functional relations—two-word utterances
4. Semantic relations
5. Three-term relations
6. Four-term relations

Miller and Yoder's (1974) approach therefore takes the child through early semantic functions to later four-term semantic relations leading to the development of syntactic structure. The approach as seen in the criteria and operating principles maintains the following relationship for the child: it gives him (1) something to say (concepts), (2) a reason for saying it (semantic intent), and (3) a way to say it (linguistic structure). Both behaviorism and mentalism guide their methodology. Mentalism provides the principles for teaching semantic concepts and intentions of language, and behaviorism provides the teaching principles and techniques for linguistic structure.

MacDonald and Blott (1974) and their colleagues have been responsible for developing a series of assessment procedures and a treatment approach generally referred to as the ELI (Environmental Language Intervention Strategy). This approach originally designed for mentally retarded children at the prelanguage or early language stages emphasizes the semantic functions of language based on normal rules underlying children's early sentences. The ELI program is now available in kit form and consists of the following:

Assessment component

1. *Oliver,* a child language assessment done by the parents prior to professional assessment
2. *Environmental Prelanguage Battery* (EPB), an assessment of skills necessary for language acquisition up to and including single-word production (Horsmeier and MacDonald, 1978)
3. *Environmental Language Inventory* (ELI), an assessment of early expressive language (two- through four-word phrases), (MacDonald, 1978)

Treatment component

1. *Ready, Set, Go—Talk to Me,* a prelanguage and early language training manual which is written for parents, teachers, and therapists (Horstmeier and MacDonald, 1978)
2. A guide to accompany the ELI program describing the use and adaptation of *Ready, Set, Go—Talk to Me* (Horstmeier and MacDonald, 1978)

Ready, Set, Go—Talk to Me (Horstmeier and MacDonald, 1978), the treatment component of the ELI, is addressed to five questions:

1. *Who* is to be taught language?
2. *When* is language training to begin?
3. *What* is to be the content of language teaching?
4. *What* procedures are to be used?
5. *Who* is to do the teaching?

The content of the program is based on semantic functions or meaning as the basic component for the social and communicative use of language whereby the child understands and expresses meaningful experiences. It follows the format of the assessment procedures from which prescriptive procedures are established for the child. The primary procedures used in this approach are based on behavioral methodology as well as other "curricular strategies" adapted to the individual needs and abilities of the child. The prescriptive levels of the program for which formats are provided are labeled as (1) preliminary skills, (2) functional play, (3) motor imitation, (4) receptive procedures, (5) following directions, (6) sound imitation, (7) single words, and (8) beginning social conversation.

These individualized procedures are used in several contexts: in regularly scheduled sessions and as part of the child's indirect learning within his personal environment. The program provides information on how to structure the language teaching sessions and, for parents, on how to utilize similar formats for providing prelanguage and language experiences in other contexts.

Generalization of language rules to new and novel conversational situations is emphasized. The ELI uses training in imitation, conversation, and play simultaneously. Thus communication and context are instrumental in this approach. MacDonald, Blott, Gordon, Spiegel, and Hartmann (1974) utilized the ELI in a parent program for six preschool children with Down's syndrome, three of whom served initially as controls. For training parents and experimenters, these authors used quite extensive protocols, which went through two phases. Results indicated marked increases in length of utterance and grammatical complexity in each phase of the program, indicating that parents that are trained can increase the functional use of language for these children as defined by the rules utilized in the ELI.

Bowerman (1976) has presented detailed information about semantic theory and has drawn from this presentation a set of semantic therapy implications. These implications derive primarily from her fundamental premise that language is categorical in nature, that words and syntax are linked to classes of events rather than to unique experiences. Some of the implications drawn are:

1. Work on semantic categorization keeping in mind that children's labels may have several meanings.
2. Eliminate activities that seem nonsensical to the child, for example, discrimination of speech sounds.
3. Capitalize on the perceptual attributes of objects.
4. Use materials that can be acted upon and that change rather than remain static.
5. Use early words that express existence and functional relations.
6. Keep in mind the different styles of learning that children have, for example, referential learning versus social learning.

These semantic orientations to treatment of child language disorders become prominent for children who exhibit little or no language output. Again, these methods focus on ways to assist the child in formulating word responses that allow him to express meaning to a listener. For the most part the processing stage being focused on is formulation; however, it is clear that when semantics is the intent of treatment, the language processing stage of integration is used also.

Pragmatic emphasis. The study of semantic relations and semantic functions during the day of psycholinguistic and linguistic description led quickly to an interest in the child's prelanguage and early language intentions and functions. The reasons that words and sentences are used for communication became the focus. Pragmatics became an intensive area of study.

As we discussed in earlier chapters, a number of schema have been derived for understanding pragmatic development in children.

Those of Halliday (1977a,b), Bates (1976a,b), and Dore (1975) stand out. Also the interest in pragmatic development occurred simultaneously with renewed interest in the cognitive development of the young child, particularly because investigators were interested in the relationship of cognition to language development and how cognitive development indicated the child's knowledge of language before the utterance of the first word.

Miller (1978) presents one of the few treatment approaches found in the literature developed directly from a pragmatic orientation. She uses two orientations to pragmatics: (1) pragmatics of language in context (Bates, 1976a), and (2) pragmatics of human interactions (Watzlawich, Beavin, Helmick, and Jackson, 1967), and she incorporates these into a pragmatic analysis and treatment program for language disordered preschool children. She describes this approach as focused on communication between people as an interactional system, taking into account the relationships among cognition, language, and social interaction.

In her article Miller (1978) describes the structure and organization of the program and the roles played by the clinicians. The overriding philosophy is on child-centered play activities rather than clinician-directed activities. The clinician's goal is to develop an interactive relationship with the child and model communicative behavior of any type within the context of play chosen by the child. The modeling by the clinician is not imposed on the child, but attempts are made to recreate communicative situations that are modeled so the child will again experience and use a similar communicative interaction. Bates's (1976a) concepts of performatives, propositions, presuppositions, and conversational postulates are used to guide the modeling. Miller provides an appendix that includes a detailed pragmatic analysis and examples of treatment goals and strategies used with one child in her group.

Blank, Rose, and Berlin (1978), concerned about the lack of material for guiding language teaching in the preschool, developed a discourse model of language in the classroom. Their approach to language teaching, although broader than a pragmatic perspective, is included here because its orientation is toward discourse as a means of facilitating children's language learning and "higher level intellectual abilities"—thinking, problem solving, concept formation, and reasoning.

Their discourse model describes three components: (1) the speaker-listener dyad, (2) the topic of discourse, and (3) the level of discussion. They present the implications of their orientation in the development of discourse in preschool children, including early discourse competence as a way to enhance these children's communicative skills. They focus on what the child does not know, structuring the speaker-listener dyad so that the child understands and can respond to the new material being presented. The discourse skills taught are utilized as a medium of exchange for gaining new information. They emphasize adapting to the individual skill level of each child and discuss how to blend their structured discourse activities to these individual skill levels.

This particular approach might not seem to be a language treatment approach, since its focus has been to understand the discourse that occurs and that can be structured to assist preschool children in acquiring the higher level intellectual abilities. It is, as the authors state, "the language of learning."

These pragmatic orientations to child language disorders we view as focusing on the language processing stage of integration where linguistic and cognitive information interact for learning and using language for communicative purposes. The reintroduction of this focus of treatment for child language disorders is interesting to compare to Myklebust's (1954) early considerations of treatment of inner language disorders of aphasic children or to the 1951 work of Backus and Beasley, titled *Speech Therapy with Children,* where they state:

> The greatest potentiality of speech therapy appears to lie in *the use of speech as an instrument for creating significant interpersonal relationships . . . The teaching situation should be structured in terms of those interpersonal relationships which involve conversational speech.*[*]

Comprehensive orientations

Although we have been presenting more narrowly focused treatment approaches, several workers in the field of child language disorders have been developing more comprehensive approaches. Some of these approaches have had a linguistic orientation, others a processing orientation. Even though some of these orientations go beyond the processing segment of language to thought to language, we are incorporating them within this segment since they principally concern this fundamental processing segment.

Comprehensive linguistic orientations. The surge of interest in communication as reflected in the study of pragmatics along with the interest in cognition-language relationships led to approaches that integrated form, content, and use of language (Bloom and Lahey, 1978) or, as stated by Muma (1978), cognitive-linguistic-communicative systems and processes. Bloom and Lahey's (1978) approach to language disorders was presented in the section on syntactic emphasis because

---

*From Backus, O., and Beasley, J., *Speech Therapy with Children.* Cambridge, Mass.: The Riverside Press, Houghton Mifflin Co., 46 (1951).

of that focus, and the reader can refer to it there.

In 1978 Muma presented his "cognitive-linguistic-communicative systems and processes" orientation to child language disorders. Detailing extensive information about normal and disordered child language, Muma (1978) interprets the relationships among cognitive systems, linguistic systems, and communicative systems in his development of an intervention model for child language disorders. His orientation to systems and processes is mentalistic and psychological as differentiated from physical and neurological processing.

Muma (1978) states his principle of intervention from which methodology flows as follows: "I propose that the best we can do is *describe (not quantify) an individual's command (knowledge and use) of cognitive-linguistic-communicative systems as he functions naturally or near naturally, then exploit his behavior.*"* He describes the basic dimensions of this natural language-learning approach as (1) content, whereby natural contexts in which the child functions are used, (2) pacing, which considers that the rate of learning is variable rather than determined by age, (3) sequencing, which utilizes the principle that stages in the emergence of the systems are highly stable, whereas sequences among the system may be highly variable, (4) reinforcement and motivation, which emphasizes that natural reinforcement is inherent in the behavior that occurs when that behavior results in expected outcomes, and (5) contexts, whereby natural language learning occurs in contexts where people participate in communicative acts.

Muma (1978) discusses six major language

intervention strategies that he believes should be used selectively according to the specific needs of the child. His strategies are:

1. First, language learning that is based on normal language development
2. Second, language learning where the treatment approach focuses on the direct comparison of the first language to the second language and direct teaching occurs
3. Intermodality transfer where one modality, for example, writing, is used to teach another, for example, speech
4. Language rehabilitation which is similar to the strategies used in teaching adult aphasics (The focus here appears to be on processes such as memory.)
5. Systematic extension of the child's available verbal repertoire, a composite of modeling and behavior modification procedures (Each task must be learned in this approach.)
6. Spontaneous exploration and variation of the child's available verbal repertoire where the intent is to have the child discover the nature and power of verbal capacities (As the child discovers this power, his range and the variability of his verbal repertoire expand.)

Muma provides specific intervention suggestions in chapters devoted to each of the systems that make up his intervention model with emphasis on techniques and procedures stemming from natural language-learning situations, as for example illustrated by *Sesame Street*. Piagetian thought guides his ideas of cognitive systems. He finds Brown's (1973) five stages of language development a useful guide for consideration of linguistic systems. As a guide to communicative systems, he discusses the development of the Parent-Child Development Center (PCDC) (Muma, 1971; Dawson and Muma, 1971).

Muma believes strongly in adopting an in-

*From Muma, J.R., *Language Handbook: Concepts, Assessment, Intervention.* Englewood Cliffs, N.J.: Prentice-Hall, Inc., 229-230 (1978).

tervention approach that utilizes other "intervention agents," including peers, parents, and relatives—what we would term the client-complex. He believes that the speech-language pathologist must first discover with the client-complex what will be productive with the individual child and then exploit that behavior.

Another guide in his intervention program relates to the "clinical groups position" and the "individual differences position." Here, Muma (1978) discusses the variability between subgroups of the language disordered population as well as the variability within a subgroup. Because of this variability, he suggests that intervention not be based on a priori assumptions about the category of the language disorder but based on the individual differences in cognitive-linguistic-communicative systems presented by the individual child, regardless of the clinical category in which he falls.

For some years in the profession of speech-language pathology, parents have been used in treatment, particularly as providers of practice of what occurred during the treatment session. However, as an outgrowth of the use of natural language teaching represented in many of these comprehensive approaches, greater use of parents as "change/intervention agents" has occurred. Parents are often thought to be instrumental in changing many of the problems presented by their children. For example, Johnson and Katz (1973) present a review of this subject for child behavior disorders ranging from speech dysfunction to self-injurious behavior. They also discuss methods of training the parents and outcomes of treatment programs.

In Chapters 3 and 4 we discussed parent-child interaction and environmental perspectives on causation, suggesting that styles of language input and interaction may be causally related to child language disorders. Much

attention has been given to this information in normal child language development and is filtering into child language disorders and their treatment.

One other comprehensive approach with a linguistic orientation will be presented here as an example of convergence from divergence, the work of McLean and Snyder-McLean (1978). These authors derived a language acquisition model based on their interpretation of information about the cognitive and social bases of language acquisition as well as data about early linguistic development. The model derived is termed a "transactional model of language acquisition" and stresses three major interacting components: (1) cognitive, (2) social, and (3) linguistic. They discuss in detail how their model accounts for the "realization process underlying the production or comprehension of a specific utterance." The model is produced in Fig. 9-1.

We have placed McLean and Snyder-McLean's (1978) implications for treatment based on their transactional model in this section because it is a clear attempt to focus intervention on what they term a "three-way matrix" for language learning, including (1) the functions of communicative acts, (2) the content of communicative acts, and (3) the structure of communicative acts. They provide an extensive discussion of the parts of the matrix in terms of treatment implications for pragmatics (function/intent), semantics (content), and syntax (structure), which enter into each communicative act.

Fig. 9-2 illustrates how the matrix can be viewed for selection of elements to be used in treatment, including references to approaches developed in the literature. These and other approaches to language treatment have been evaluated by McLean and Snyder-McLean (1978) in the context of their transactional approach. An interesting part of their evaluation of these other approaches has been a

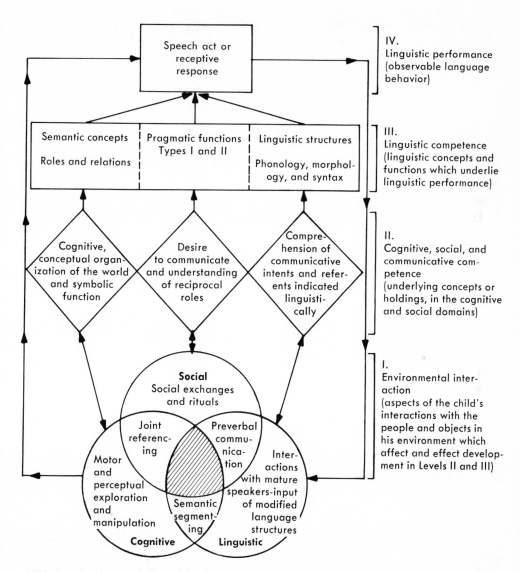

FIG. 9-1. A transactional model of language acquisition. (From McLean, J.E., and Snyder-McLean, L.K., *A Transactional Approach to Early Language Training.* Columbus, Ohio: Charles E. Merrill Publishing Co. [1978].)

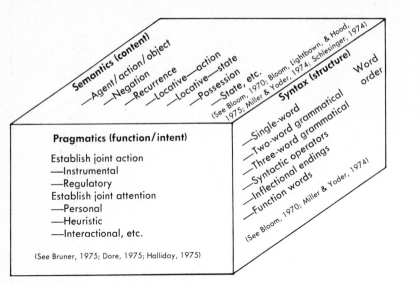

FIG. 9-2. Selected examples of possible elements of a three-way matrix for selection of language intervention targets. (From McLean, J.E., and Snyder-McLean, L.K., *A Transactional Approach to Early Language Training.* Columbus, Ohio: Charles E. Merrill Publishing Co. [1978].)

statement of whether the approach has the potential for continued evolution based on new information that may be forthcoming. They offer no specific treatment approach based on their model, stating instead that there are enough approaches and that what is needed is the development of intervention strategies that allow for a variety of available methods.

McLean and Snyder-McLean summarize their implications for treatment in eight major points:

1. Language-intervention programs for young, significantly language-deficient children which apply only the dependent and independent variables suggested by either transformational grammar systems or radical behavioral modification systems appear inadequate to the task of attaining productive language repertoiries for such children.

2. Language-intervention programs which would attain adequacy with such children must, instead, apply variables derived from theoretical language models which include consideration of a child's cognitive functions and holdings, social functions, and both the physical and human elements and functions in the intervention environment.

3. Language-intervention programs for such children must target the development of expanded cognitive bases for language and specific language targets which represent semantic-linguistic "maps" of the child's demonstrated existing cognitive holdings.

4. Similarly, the treatment program for many severely language-delayed or deficient young children will need to target the expansion of social-interaction repertoeis and the development of preverbal communication exchange rituals which can later be mapped linguistically.

5. In designing treatment programs for verbal children, the clinician/teacher must target not only a broad and generative repertoire of linguistic structures, but also—and primarily—a full and functional repertoire of semantic relationships or meanings and pragmatic functions or intents.

6. In the light of the multidimensional and pervasive nature of the language-intervention model suggested here, it is unrealistic to expect such treatment to be implemented effectively through short, infrequent and isolated language-training sessions. Rather, such treatment must be generated and implemented in a

contexts in which the child has natural opportunities for interaction and communication.

7. A review of existing treatment programs revealed a few which are consonant with some of the implication of this model—particularly for verbal children whose deficits are primarily in the area of linguistic structure or even semantic mapping. However, for the nonverbal child with deficient social and cognitive bases for language, no existing programs were identified which would be consistent with the intervention model described in this book.

8. Language-intervention programs for handicapped children must be designed to reflect the ethological and transactional variables of normal language development and the child-perspective orientation inherent in that process.*

Comprehensive processing orientations.
We are including here those multistage processing orientations that go beyond a focus on auditory processing. Our intent in placing them here is to demonstrate that some of the concepts presented in these orientations can help bring a processing perspective to treatment. Some of the processing concepts presented, although heavily criticized, can be useful in orienting treatment approaches within the Language to Thought to Language Processing Segment.

Bangs (1968) developed a complete curriculum guide for the preacademic child with language and learning disorders. She cites sensation, perception, memory-retrieval, attention, and integration in both auditory and visual modalities as the avenues by which the child learns, including language learning. Throughout the development of her curriculum guides and descriptions of techniques and procedures for various types of language disordered children, Bangs (1968) utilizes these avenues of learning along with a variety of other natural language activities and techniques that present specific linguistic stim-

---

*From McLean, J.E., and Snyder-McLean, L.K., *A Transactional Approach to Early Language Training.* Columbus, Ohio: Charles E. Merrill Pub. Co., 253-254 (1978).

ulation. Her approach therefore goes beyond the specifics of the avenues of learning she proposes and is not considered to be simply a prescriptive perceptual approach. However, there is an inconsistency in her approach, since she deviates significantly from her "model" of avenues of learning. While there is much interesting and useful information in her book that can be adopted for treatment of child language disorders, one does not obtain an overall consistency in her orientation to language disorders and their treatment.

The development of the *Illinois Test of Psycholinguistic Abilities* (Kirk, McCarthy, and Kirk, 1968) has led to the extensive development of treatment methods for children with language disorders. This test, together with the orientation from which it stems (Osgood, 1957), is considered here as a multi-stage process. It has been widely used as an assessment tool for child language disorders, and many treatment tasks have been designed to remedy the specific levels where the child failed on the test. Prescriptive teaching to failed tasks was developed and has gone under the general name of "psycholinguistic training."

Several examples of this approach will suffice here. The first, a specific application of teaching psycholinguistic skills as identified by the ITPA, is *Target on Language,* produced by Novakovich and her colleagues at Christ Church Child Center (1973, 1977). The manual is a compilation of therapy techniques based on each of the processes identified in the ITPA. Each process is defined; sampling procedures for gathering data about the child's abilities are discussed; and remedial techniques are provided. The tasks for remediation are essentially tasks comparable to the ITPA test items.

A second example, although broader in scope and bringing in other information about language development, is still based on the

ITPA, according to the author. The *Source-book of Language Learning Activities* prepared by Worthley (1978) describes techniques and methods within what the author calls language sets, including (1) basic skills, (2) receptive vocabulary building, (3) expressive syntax—words and phrases, (4) expressive syntax—sentences, (5) communication skills—cognitive analysis, (6) reading, and (7) writing-spelling. The approach the author uses for developing this source book stems from his premise that words and word symbols are the building blocks of language and that since words are learned, they must be taught from a psycholinguistic view, specifically that described by Kirk, McCarthy, and Kirk (1968) in the ITPA.

Bloom and Lahey (1978) critically evaluate the information available about teaching psycholinguistic abilities, what they term "specific abilities." They rely heavily on the review of studies of this type done by Hammill and Larsen (1974), who in their review of 38 studies of the effectiveness of treatment from this approach concluded that the studies did not validate that the child's abilities measured by the ITPA can be trained. Bloom and Lahey (1978) conclude:

> We are not aware of any studies that have found improvement in general language development after the remediation of specific abilities—perhaps because few have looked for such transfer of improvement in language use. Without such evidence, however, and without evidence that such abilities are necessary for the development and use of oral language, it is questionable that the remediation of specific abilities should dominate a remedial program for children who are learning language slowly and with difficulty.*

In their two works Wiig and Semel (1976, 1980) present various kinds of information on language and learning disorders, including

*From Bloom, L., and Lahey, M., *Language Development and Language Disorders*. New York: John Wiley and Sons, 547 (1978).

assessment and intervention. They take a processing orientation to language disabilities. The processes they discuss are auditory perceptual processing, cognitive and linguistic processing, and language formation and production. Their models illustrating the relationship among these processes have been presented in Chapter 2 of this book where we discussed Wiig and Semel (1976) as representing a multi-stage processing approach to language disorders. However, in the 1980 work that focuses on assessment and intervention, no processing model is presented as a guide, although it is clear that the presentation of material in the 1980 book is guided by the 1976 work.

The methodology presented by Wiig and Semel in their two works is one of task analysis for each processing component as it relates to levels of language. They draw upon the literature in language and learning to demonstrate specific tasks that can be used both to assess and treat language-learning disordered children and adolescents. For example, in the 1980 work they illustrate tasks for forming words, forming sentences, understanding words and word relationships, remembering spoken messages, word finding, fluency, and flexibility. Or similarly, in the earlier work of 1976, they present tasks designed for remediation of auditory-perceptual processing deficits, such as auditory attention and identification of nonsymbolic stimuli, localization of sounds, auditory figure-ground, auditory discrimination of phonemes, and auditory sequencing. They provide extensive suggestions for techniques and procedures for carrying out these tasks, often supplying underlying principles for guiding this type of intervention.

All in all, the overriding methodology proposed by Wiig and Semel (1976, 1980) for treatment of language and language-learning disorders is to define a specific process, level of language, subcomponent of language, and so forth, and then isolate tasks that assess the child's abilities in those areas, finally providing specific intervention techniques, often quite similar to the tasks used to assess the ability.

Even though the two works of Wiig and Semel are comprehensive, they leave the reader with an overwhelming feeling that language and language-learning disorders are fundamentally resolved through applying specific tasks that in some way are presumed to be related to language. We have raised precautions regarding this approach as related to auditory processing disruptions, and again the analysis of teaching to psycholinguistic abilities by Bloom and Lahey (1978) is appropriate to consider here.

In her early work, which we discussed in Chapter 2, Berry (1969) was instrumental in developing the principle that child language disorders are reflections of underlying physical processing, and she has followed this up in her later work (1980). She states:

> The taproots of oral language are embedded in neurobiology, but we cannot define exactly all the mechanisms by which it emerges from these taproots. How does the nervous system order and integrate the oral information to which we attend? How do we make those connections between comprehension and verbalization, between the understanding and the telling? . . . In order to find answers, even partial answers, we must understand the operation of certain systems of neural organization and integration although we may not understand the intricacies of structure.[*]

Berry goes on to present an extensive discussion of "the mediation of oral language in the central nervous system" and the "neuropsychosocial substrates of oral language," concluding with her transactional orientation to neurologic processing for language, an orientation very like that presented in 1969 and discussed here in Chapter 2.

Berry (1980) discusses "hallmarks of oral language acquisition" as "ontogenic" schedules and principles that follow the natural course of normal language development. The first is perceptual-semantic development to which all other hallmarks are subordinate. Second is the phonatory (prosodic) hallmark seen in infancy in the child's prosodic, emotional intent vocalizations. This is followed by the third hallmark, phonologic development, and the fourth, syntactic development. All these hallmarks continually reflect the child's development of comprehension-expression of oral language—"language grows as thought develops."

Berry (1980) calls her approach to teaching language disordered children A Global-Ontogenic Teaching Program. Her concept of *global* means that treatment (teaching) must be interlocking, developing constant relationships among all facets of language, verbal and nonverbal. It is ontogenic in that it follows the normal course of language development as expressed in her hallmarks of oral language development. Basically her methodology is communicative, situational, and pragmatic; the goal is spontaneous talking that serves a purpose for the child. She states:

> . . . what we mean by the pragmatic approach to teaching: teaching language in the context and environment in which it is generated. It involves the interpretation of the child's utterance; the meaning intended by the child; his sensorimotor actions that precede, accompany, and follow the utterance; the knowledge shared by the communicative dyad. The pragmatic approach makes use of speaker-listener intentions and relations and all the elements in the environment surrounding the message. From this explanation, it is clear that pragmatics cannot be limited to the intent of word meanings in structured units. . . .[*]

---

[*]From Berry, M.F., *Teaching Linguistically Handicapped Children*. Englewood Cliffs, N.J.: Prentice-Hall, Inc., 25, 27 (1980).

[*]From Berry, M.F., *Teaching Linguistically Handicapped Children*. Englewood Cliffs, N.J.: Prentice-Hall, Inc., 18 (1980).

Her treatment approach therefore falls into the category of natural language teaching, and structured exercises and drills in phonology, syntax, and semantics are seldom used. Berry makes it quite clear that she feels these approaches for the most part do not teach children what they need to know about language. Instead, situational teaching provides the child with experiences from which he can build hypotheses, test them, and change them based on a total set of situational and environmental circumstances.

Berry provides example teaching units and illustrative case examples and suggests ideas and materials for teaching, but she cautions the language teacher that these examples are not prescriptive but only aids to the teacher's own creativity. She also uses parents and peers heavily to carry out her global-ontogenic teaching program.

Even though the reader will recognize that Berry (1980) does not prescribe a treatment approach based directly on specified neurologic processes for language, her approach has been included here because of her tenet that the ontogenic development of language based on her hallmarks of language is mediated by the structure and function of the nervous system in an orderly, developmental way. Thus, this processing approach varies strikingly from those following the ITPA or Wiig and Semel (1976, 1980).

LANGUAGE TO SPEECH PROCESSING
Phonologic orientations

The child's ability to be understood by those around him is ultimately dependent upon his appropriate use of the sound system. One part of that system is his learning of the sounds and sound sequences that represent the words and sentences of his language. In Chapters 2 and 3 we discussed the normal and disordered development of the sound system (phonology) as it relates to the overall development of other levels of language. We emphasized that this information is needed by professionals working with child language disorders.

However, phonologic disorders in children with and without disorders of other aspects of language have usually been treated apart from rather than incorporated into child language disorders. It is interesting to note in the comprehensive approaches to treatment of child language disorders that Berry (1980) is the only one who advocates significant attention to phonology as a part of the treatment approach.

In keeping with the overall professional orientation in speech-language pathology we will not discuss treatment approaches to phonologic disorders as a part of child language disorders. In Chapter 3 we pointed out how phonologic disorders may be in hierarchical relationship to disorders at other levels (Aram and Nation, 1975). We caution the reader that more attention must be paid to the relationship of phonologic development and disorders as one part of child language disorders. The student is referred to previous chapters for literature references that provide information about treatment approaches available.

In Chapter 7 phonology was discussed as a function of the speech programming processing stage within the Language to Speech Processing Segment of the CLPM, and we distinguished phonologic disorders from articulation disorders. In that chapter we concentrated on developmental verbal apraxia, and likewise here we will focus on treatment approaches for this disorder.

Childhood apraxia. Childhood apraxia has been much written about in terms of classification, differentiation, and description, but little has been said regarding treatment approaches for it. McGinnis's (1963) association method, which developed from her orientation to childhood aphasia (McGinnis, Kleffner, and Goldstein, 1956), has more often been adopted for use with childhood apraxia. In essence the association method is a highly structured, elemental approach to teaching based on the idea of language output as the starting point for all aphasic children. The method relies on teaching sound elements individually through phonetic placement and then moving on to sequencing these sounds into words. The approach emphasizes a combined auditory-visual-phonetic placement for building the motor patterns for speech sounds and sound sequences. Much drill work is necessary.

Systematic sensory-motor association through auditory, visual, and motor matching is the hallmark of the approach. McGinnis and her associates provide a sequence of steps for teaching each of the tasks believed to go into the learning of words and sentences. For example, she specifies seven steps for teaching a noun. The teacher should have the child:

1. Produce in sequence from the written form the sounds composing a noun.
2. Match the picture of the object represented by this word to the written form of the word.
3. Copy the word and articulate each sound as the letter(s) for it are written.
4. Repeat the word aloud after watching the teacher say it and match the object or picture to the written form of the word.
5. Say the name of the object from memory.
6. Write the word for the object from memory, articulating each sound as the letter(s) for it are written.
7. Repeat the word as the teacher speaks it into his ear and match the picture to the written form of the word.

Much rote learning is a part of the method. In essence this approach builds language from isolated speech sounds to sound sequences, then to words and to sentences. Meaning generally is not applied in the early stages.

While McGinnis was to receive criticism from many camps for her insistence upon starting with expression for all aphasic children, both she and her followers reported impressive gains for the children taught in this manner. Speech-language pathologists continue to draw from her approach. Work with the apraxic child is very similar to and much indebted to the McGinnis approach.

One of McGinnis' major later supporters is DuBard (1974), who presented a work on the theory and application of the association method to teaching aphasic and other language disordered children. Her handbook provides a discussion of childhood aphasia, support for the association method through her personal use and conviction, and material and procedures designed for application of the method.

Eisenson (1972) describes a small number of children who understood language but were unable to produce it as children with congenital (articulatory) apraxias. In very severe forms the child was unable to imitate isolated movements of the articulators. His treatment approach is based on teaching the child to produce a sequential set of articulatory movements necessary for speech. The approach begins with teaching the child isolated sounds, then sound sequences, then words from the sequences, and ultimately sentences constructed from the words. The approach requires modeling and imitation using combined auditory and visual stimulation and is not unlike McGinnis's method.

Logue and McClumpha (1970) present a slight adaptation of the McGinnis approach. Instead of beginning with speech sound production, Logue and McClumpha (1970) begin treatment focusing on movement of the articulators isolated from sound production. The child is asked to model/imitate articulatory movements from visual stimulation with no sound production. Once these oral movement patterns are established, Logue and McClumpha then introduce production of speech sounds, and the remainder of the approach is much like that of McGinnis and Eisenson. They do pay greater attention to phonologic concepts, particularly in terms of the features inherent in speech sounds as well as the place of articulation. For example, in one case study presented, Logue and McClumpha introduced the /ʃ/ sound after having worked on /b/ because of the distinctly different features and place and manner of articulation between the two sounds.

In a recent review of symptomatology and treatment of developmental apraxia, Macaluso-Haynes (1978) has summarized many of the approaches to this therapeutically resistant disorder. Among the methods and techniques suggested are:

1. Concentration on performance drill, both in imitation and on command, of tongue and lip movements
2. Imitation of sustained vowels and consonants followed by production of simple syllable shapes
3. Development of movement patterns and sequences of sounds
4. Use of slow rate and self-monitoring
5. Pairing rhythm, intonation, and stress with motor activity
6. Development of orosensory perceptual awareness
7. Use of core vocabulary and carrier phrases

Our general guidelines for treating childhood apraxia are similar:

1. Begin with associating written symbols to oral movements.
   a. Begin with or without phonation.
   b. Use 2 or 3 contrasting consonants (suggest /p/ /m/ /s/).
   c. Start with neutral vowel (/ʌ/).
2. Immediately begin sequence practice (/pʌm/, /pʌp/, /mʌp/, etc.) while reading symbols.
   a. Read initially without meaning.
   b. Introduce meaning.
3. Use aural imitation drill.
4. Incorporate semantic and syntactic goals.
   a. Vocabulary development.
   b. Lexical retrieval.
   c. Syntax development—especially verb tenses, prepositional phrases.
5. Think *rules* and *sequencing* on all language/motor speech levels.

Alternate forms of expression

A final comment is in order regarding the use of alternate forms of expression, some of which were discussed earlier. Communication boards, sign language, and other forms of nonverbal communication have been used with a number of categories of children unable to or limited in their ability to speak, for example, children with cerebral palsy, children with multiple handicaps affecting speech production abilities, those who are deaf and hard-of-hearing, and those who are mentally retarded, autistic, and apraxic. Davis (1973) has described an apparatus called the sentence construction board developed from linguistic principles and from Fitzgerald's (1949) method of teaching language to the deaf. McDonald and Schultz (1973) discuss the use of communication boards designed for cerebral palsied children, as have Hagen, Porter, and Brink (1973). The literature in this area is growing, and the area is becoming a specialization in our profession even though some professionals are expressing concern over the unjustified use of nonverbal communication with children who may (or do) have the potential for verbal language. We will not be discussing these approaches to language treatment in this book because our intent here is to focus on the use of speech, although we recognize that alternative forms must be used with some language disordered children. For further information regarding nonverbal communication we suggest Silverman (1980).

•   •   •

It is evident from the foregoing discussion that treatment approaches for child language disorders have followed our heritage in normal and disordered child language. We see divergent perspectives presented; however, common threads of information exist within the treatment approaches developed. First, the approaches reflect the state of knowledge and theory that existed at the time. Second, normal language development is used heavily as an underlying orientation to the approaches. Third, intervention strategies are based on either direct language teaching, behavior modification procedures, or natural language learning activities.

We, like McLean and Snyder-McLean (1978), do not believe new approaches to treatment need to be developed. What is available can be brought into the perspectives we have developed. We have done this in the preceding section by placing the various approaches, procedures, and methods into the processing segments of the CLPM. Thus, our model can guide the selection of available treatment approaches. The major emphasis in our perspective is on language processing and performance rather than on levels of language behavior or on the pragmatic/communicative/cognitive perspectives so prevalent at this time. Our perspective is based more on

how children receive, comprehend, integrate, formulate, and produce language than on the language behavior itself.

We believe there is a need to continue exploring the basis and rationale for developing a comprehensive model for language treatment of young children, a model based on a set of principles and oriented toward formulating management and treatment plans. Even though not designed for child language disorders, the questions raised by Shames and Egolf (1976) seem applicable as a guide. Restated here as principles they are:

1. The treatment method must derive from a theoretical point of view.
2. The theoretical orientation should lead to a set of treatment strategies and descriptions of procedures for accomplishing those strategies.
3. The treatment approach should result in a change of the disorder and the behaviors that are characteristic of the disorder.
4. The treatment approach and results should be able to be evaluated.
5. Revision of the treatment approach should be possible and associated activities modifiable in a systematic and orderly fashion.
6. The treatment should be responsive to the social and emotional content of the disorder.

THE DOMAIN OF MANAGEMENT AND TREATMENT

Treatment of a child's language disorder must be cast into the broader context of management, a superordinate clinical concern of the speech-language pathologist not limited solely to the language disorder. The development of management plans is based on a comprehensive understanding of the total set of circumstances that characterize the child: environmental, physical, educational, social, familial, and others. These plans require that the speech-language pathologist address a number of issues, some related to the nature of the disorder, others related to the child's family, some related to other professionals, and still others related to the community at large. Development of management plans involves a number of decisions that reflect both the idealistic and the practical.

Nation (1982) addresses management and treatment issues and arrives at four components that serve as the basis for decision making in the development of management plans. These four components are:

1. A "rehabilitation" philosophy that guides the objectives of the management plan
2. The professional services required to meet the objectives
3. The role of the child's family in the plan
4. Implementation and monitoring of the plan

Rehabilitation philosophy guides management objectives

To formulate management objectives, the speech-language pathologist must have a well-reasoned philosphy of rehabilitation of child language disorders. Our profession at this time, however, has not yet arrived at a consistent philosophy of rehabilitation that guides the decisions we make in formulating these objectives. There are still many unresolved issues regarding management and treatment of child language disorders, for example, the relationship between early language intervention and maturation.

At this time we believe that a rehabilitation philosophy for guiding management objectives should take into account the following. First, all children diagnosed as having a language disorder can benefit to some degree from speech-language pathology services.

Second, the overall objective for these children should be to provide them with the best possible communicative abilities they can achieve within the limitations imposed by the nature and cause of their language disorder. Third, the objectives should be determined within a comprehensive perspective that takes into account all aspects of the child and his family. Fourth, the role of other professionals must be considered within the management objectives. Fifth, a longitudinal, interactive developmental perspective that takes into account the relationship of maturation to treatment is essential in formulating management plans. Sixth, the plan of action must have a means by which it can be evaluated for effectiveness, for determining the outcome if the plan of action is carried out. Seventh, it should be clear how speech-language pathology services relate to the overall management objectives.

The formulation of management objectives from these seven ingredients stems from a crucial issue: Can child language disorders be changed? This is an issue that must consider the nature and cause of the disorder, its severity, and the prediction for change. Of all the child language disorders, which are most amenable to change? The information needed by the speech-language pathologist is embedded in the knowledge he acquires about child language disorders. In addition, he must be able to integrate the various theoretical orientations he studies. The previous chapters of this book have focused on bringing together this information through a processing orientation. This material can serve as a primary resource for understanding child language disorders in order to raise questions and provide tentative answers as to whether child language disorders can be changed.

At this point we feel the need to emphasize causation as it relates to expectations for change in child language disorders. In Chapter 4 we saw that causation in speech-language pathology has had a stormy history, and there are strong adherents to the "causation does not matter" school, as well as to the "causation does matter" philosophy. We, of course, belong to the latter and wish to reemphasize that point in its relationship to determining management objectives.

Certain causal factors and processing deficits have a limiting effect on the success of management and treatment programs for some groups of children with language disorders. Normal language processing is not readily acquired in the presence of physical, biologic, and mental abnormalities. Brain injury, structural deficits, neuromuscular problems, hearing loss, and other causal factors of this type can prevent a child from receiving and processing language information.

Therefore, the intactness of the child guides the establishment of management objectives. If normal development of language is not possible because of physical limitations, then management objectives must be set in line with the imposed limitations. Our understanding of behavioral change resides in our knowledge of how these causal factors limit the ability of the child to learn and use language. For example, children with severe sensorineural hearing losses, uncontrolled seizures, or mental retardation can learn language only within the limits of the damaged nervous system.

Similarly, when viewing environmental causal factors in relation to the development of language, the speech-language pathologist must determine if changes can be made in the environmental circumstances and, if not, how much change can be expected from treatment. For example, if a child is receiving little language stimulation, this causal factor must be altered if the management objective is normal language development and usage. If it is not possible to alter this circumstance, then the management objective will have to consider the range and type of treatment necessary to offset this lack of stimulation.

As we pointed out in Chapter 4 and when discussing the developmental-interactive view of child language disorders, it is more likely that there will be several causal factors interacting over time. If management objectives are to be set in terms of expectations for change, these factors require analysis in relation to proposed objectives.

The severity of each child's language disorder must be considered in developing management plans. It is generally agreed that each child's language disorder will vary in severity in some aspect from any other child's language disorder. For example, 3-year-old David, who is only beginning to use four- and five-word sentences with inconsistent use of inflectional markers, presents a mild disorder of syntax, whereas 8-year-old Brian at the same stage would be more severe. Or similarly, 4-year-old Eric, who uses only four words spontaneously, presents a markedly more severe disorder than 4-year-old Erica, who speaks in complete sentences but whose lexicon is underdeveloped.

In arriving at a statement of the severity of a given language disorder, probably the level of language behavior in contrast with the child's chronologic and mental age is a chief measuring stick. Two children with similar semantic problems, one age 4 and the other 10, would certainly be considered differently in terms of severity. Similarly, a 2-year-old nonverbal child likely presents a less severe problem than a 5-year-old child with limited language output. Therefore, age vis-a-vis language behavior represents a chief determinant of severity and an important dimension to consider when developing management objectives for the individual child.

Generally, the more prevasive the language disorder across processes and behavior, the more severe it is likely to be. For example, 5-year-old Traci, who has difficulty with comprehension, formulation, and repetition of phonologic, syntactic, and semantic aspects of language, is relatively worse off than 5-year-old Troy, whose problems are confined primarily to syntactic formulation. For a given age group, the more pervasive the disorder, the more severe the disorder. However, a very young child 2 or 3 years of age with a pervasive language disorder can change rapidly, and therefore his problem ends up being less severe than if present in an older child. Four- and five-year-old children with similar problems tend not to undergo the rapid change we see in younger children. By these ages pervasiveness of the disorder is an important indicator of severity. Thus, pervasiveness of the language disorder is an important yardstick of severity but cannot be a measurement made without consideration of age and requires that, when planning management objectives, the speech-language pathologist maintain a longitudinal perspective on severity, incorporating the interaction of maturation with treatment.

However, it has been found that some types of circumscribed disorders are more resistent to change than others and therefore tend to be judged as more severe. For example, childhood apraxia, while presenting a relatively circumscribed language to speech processing disruption, is a disorder typically requiring intensive, long-term treatment. Therefore, because of the nature of apraxia, it is generally considered to be one of the more severe forms of childhood language disorders. Likewise, it has been shown that comprehension deficits (Wolpaw, Nation, and Aram, 1977) have a more pronounced effect on later school performance than do formulation deficits. Because of this relationship to later learning requirements, comprehension disorders would

be judged as more severe than comparable formulation disorders. Similarly, a profound peripheral hearing loss would produce a more severe language disorder than would an intermittent conductive hearing loss. There is, then, a cause-effect issue in determining severity in relationship to management objectives and planning.

The static quality of the disorder also enters into consideration of severity. If a deficit is showing improvement and is in a process of change, the disorder carries a better prediction for change and thus is not considered as severe as a disorder highly resistant to change.

Finally, the personal characteristics of the child and his family affect judgments of change. The child's motivation to change, his acceptance of responsibility for change, and the attitudes and resources of others in his environment all affect the amount of change that can be expected. Thus, a neurologically intact, motivationally energized child brings more equipment for potential change. His language disorder would be judged as less severe than a similar problem found in another child whose motivational mechanisms are not optimal.

In determining management objectives the severity of the disorder and predictions for change must be considered. However, this information is not always immediately apparent at the beginning of treatment, and management objectives may have to be altered as more information accrues about the nature of the child's language disorder.

Professional services required

To develop his management plan, the speech-language pathologist must consider the range and type of professional services needed by children with language disorders. Consideration of needed professional services stems from the management objectives determined for each client, which in turn are based on the nature, cause, severity, and prognosis of the language disorder. Therefore, consideration must be given to the relationship between the services offered by speech-language pathologists and the services offered by other professionals. The time at which these various services are needed during the course of treatment must be part of the management plans as well.

Speech-language pathology services. Speech-language pathology services, as we stated earlier, are assumed to be needed in each instance of child language disorders and therefore are a part of the management objectives. The approaches to language treatment for children were taken up in greater detail earlier in this chapter.

Here, assuming a treatment approach has been selected, the speech-language pathologist must determine how to carry out the treatment approach. Nation (1982), in an earlier review of management and treatment, presented a series of topics usually discussed in this regard. They are:

1. Determining the most appropriate treatment schedule that will accomplish the management objectives in the shortest amount of time
2. Establishing specific long-term and short-term operational goals over time
3. Selecting techniques and procedures that will meet the operational goals
4. Measuring and evaluating progress; revising and restating goals as required
5. Determining when maximum benefit has been derived from treatment and establishing termination criteria
6. Conducting follow-up evaluations to determine if treatment effects have been maintained

Other professional services. The treatment of child language disorders often requires the services of other professionals in conjunction with the speech-language pathologist. Therefore, the management plan must take into account when medical, dental, social, educational, psychologic, and other services may be needed in the course of treatment. Seldom do children with language disorders fall only into the hands of the speech-language pathologist, since these disorders are not circumscribed; rather, they are long term, developmental, and interactive with other aspects of the child's development and growth. The speech-language pathologist must remain highly aware of the need of other services and must know when these services should be called upon in the resolution of the disorder.

In addition to the knowledge of what services are needed in conjunction with speech-language pathology services, the speech-language pathologist must be aware of the availability of these services in the professional community. The lack of available specialty services may require changes in the management plan to achieve the management objectives. Alternatives may be required. For example, in a limited resources community there may be no special class for the aphasic child, and his language and educational needs may have to be met by other alternatives. Or similarly there may be no class for the hard-of-hearing or deaf child. Other options, although not optimal for meeting the management objectives, may have to be instituted.

The speech-language pathologist must know the professionals in his community for making referrals for other services: the psychologist who works well with disturbed preschoolers, the physician who understands childhood aphasia, the social worker who understands dialectal differences, and so forth. The speech-language pathologist must give careful consideration to (1) when a referral is needed, (2) the professional to whom the referral is made, (3) the process of making the referral, and (4) what to expect from the referral source. Nation and Aram (1977) have provided a guide for consideration of referrals.

Role of the child's family

The role to be played by the child's family in determining and carrying out the management objectives must be considered. While the speech-language pathologist can specify his professional services and call upon other professionals, he cannot carry out the role expected of the child's family in meeting the management objectives, something as concrete, for example, as meeting appointments. The child's family, including parents, extended family members, and guardians, must be viewed in a broad perspective; their educational, social, cultural, personal, and communicative background and expectations for the child must be considered. Do they view the problem in the same way and have the same expectations as does the professional? Are their priorities for management and treatment different from the professional's? The speech-language pathologist may have to modify his management plan based on the characteristics and concerns of the family, particularly in those treatment approaches now expecting a great deal from parents in the intervention process.

Children cannot take responsibility for the management of their disorders; therefore it is vital to arrive at decisions in cooperation with the family. It may require that the family's role in the management plan be established over time rather than at the outset of treatment. Some families are better able to handle the process one step at a time instead of having to confront a wide range of objectives at once. Their response to the needs of the management plan is vital to successful treatment

of child language disorders. Committment to the objectives and a desire for carrying them out must be nurtured in the child's family.

Implementing and monitoring the plan

Decisions must be made as to the best way the management plan is to be initiated, co-ordinated, and monitored. We will address this issue from the point of view of who may be best suited to monitor the plan of action that brings together the management objectives, the professional services required, and the role of the family.

It is our belief that the speech-language pathologist takes on different roles depending on the nature and cause of the language disorder and depending on the work setting in which he provides service. It is crucial that the speech-language pathologist understand his role in relation to all the needs of the child with a language disorder. In our profession much emphasis is placed on the concept of client management, which implies the responsibility for carrying out the management objectives and plans, coordinating the efforts of all involved, For convenience, the role of the speech-language pathologist in managing child language disorders can be broken down into the following categories (Nation, 1982):

1. Speech-language pathologist as the primary manager
2. Shared management
3. Team management
4. Speech-language pathology as a related service

Speech-language pathologist as the primary manager. When direct language treatment is the only service required, the speech-language pathologist may be the child's primary manager although he may utilize adjunct consultative professional services. Adjunct services are considered to be services that may be needed during the course of treatment, some simply related to the fact that the client is a child, for example, pediatric services; others related to the need for further information, for example, a consultation from a psychologist to gain better understanding of the child's mental abilities; or others related to assistance with a specific problem, for example, calling upon the social worder to assist with financial matters. However, the speech-language pathologist in these contexts is considered the primary manager of the language disorder and would be expected to coordinate and monitor the use of these adjunct services and relate the effectiveness of all services to the overall management objectives and plan of action.

Shared management. In some instances the management of the child and his language disorder is shared by several specialists and agencies, particularly management of those children requiring ongoing services from several professionals because of their multiple problems. For example, children with language disorders may also be emotionally disturbed, requiring treatment from both the speech-language pathologist and the psychologist or psychiatrist. Many mentally retarded children have language disorders and educational problems, and they may have parents unable to cope with these circumstances. Management for these children is often shared and includes placement in a preschool for the retarded, treatment by a speech-language pathologist, and parental counseling by a psychologist or social worker.

Many management plans therefore are jointly shared. In these instances careful coordination of the various services and progress made is important. Shared management without coordination results in a weak link in reaching management objectives.

Team management. At times management of the child with a language disorder will specify that the child be seen in an agency where a formalized team is available to provide services. Teams have been formed to manage children with certain medical conditions that include a language disorder as a possible concomitant; for example, there are craniofacial anomalies teams, pediatric neurology teams, and mental retardation teams. Team management is distinguished from shared management primarily by its formalization and designation as a team and its specification of location, participants, functions, and coordination. In these formalized teams there is generally a team leader, who may be any one of the team members, who is responsible for coordinating and monitoring the team activities for each child. Teams also will use adjunct services as needed.

Speech-language pathology as a related service. Many children with language disorders have other conditions that require primary care from professionals other than speech-language pathologists. Children with certain conditions come to mind—children with neurologic disease, with profound mental retardation, with severe psychiatric disturbances, and so forth. The service provided by the speech-language pathologist in these instances may best be considered a related service, since the primary management of the child is the role of another professional.

Significant issues have arisen in this regard about the role of the speech-language pathologist in treating children in need of special education, particularly children who have learning disabilities. Who is the professional best suited for managing the overall needs of these children—the special educator (learning disabilities teacher) or the language specialist (speech-language pathologist)? Differences of opinion on this issue arise from political, legislative, and financial considerations as well as from educational and language treatment perspectives.

Summary

In this section we have discussed the domain of management in relation to treatment of child language disorders. The focus here has been on superordinate management decisions, including (1) formulation of management objectives guided by a rehabilitation philosophy, (2) determination of professional services needed to carry out the management plan, (3) consideration of the role the family is to take in the plan of action, and (4) determination of the roles to be taken by the various professionals in implementing and monitoring the plan. Consideration of these superordinate clinical concerns will assist the speech-language pathologist in selecting appropriate treatment approaches for children with language disorders.

STUDY QUESTIONS

1. What do the following resources offer regarding treatment approaches for childhood aphasia (Barry, 1961, 1969; Bliss and Peterson, 1975; Morley, 1973; Petrie, 1975)?

2. How might the information provided in the following resources be applied to the treatment of language in autistic children (Dalgleish, 1975; Miller and Miller, 1973; Stevens-Long and Rasmussen, 1974; Sulzbacher and Costello, 1970)?

3. How did Ratusnik and Ratusnik (1976) utilize the Lee and others (1975) interactive language development teaching approach with psychotic children?

4. In her article discussing selection of grammatical structures to use in language training, Rees (1972) presents six bases for decision making derived from differing theoretical approaches. What does she see as the bases for decision making, and what conclusions does she draw? How could her discussion be interpreted in relation to the delay versus deviant models of child language disorders?

5. How does Miller and Yoder's (1972) syntax teaching program, developed earlier than their semantic

approach, relate to their semantic approach to treatment? Are the criteria and operating principles compatible? Would you suggest that the two programs can be used sequentially?

6. Holland (1975) discusses the context and content of language therapy with children considering how a core lexicon might be presented as a psycholinguistic strategy. Drawing upon Holland's suggestions, devise a 50-word core lexicon for a preschool language disordered child with whom you have contact.

7. Muma (1975) has developed a communication game that he calls "Dump and Play." Analyze this game as an approach to language disordered children. (See Anderson, 1976; Knight, 1976; Muma, 1976).

8. Review the articles discussed in Chapters 3 and 4 and the following with the intent of determining how this information might be used in parent intervention/treatment programs for child language disorders: Abrams and Kaslow, 1976; Buium, Rynders, and Turnure, 1974; Cramblit and Siegel, 1977; Doleys, Cartelli, and Doster, 1976; Goldfarb, Levy, and Myers, 1972; Guralnick and Paul-Brown, 1977; Kogan, Wimberger, and Bobbitt, 1969; Schachter, Fosha, Stemp, Brotman, and Ganger, 1976; Schiff, 1979.

9. Approaches to treatment of child language disorders that are based on a delay model or a model of arrested development imply a certain teaching approach. Would these be applicable to children who have a deviant system of language? (See Cromer, 1974a,b; Morehead and Ingram, 1973).

10. Kirk and Kirk (1971) report improvement from treatment following the ITPA model. How can their results be reconciled with those of Hammill and Larsen (1974) and the conclusions of Bloom and Lahey (1978)?

11. What are the similarities and differences in the approach to treatment of childhood verbal apraxia offered by Chappell (1973) compared with those of Eisenson (1972), McGinnis (1963), and Rosenbek, Hanson, Baughman, and Lemme (1974)?

12. What suggestions do Connell, Spradlin, and McReynolds (1977) make for selection of treatment approaches for child language disorders and for determining the effectiveness of these procedures?

References and recommended readings

Abbs, J.H., and Sussman, H.M., Neurophysiological feature detectors and speech perception: A discussion of theoretical implications. *Journal of Speech and Hearing Research*, **14,** 23-36 (1971).

Abrams, J., and Kaslow, F., Learning disability and family dynamics: A mutual interaction. *Journal of Clinical Child Psychology*, Spring, 35-40 (1976).

Adler, S., *The Non-Verbal Child*. Springfield, Ill.: Charles C Thomas, Publisher (1964).

Alajouanine, T., and Lhermitte, F., Acquired aphasia in children. *Brain*, **88,** 653-662 (1965).

Ammons, R.B. and Ammons, H.S., *Full-Range Picture Vocabulary Test*. Missoula, Mont.: Psychological Test Specialists (1958).

Anderson, N.B., "The communication game" and beyond. Letter to the Editor, *Journal of Speech and Hearing Disorders*, **41,** 423 (1976).

Aram, D.M., Developmental apraxia of speech. Paper presented at the Annual Convention of the American Speech-Language and Hearing Association, Atlanta (1979).

Aram, D.M., Developmental language disorders: Patterns of language behavior. Doctoral dissertation, Cleveland, Ohio: Case Western Reserve University (1972).

Aram, D.M., Developmental language disorders related to pediatric syndromes: Heller's syndrome. Paper presented at the Annual Convention of the American Speech-Language and Hearing Association, San Francisco (1978).

Aram, D.M., Predicting learning disabilities from preschool language performance. Ohio Association for Children with Learning Disabilities Convention, Cleveland, Ohio (1977).

Aram, D.M., and Glasson, C., Developmental apraxia of speech. Mini-seminar presented at the Annual Convention of the American Speech-Language and Hearing Association, Atlanta (1979).

Aram, D.M., and Nation, J.E., Intelligence tests for children: A language analysis. *Ohio Journal of Speech and Hearing*, **6,** 22-43 (1971).

Aram, D.M., and Nation, J.E., Patterns of language behavior in children with developmental language disorders. *Journal of Speech and Hearing Research*, **18,** 229-241 (1975).

Aram, D.M., and Nation, J.E., Preschool language disorders and subsequent language and academic difficulties. *Journal of Communication Disorders*, **13,** 159-170 (1980).

Arthur, G., *The Arthur Adaptation of the Leiter International Performance Scale*. Washington, D.C.: Psychological Service Center Press (1952).

Atchison, M.J., and Canter, G.J., Variables influencing phonemic discrimination performance in normal and learning-disabled children. *Journal of Speech and Hearing Disorders*, **44,** 543-556 (1979).

Aten, J., Auditory memory and auditory sequencing. *Acta Symbolica*, **5,** 37-65 (1974).

Aten, J., and Davis, J., Disturbances in the perception of auditory sequence in children with minimal cerebral dysfunction. *Journal of Speech and Hearing Research*, **11,** 236-245 (1968).

Austin, J.L., *How To Do Things With Words*. London: Oxford University Press (1962).

Backus, O., and Beasley, J., *Speech Therapy with Children*. Cambridge, Mass.: The Riverside Press, Houghton Mifflin Co. (1951).

Baker, D.C., and Savetsky, L., Congenital partial atresia in the larynx. *Laryngoscope*, **76,** 616-620 (1966).

Baker, H.J., and Leland, B., *Detroit Test of Learning Aptitude: Examiner's Handbook*. Indianapolis: The Bobbs-Merrill Co., Inc. (1967).

Baker, H.J., and Leland, B., *Detroit Tests of Learning Aptitude*. (Rev. Ed.) Indianapolis: The Bobbs-Merrill Co., Inc. (1967).

Baltaxe, C.A.M., and Simmons, J.Q., Language in childhood psychosis: A review. *Journal of Speech and Hearing Disorders*, **40,** 439-458 (1975).

Bangs, J., A clinical analysis of the articulatory defects of the feebleminded. *Journal of Speech and Hearing Disorders*, **7,** 343-356 (1942).

Bangs, T.E., *Language and Learning Disorders of the Pre-Academic Child*. New York: Appleton-Century-Crofts (1968).

Bankson, N.W., *Bankson Language Screening Test*. Baltimore: University Park Press (1977).

Barry, H., *The Young Aphasic Child*. Washington, D.C.: The Alexander Graham Bell Association for the Deaf, Inc. (1969).

Barry, H., *The Young Aphasic Child: Evaluation and Training*. Washington, D.C.: The Volta Bureau (1961).

Basser, L.S., Hemiplegia of early onset and the faculty of speech with special reference to the effects of hemispherectomy. *Brain*, **85**, 427-460 (1962).

Bateman, R. Discussion summary—language intervention for the mentally retarded. In R.L. Schiefelbusch and L.L. Lloyd (Eds.), *Language Perspectives—Acquisition, Retardation, and Intervention*. Baltimore: University Park Press (1974).

Bates, E., *Language and Context: The Acquisition of Pragmatics*. New York: Academic Press, Inc. (1976a).

Bates, E., Pragmatics and sociolinguistics in child language. In D. Morehead, and A. Morehead (Eds.), *Normal and Deficient Child Language*. Baltimore: University Park Press (1976b).

Bateson, M.C., Mother-infant exchanges: The epigenesis of conversational interaction. *Annals of the New York Academy of Sciences*, **263**, 101-113 (1975).

Beasley, D.S., Forman, B., and Rintelmann, W., Perception of time-compressed CNC monosyllables by normal listeners. *Journal of Auditory Research*, **12**, 71-75 (1973).

Beasley, D.S., and Freeman, B.A., Time-altered speech as a measure of central auditory processing. In R.W. Keith (Ed.), *Central Auditory Dysfunction*. New York: Grune & Stratton, Inc. (1977).

Beasley, D.S., and Maki, J.E., Time- and frequency-altered speech. In N.J. Lass (Ed.), *Contemporary Issues in Experimental Phonetics*. New York: Academic Press, Inc. (1976).

Beasley, D.S., Maki, J.E., and Orchik, D.J., Children's perception of time compressed speech on two measures of speech discrimination. *Journal of Speech and Hearing Disorders*, **41**, 216-225 (1976).

Beasley, D.S., Schwimmer, S., and Rintelmann, W., Intelligibility of time-compressed CNC monosyllables. *Journal of Speech and Hearing Research*, **15**, 340-350 (1972).

Bedrosian, J.L., and Prutting, C.A., Communicative performance of mentally retarded adults in four conversational settings. *Journal of Speech and Hearing Research*, **21**, 79-95 (1978).

Benedict, H., Early lexical development: Comprehension and production. *Journal of Child Language*, **6**, 183-200 (1979).

Benton, A.L., Aphasia in children. *Education*, **79**, 408-412 (1959).

Benton, A.L., Developmental aphasia and brain damage. *Cortex*, **1**, 40-52 (1964).

Berg, F.S., *Educational Audiology: Hearing and Speech Management*. New York: Grune & Stratton, Inc. (1976).

Berg, F.S., Educational audiology. Short course presented at the Annual Convention of the American Speech-Language Hearing Association, Atlanta (1979).

Berg, F.S., and Fletcher, S. (Eds.), *The Hard of Hearing Child: Clinical and Educational Management*. New York: Grune & Stratton, Inc. (1970).

Berko, J., The child's learning of English morphology. *Word*, **14**, 150-177 (1958).

Berry, M.F., *Language Disorders of Children*. New York: Appleton-Century-Crofts (1969).

Berry, M.F., *Teaching Linguistically Handicapped Children*. Englewood Cliffs, N.J.: Prentice-Hall, Inc. (1980).

Berry, M.F., and Eisenson, J., *Speech Disorders: Principles and Practices of Therapy*. New York: Appleton-Century-Crofts (1956).

Berry, M.F., and Erickson, R.L., Speaking rate: Effects on children's comprehension of normal speech. *Journal of Speech and Hearing Research*, **16**, 367-374 (1973).

Bidder, R.T., Bryant, G., and Gray, O.P., Benefits to Down's syndrome children through training their mothers. *Archives of Disease in Childhood*, **50**, 383-386 (1975).

Blank, M., Gessner, M., and Esposito, A., Language without communication: A case study. *Journal of Child Language*, **6**, 329-352 (1979).

Blank, M., Rose, S.A., and Berlin, L., *The Language of Learning: The Pre-school Years*. New York: Grune & Stratton, Inc. (1978).

Bliss, L., and Peterson, D., Performance of aphasic and nonaphasic children on a sentence repetition task. *Journal of Communication Disorders*, **8**, 207-212 (1975).

Bloodstein, O., The rules of early stuttering. *Journal of Speech and Hearing Disorders*, **39**, 379-394 (1974).

Bloodstein, O., and Gantwerk, B.F., Grammatical function in relation to stuttering in young children, *Journal of Speech and Hearing Research*, **10**, 786-789 (1967).

Bloom, L., *Language Development: Form and Function of Emerging Grammars*. Cambridge, Mass.: MIT Press (1970).

Bloom, L., *One Word at a Time: The Use of Single-Word Utterances Before Syntax*. The Hague: Mouton (1973).

Bloom, L., Talking, understanding and thinking. In R. Schiefelbusch and L. Lloyd (Eds.), *Language Perspec-*

tives—Acquisition, Retardation and Intervention. Baltimore: University Park Press (1974).

Bloom, L., Hood, L., and Lightbrown, P., Imitation in language development: If, when, and why. *Cognitive Psychology,* **6,** 380-420 (1974).

Bloom, L., and Lahey, M., *Language Development and Language Disorders.* New York: John Wiley & Sons, Inc. (1978).

Bloom, L., Rocissano, L., and Hood, L., Adult-child discourse: Developmental interaction between information processing and linguistic knowledge. *Cognitive Psychology,* **8,** 521-552 (1976).

Blount, W.R., Concept usage research with the mentally retarded. *Psychological Bulletin,* **6,** 281-293 (1968).

Blumstein, S., *A Phonological Investigation of Aphasia in Speech.* The Hague: Mouton (1973).

Boehm, A.E., *Boehm Test of Basic Concepts Manual.* New York: Psychological Corporation (1971).

Bonvillian, J.D., and Nelson, K.E., Sign language acquisition in a mute autistic boy. *Journal of Speech and Hearing Disorders,* **41,** 339-347 (1976).

Bonvillian, J.D., Raeburn, V.P., and Horan, E.A., Talking to children: The effect of rate, intonation, and length on children's sentence imitation. *Journal of Child Language,* **6,** 459-467 (1979).

Boone, S.R., *Cerebral Palsy.* Indianapolis: Bobbs Merrill Co., Inc. (1975).

Borden, G.J., and Harris, K.S., *Speech Science Primer: Physiology, Acoustics, and Perception of Speech.* Baltimore: The Williams & Wilkins Co. (1980).

Bowerman, M., Semantic factors in the acquisition of rules for word use and sentence construction. In D.M. Morehead, and A.E. Morehead (Eds.), *Normal and Deficient Language.* Baltimore: University Park Press (1976).

Braine, M.D.S., The ontogeny of English phrase structure: The first phrase. *Language,* **39,** 1-13 (1963).

Brannon, J.B., and Murry, T., The spoken syntax of normal, hard-of-hearing, and deaf children. *Journal of Speech and Hearing Research,* **9,** 604-610 (1966).

Brennan, D., and Cullinan, W., Object identification and naming in cleft palate children. *Cleft Palate Journal,* **11,** 188-195 (1974).

Bricker, W.A., and Bricker, D.D., A program of language training for the severely language handicapped child. *Exceptional Children,* **36,** 101-111 (1970).

Broca, P., Nouvelle observation d'aphémie produite par une lésion de la mortié posterieure des deuxième et troisième circonvolutions frontales. *Bull. Soc. Anat. Paris,* 398-407 (1861a).

Broca, P., Remarques sur le siège de la faculté du language articulé, suivés d'une observation d'aphémie. *Bull. Soc. Anat. Paris,* 330-357 (1861b).

Broen, P.A., The verbal environment of the language-learning child. *Monographs of the American Speech and Hearing Association,* 17 (1972).

Brookhouser, P.E., Hixson, P.K., and Matkin, N.D., Early childhood language delay: The otolaryngologist's perspective. *The Laryngoscope,* **89,** 1898-1913 (1979).

Brooks, D.N., Otitis media and child development: Design factors in the identification and assessment of hearing loss. In D.G. Hanson and R.F. Ulvestad (Eds.), Otitis media and child development: Speech, language and education. *The Annals of Otology, Rhinology and Laryngology,* **88,** Supp. 60, 29-47 (1979).

Brotsky, S., Auditory figure-ground perception in neurologically impaired children. *Journal of Auditory Research,* **10,** 5-10 (1970).

Brown, J., *Mind, Brain and Consciousness: The Neuropsychology of Cognition.* New York: Academic Press (1977).

Brown, J.W., *Aphasia, by Arnold Pick.* Springfield, Ill.: Charles C Thomas, Publisher (1973).

Brown, R., *A First Language.* Cambridge, Mass.: Harvard University Press (1973).

Brown, R., and Bellugi, U., Three processes in the child's acquisition of syntax. *Harvard Educational Review,* **34,** 133-150 (1964).

Brown, R., and Fraser, C., The acquisition of syntax. Child Development Monographs, **29,** 43-79 (1964).

Bruner, J.S., The ontogenesis of speech acts. *Journal of Child Language,* **2,** 1-19 (1975).

Buffery, A.W., and Gray, J.A., Sex differences in development of spatial and linguistic skills. In C. Ounsted and D.C. Taylor (Eds.), *Gender Differences: Their Ontogeny and Significance.* Baltimore: The Williams & Wilkins Co. (1972).

Buium, N., Rynders, J., and Turnure, J., Early maternal linguistic environment of normal and Down's syndrome language-learning children. *American Journal of Mental Deficiency,* **79,** 52-58 (1974).

Butler, K., Short-course on auditory perception taught at the American Speech-Language and Hearing Association Convention, Washington, D.C. (1975). As cited in Willeford, J.A., and Billger, J.M., Auditory perception in children with learning disabilities. In J. Katz (Ed.) *Handbook of Clinical Audiology.* (2nd ed.) Baltimore: The Williams & Wilkins Co. (1978).

Cairns, H.S., and Williams, F., An analysis of the substitution errors of a group of standard English-speaking children. *Journal of Speech and Hearing Research,* **15,** 811-820 (1972).

Carpenter, R.L., and Freedman, P.P., Semantic relations used by normal and language-impaired children at Stage I. *Journal of Speech and Hearing Research,* **19,** 784-795 (1976).

Carrow, E., *Test for Auditory Comprehension of Language* (5th Ed.). Boston: Teaching Resources Corp. (1973).

Carrow-Woolfork, E., *Test for Auditory Comprehension of Language*. Austin, Texas: Learning Concepts (1970).

Cazden, C., Programs for promoting language skills in early childhood. Panel discussion at the Convention of the National Association for the Education of Young Children, Boston (1970).

Chalfant, J.C., and Scheffelin, M., *Cerebral Processing Dysfunctions in Children*. U.S. Department of Health, Education and Welfare, National Institute of Neurological Diseases and Stroke (1969).

Chapman, R.S., Developmental relationship between receptive and expressive language. In R.L. Schiefelbusch, and L.L. Lloyd (Eds.), *Language Perspectives-Acquisition, Retardation and Intervention*. Baltimore: University Park Press (1974).

Chappell, G.E., Childhood verbal apraxia and its treatment. *Journal of Speech and Hearing Disorders*, **38,** 362-368 (1973).

Chappell, G.E., Developmental aphasia revisited. *Journal of Communication Disorders*, **3,** 181-197 (1970).

Chappell, G.E., Generalized auditory agnosia: The first phase of treatment. *Journal of Speech and Hearing Disorders*, **37,** 152-161 (1972).

Chomsky, C., *The Acquisition of Syntax in Children from 5 to 10*. Cambridge, Mass.: MIT Press (1969).

Chomsky, N., *Aspects of the Theory of Syntax*. Cambridge, Mass.: MIT Press (1965).

Chomsky, N., *Syntactic Structures*. The Hague: Mouton (1957).

Chomsky, N., and Halle, M., *The Sound Pattern of English*. New York: Harper & Row, Publishers, Inc. (1968).

Clark, E.V., What's in a word: On the child's acquisition of semantics in his first language. In T. Moore (Ed.), *Cognitive Development and the Acquisition of Language*. New York: Academic Press, Inc. (1973).

Clark, H.H., and Clark, E.V., *Psychology and Language: An Introduction to Psycholinguistics*. New York: Harcourt Brace Jovanovich, Inc. (1977).

Clark, R., What's the use of imitation? *Journal of Child Language*, **4,** 341-358 (1977).

Clarren, S.K., and Smith, D.W., The fetal alcohol syndrome. *The New England Journal of Medicine*, **298,** 1063-1067 (1978).

Coggins, T.E., Relational meaning encoded in the two word utterances in Stage I Down's syndrome children. *Journal of Speech and Hearing Research*, **22,** 166-178 (1979).

Cohen, S.R., Congenital atresia of the larynx with endolaryngeal surgical correction: A case report. *Laryngoscope, 81,* 1607-1615 (1971).

Cole, M.F., and Cole, M., *Pierre Marie's Papers on Speech Disorders*. New York: Hafner Pub. Co. (1971).

Cole, R.A., Invariant features and feature detectors: Some developmental implications. In S.J. Segalowitz and F.A. Gruber, (Eds.), *Language Development and Neurological Theory*. New York: Academic Press, Inc. (1977).

Compton, A.J., Generative studies of children's phonological disorders. *Journal of Speech and Hearing Disorders*, **35,** 315-339 (1970).

Compton, A.J., and Hutton, J.S., *Compton-Hutton Phonological Assessment*. San Francisco: Carousel House (1978).

Condon, W.S., and Sander, L.W., Neonate movement is synchronized with adult speech: Interactional participation and language acquisition. *Science, 183,* 99-101 (1974).

Connell, P.J., Spradlin, J.E., and McReynolds, L.V., Some suggested criteria for evaluation of language programs. *Journal of Speech and Hearing Disorders*, **42,** 563-567 (1977).

Cooper, J.A., and Ferry, P.C., Acquired auditory verbal agnosia and seizures in childhood. *Journal of Speech and Hearing Disorders*, **43,** 176-184 (1978).

Costello, M.R., Evaluation of auditory behavior using the Flowers-Costello Test for Central Auditory Abilities. In R.W. Keith (Ed.), *Central Auditory Dysfunction*. New York: Grune & Stratton, Inc. (1977).

Courtney, D.P., Developmental language disorders related to pediatric syndromes. Paper presented at the Annual Convention of the American Speech-Language and Hearing Association, San Francisco (1978).

Courtright, J.A., and Courtright, I.C., Imitative modeling as a language intervention strategy: The effects of two mediating variables. *Journal of Speech and Hearing Research*, **22,** 389-402 (1979).

Courtright, J.A., and Courtright, I.C., Imitative modeling as a theoretical base for instructing language-disordered children. *Journal of Speech and Hearing Research*, **19,** 655-663 (1976).

Crabtree, M., *Houston Test for Language Development*. Houston: Houston Test Co. (1963).

Cramblit, N.S., and Siegel, G.M., The verbal environment of a language-impaired child. *Journal of Speech and Hearing Disorders*, **42,** 474-482, (1977).

Crocker, J.R., A phonological model of children's articulation competence. *Journal of Speech and Hearing Disorders*, **34,** 203-213 (1969).

Cromer, R.F., Receptive language in the mentally retarded: Processes and diagnostic distinctions. In R.L. Schiefelbusch, and L.L. Lloyd (Eds.), *Language Perspectives-Acquisition, Retardation, and Intervention.* Baltimore: University Park Press (1974b).

Cromer, R.F., The basis of childhood dysphasia: A linguistic approach. In M.A. Wyke (Ed.), *Developmental Dysphasia.* New York: Academic Press, Inc., 104-105 (1978).

Cromer, R.F., The cognitive hypothesis of language acquisition and its implications for child language deficiency. In D. Morehead, and A. Morehead (Eds.), *Normal and Deficient Child Language.* Baltimore: University Park Press (1976).

Cromer, R.F., The development of language and cognition: The cognition hypothesis. In B. Foss (Ed.), *New Perspectives in Child Development.* Harmondsworth, Middlesex: Penguin Books (1974a).

Cross, T., Some relationships between mothers and linguistic level in accelerated children. In E. Clark (Ed.), *Papers and Reports on Child Language Development* (No. 10). Stanford, Calif.: Stanford University Department of Linguistics (1975).

Crystal, D., Fletcher, P., and Garman, M., *The Grammatical Analysis of Language Disability.* New York: Elsevier North-Holland, Inc. (1976).

Cutting, J., and Eimos, P.D., Phonetic feature analyzers and the processing of speech in infants. In J.F. Kavanaugh and J.E. Cutting (Eds.), *The Role of Speech and Language.* Cambridge, Mass.: MIT Press (1975).

Dabul, B.L., Lingual incoordination—language delay—a case of a lazy tongue? *California Journal of Communication Disorders,* 30-33 (1971).

Dale, P.S., Is early pragmatic development measurable? *Journal of Child Language,* **7,** 1-12 (1980).

Dale, P.S., *Language Development: Structure and Function.* (2nd Ed.) New York: Holt, Rinehart & Winston, Inc. (1976).

Dalgleish, B., Cognitive processing and linguistic reference in autistic children. *Journal of Autism and Childhood Schizophrenia,* **5,** 353-361 (1975).

Daly, D.A., Cantrell, R.P., Cantrell, M.L., and Aman, L.A., Structuring speech therapy contingencies with an oral apraxic child. *Journal of Speech and Hearing Disorders,* **37,** 22-32 (1972).

DaMasio, A.R., Maurer, R.G., A neurological model for childhood autism. *Archives of Neurology,* **35,** 777-786 (1978).

Daniloff, R., Schuckers, G., and Feth, L., *The Physiology of Speech and Hearing: An Introduction.* Englewood Cliffs, N.J.: Prentice-Hall, Inc. (1980).

Darley, F.L., *Diagnosis and Appraisal of Communication Disorders.* Englewood Cliffs, N.J.: Prentice-Hall, Inc. (1964).

Darley, F.L. (Ed.), *Evaluation of Appraisal Techniques in Speech and Language Pathology.* Reading, Mass.: Addison-Wesley Publishing Co., Inc. (1979).

Darley, F.L., Aronson, A.E., and Brown, J.R., *Motor Speech Disorders.* Philadelphia: W.B. Saunders Co. (1975).

Darley, F.L., and Spriestersbach, D.C., *Diagnostic Methods in Speech Pathology.* (2nd ed.) New York: Harper & Row, Publishers, Inc. (1978).

Darwin, C., The perception of speech. In E.C. Carterette and M.P. Friedman (Eds.), *Handbook of Perception: Language and Speech.* Vol. 7. New York: Academic Press, Inc. (1976).

Davis, G.A., Linguistics and language therapy. The sentence construction board. *Journal of Speech and Hearing Disorders,* **38,** 205-214 (1973).

Davis, J., Performance of young hearing-impaired children on a test of basic concepts. *Journal of Speech and Hearing Research* **17,** 342-351 (1974).

Davis, S.M., Audition and speech perception. In R.L. Schiefelbusch (Ed.), *Bases of Language Intervention.* Vol. 1. Baltimore: University Park Press (1978).

Dawson, B., and Muma, J.R., *Parent-Child Development Center Curriculum.* Birmingham, Alabama: Parent-Child Development Center (1971).

DeAjuriaguerra, J., Jaeggi, A., Guignard, F., Kocker, F., Maquard, M., Roth, S., and Schmid, E., The development and prognosis of dysphasia in children. In D.M. Morehead and A.E. Morehead (Eds.), *Normal and Deficient Child Language.* Baltimore: University Park Press (1976).

Deal, J.L., and Darley, F.L., The influence of linguistic and situational variables on phonemic accuracy in apraxia of speech. *Journal of Speech and Hearing Research,* **15,** 639-653 (1972).

deHirsch, K., Jansky, J.J., and Langford, W.S., The oral language performance of premature children and controls. *Journal of Speech and Hearing Disorders,* **29,**60-69 (1964).

Delong, G.R., A neuropsychologic interpretation of infantile autism. In M. Rutter and E. Schopler (Eds.), *Autism: A Reappraisal of Concepts and Treatment.* New York: Plenum Press (1978).

Denckla, M.B., and Rudel, R.G., Naming of object-drawings by dyslexic and other learning disabled children. *Brain and Language,* **3,** 1-15, (1976).

Dennis, M., Language acquisition in a single hemisphere: Semantic organization. In D. Caplan (Ed.), *Biological Studies of Mental Processes.* Cambridge, Mass.: MIT Press (1980).

Dennis, M., and Kohn, B., Comprehension of syntax in infantile hemiplegics after cerebral hemidecortication: Left hemisphere superiority. *Brain and Language,* **2,** 472-482 (1975).

Dennis, M., and Whitaker, H.A., Hemispheric equipotentiality and language acquisition. In S.J. Segalowitz and F. A. Gruber (Eds.), *Language Development and Neurological Theory*. New York: Academic Press, Inc. (1977).

Dennis, M., and Whitaker, H.A., Language acquisition following hemidecortication: Linguistic superiority of the left over the right hemisphere. *Brain and Language*, **3**, 404-433 (1976).

DeRenzi, E., and Ferrari, C., The reporter's test: A sensitive test to detect expressive disturbances in aphasics. *Cortex*, **14**, 279-293 (1978).

DeRenzi, E., and Vignolo, L.A., The Token Test: A sensitive test to detect receptive disturbances in aphasics. *Brain*, **85**, 665-678 (1962).

Dever, R.B., *TALK: Teaching the American Language to Kids*. Columbus, Ohio: Charles E. Merrill Publishing Co. (1978).

de Villiers, J., and de Villiers, P., A cross-sectional study of the acquisition of grammatical morphemes in child speech. *Psycholinguistic Research*, **2**, 267-278 (1973).

de Villiers, J.G., and de Villiers, P.A., *Language Acquisition*. Cambridge, Mass.: Harvard University Press (1978).

DiSimoni, F., *The Token Test for Children*. Boston: Teaching Resources Corporation (1978).

Doleys, D.M., Cartelli, L.M., and Doster, J., Comparison of patterns of mother-child interaction. *Journal of Learning Disabilities*, **9**, 371-375 (1976).

Dore, J., A pragmatic description of early language development. *Journal of Psycholinguistics Research*, **3**, 3, 343-350 (1974).

Dore, J., Holophrases, speech acts and language universals. *Journal of Child Language*, **2**, 21-40 (1975).

Downs, M.J., and Silver, H., The A.B.C.D.'s to H.E.A.R. *Clinical Pediatrics*, **11**, 563-566 (1972).

DuBard, E., *Teaching Aphasics and Other Language Deficient Children: Theory and Application of the Association Method*. Jackson, Miss.: University Press of Mississippi (1974).

Dubos, R., Health and creative adaptation. *Human Nature*, **1**, 2-10 (1978).

Duchan, J., and Erickson, J.G., Normal and retarded children's understanding of semantic relations in different verbal contexts. *Journal of Speech and Hearing Research*, **19**, 767-777 (1976).

Dunn, L.M., *Expanded Manual for the Peabody Picture Vocabulary Test*. (Rev. Ed.) Circle Pines, Minn.: American Guidance Service, Inc. (1965).

Dunn, L.M., *Manual for the Peabody Picture Vocabulary Test*. Nashville, Tenn.: American Guidance Service (1959).

Dunn, L.M. *Peabody Picture Vocabulary Test*. Circle Pines, Minn.: American Guidance Service (1965).

Dunn, L.M., and Markwadt, F.C., *Peabody Individual Achievement Test*. Circle Pines, Minn.: American Guidance Service (1970).

Dworkin, J.P. and Culatta, R.A., *D-COME: A Practical Tool for the Clinical Examination of the Oral Mechanism*. Nicholasville, Ky.: Edgewood Press, Inc. (1980).

Edwards, M., Developmental verbal dyspraxia. *British Journal of Disorders of Communication*, **8**, 64-70 (1973).

Edwards, M.L., Perception and production in child phonology: The testing of four hypotheses. *Journal of Child Language*, **1**, 205-219 (1974).

Edwards, M.L., Phonological analysis of children's speech. Miniseminar presented at the Annual Convention of the American Speech-Language and Hearing Association, Detroit (1980a).

Edwards, M.L., The use of "favorite sounds" by children with phonological disorders. Paper presented at the Fifth Annual Boston University Conference On Language Development, Boston (1980b).

Efron, R., Temporal perception, aphasia and deja vu. *Brain*, **86**, 403-424 (1963).

Ehrlich, C., Shapiro, E., and Huttner, K., Communication skills in five-year old children with high-risk neonatal histories. *Journal of Speech and Hearing Research*, **16**, 522-529 (1973).

Eilers, R.E., and Minifie, F.D., Fricative discrimination in early infancy. *Journal of Speech and Hearing Research*, **18**, 158-167 (1975).

Eilers, R.E., and Oller, D.K., The role of speech discrimination in developmental sound substitutions. *Journal of Child Language*, **3**, 319-329 (1976).

Eilers, R.E., Wilson, W.R., and Moore, J.M., Developmental change in speech discrimination in infants. *Journal of Speech and Hearing Research*, **20**, 766-780 (1977).

Eimas, P.D., Auditory and linguistic processing of cues for place of articulation by infants. *Perception and Psychophysics* **16**, 513-521 (1974a).

Eimas, P.D., Linguistic processing of speech by young infants. In R.L. Schiefelbusch and L.L. Lloyd (Eds.), *Language Perspectives—Acquisition, Retardation and Intervention*. Baltimore: University Park Press (1974b).

Eimas, P.D., Speech perception in early infancy. In L.B. Cohen and P. Salapatek (Eds.), *Infant Perception: From Sensation to Cognition*. New York: Academic Press, Inc. (1975).

Eimas, P.D., Siqueland, E.R., Jusczyk, P., and Vigorito, J., Speech perception in infants. *Science*, **171**, 303-306 (1971).

Eisenberg, R.B., *Auditory Competence in Early Life: The Roots of Communicative Behavior.* Baltimore: University Park Press (1976).

Eisenberg, R.B., The organization of auditory behavior. *Journal of Speech and Hearing Research,* **13,** 453-471 (1970).

Eisenson, J., Aphasia in adults—classification and examination procedures. In L.E. Travis (Ed.), *Handbook of Speech Pathology.* New York: Appleton-Century-Crofts (1957a).

Eisenson, J., *Aphasia in Children.* New York: Harper & Row, Publishers, Inc. (1972).

Eisenson, J., Correlates of aphasia in adults. In L.E. Travis (Ed.), *Handbook of Speech Pathology.* New York: Appleton-Century-Crofts (1957b).

Eisenson, J., Developmental aphasia: A speculative view with therapeutic implications. *Journal of Speech and Hearing Disorders,* **33,** 3-13 (1968).

Eisenson, J., Developmental aphasia (dyslogia): A postulation of a unitary concept of the disorder. *Cortex,* **2,** 184-200 (1968).

Eisenson, J., *Examining for Aphasia.* (Rev. ed.) New York: The Psychological Corp. (1954).

Eisenson, J., Therapeutic problems and approaches with aphasic adults. In L.E. Travis (Ed.), *Handbook of Speech Pathology.* New York: Appleton-Century-Crofts (1957c).

Emerick, L.L., and Hatten, J.J., *Diagnosis and Evaluation in Speech Pathology.* (2nd ed.) Englewood Cliffs, N.J.: Prentice-Hall, Inc. (1979).

Engler, L., Hannah, E., and Longhurst, T., Linguistic analysis of speech samples: A practical guide for clinicians. *Journal of Speech and Hearing Disorders,* **38,** 192-204 (1973).

Erber, N.P., Speech perception by profoundly hearing-impaired children. *Journal of Speech and Hearing Disorders,* **44,** 255-270 (1979).

Ervin-Tripp, S.M., Imitation and structural change in children's language. In E.H. Lenneberg (Ed.), *New Directions in the Study of Language.* Cambridge, Mass.: MIT Press, 163-189 (1964).

Ervin-Tripp, S.M., and Mitchell-Kernan, C. (Eds.), *Child Discourse.* New York: Academic Press, Inc. (1977).

Everhart, R.W., Literature survey of growth and developmental factors in articulatory maturation. *Journal of Speech and Hearing Disorders,* **25,** 59-69 (1960).

Ewing, A., *Aphasia in Children.* London, England: Oxford University Press (1930).

Fadiman, A., The expanding world of Bill Rush. *Life,* **3,** 90-98 (1980).

Fairbanks, G., Everitt, W.L., and Jaeger, R.P., Methods for time or frequency compression-expansion of speech. *Transact of I.R.E.-P.G.A.,* AU-2, 7-12 (1954).

Falck, V.T., Auditory processing for the child with language disorders. *Exceptional Child,* **39,** 413-416 (1973).

Fay, W.H., Childhood echolalia: A group study of late abatement. *Folia Phoniatrica,* **19,** 297-306 (1967a).

Fay, W.H., Childhood echolalia in delayed, psychotic and neuropathologic speech patterns. *Folia Phoniatrica,* **18,** 68-71 (1966).

Fay, W.H., Mitigated echolalia of children. *Journal of Speech and Hearing Research,* **10,** 305-310 (1967b).

Fay, W.H., On the echolalia of the blind and of the autistic child. *Journal of Speech and Hearing Disorders,* **38,** 478-489 (1973).

Fay, W.H., and Butler, B.V., Echolalia, I.Q. and the developmental dichotomy of speech and language systems. *Journal of Speech and Hearing Research,* **11,** 365-371 (1968).

Fay, W.H., and Coleman, R.O., A human sound transducer/reproducer: Temporal capabilities of a profoundly echolalic child. *Brain and Language,* **4,** 396-402 (1977).

Fay, W.H., and Schuler, A.L., *Emerging Language in Autistic Children.* Baltimore: University Park Press (in press).

Ferry, P., Hall, S., and Hicks, J., "Dilapidated" speech: Developmental verbal dyspraxia. *Developmental Medicine and Child Neurology,* **17,** 749-756 (1975).

Fillmore, C., Some problems for case grammar. *Georgetown University Monographs for Language and Linguistics,* **24,** 35-56 (1971).

Fillmore, C., The case for case. In E. Bach and R. Harms (Eds.), *Universals in Linguistic Theory.* New York: Holt, Rinehart & Winston, Inc. (1968).

Fitzgerald, E., *Straight Language for the Deaf.* Washington, D.C.: Volta Bureau (1949).

Flowers, A., and Costello, M.R., The responses to distorted speech of children with severe articulation disorders. *Journal of Auditory Research,* **3,** 133-140 (1963).

Flowers, A., Costello, M., and Small, V., *Flowers-Costello Test of Central Auditory Abilities.* Dearborn, Mich.: Perceptual Learning Systems (1970).

Foster, R., Giddan, J.J., and Stark, J., *Assessment of Children's Language Comprehension.* Palo Alto, Calif.: Consulting Psychologists Press (1973).

Foster, R., Giddan, J.J., and Stark, J., *Manual for the Assessment of Children's Language Comprehension.* Palo Alto, Calif.: Consulting Psychologists Press (1972).

Fourcin, A.J., Language development in the absence of expressive speech. In E.H. Lenneberg and E. Lenneberg (Eds.), *Foundations of Language Development: A Multidisciplinary Approach.* (Vol. 2). New York: Academic Press, Inc. (1975).

Fraiberg, S., and Adelson, E., Self-representation in language and play: Observations of blind children. *The Psychoanalytic Quarterly*, **42**, 539-562 (1973).

Fraiberg, S. and Adelson, E., Self-representation in language and play: Observation of blind children. In E.H. Lenneberg, and E. Lenneberg (Eds.), *Foundations of Language Development* (Vol. 2). New York: Academic Press (1975).

Fraser, C., Bellugi, U., and Brown, R., Control of grammar in imitation, comprehension, and production. *Journal of Verbal Learning and Verbal Behavior*, **2**, 121-135 (1963).

Freedman, P.P., and Carpenter, R.L., Semantic relations used by normal and language impaired children in Stage I. *Journal of Speech and Hearing Research*, **19**, 784-795 (1976).

Freeman, B.A., and Beasley, D.S., Discrimination of time-altered sentential approximations and monosyllables by children with reading problems. *Journal of Speech and Hearing Research*, **21**, 497-506 (1978).

Fristoe, M., Appendix D/Language intervention systems: Programs published in kit form. In L.L. Lloyd (Ed.), *Communicative Assessment and Intervention Strategies*. Baltimore: University Park Press (1976).

Fristoe, M., *Language Intervention Systems for the Retarded: A Catalogue of Original Structured Language Programs in Use in the U.S.* Montgomery, Ala.: State of Alabama Department of Education (1975). (Available from: Language Intervention Systems for the Retarded, L.B. Wallace Development Center, P.O. Box 2224, Decatur, Alabama 35601.)

Fromkin, V.A., Krashen, S., Curtiss, S., Rigler, D., and Rigler, M., The development of language in Genie: A case of language acquisition beyond the "critical period." *Brain and Language*, **1**, 81-107 (1974).

Galaburda, A.M., LeMay, M., Kemper, T.L., and Geschwind, N., Right-left asymmetries in the brain. *Science*, **199**, 852-856 (1978).

Galaburda, A.M., Sanides, F., and Geschwind, N., Human brain: Cytoarchitectonic left-right asymmetries in the temporal speech region. *Archives of Neurology*, **35**, 812-817 (1978).

Gallagher, T.M., Revision behaviors in the speech of normal children developing language. *Journal of Speech and Hearing Research*, **20**, 303-318 (1977).

Gallagher, T.M., and Darnton, B.A., Conversational aspects of the speech of language-disordered children: Revision behaviors. *Journal of Speech and Hearing Research*, **21**, 118-135 (1978).

Garstecki, D.C., Borton, T.E., Stark, E.W., and Kennedy, B.T., Speech, language, and hearing problems in the Laurence-Moon-Biedl syndrome. *Journal of Speech and Hearing Disorders*, **37**, 407-413 (1972).

Gascon, C., Victor, D., Lombroso, D., and Goodglass, H., Language disorder, convulsive disorder and electroencephalographic abnormalities. *Archives of Neurology*, **28**, 156-162 (1973).

Geschwind, N., The clinical syndromes of the cortical connections. In D. Williams (Ed.), *Modern Trends in Neurology*, No. 5. London: Whitefriars Press (1964).

Geschwind, N., and Levitsky, W., Human brain: Left-right asymmetries in temporal speech region. *Science*, **161**, 186-187 (1968).

Geschwind, N., Segarra, J., and Quadfasel, F.A., Isolation of the speech area. *Neuropsychologia*, **7**, 327-340 (1968).

Gesell, A., *The First Five Years of Life*. New York: Harper & Row (1940).

Gleason, J.B., Code switching in children's language. In T. Moore (Ed.), *Cognitive Development and the Acquisition of Language*. New York: Academic Press, Inc. (1973).

Goldfarb, W., Levy, D., and Myers, D., The mother speaks to her schizophrenic child. Language in childhood schizophrenia. *Psychiatry*, **35**, 217-226 (1972).

Goldstein, K., *Aftereffects of Brain Injuries in War: Their Evaluation and Treatment*. New York: Grune & Stratton, Inc. (1942).

Goldstein, K., *Language and Language Disturbances*. New York: Grune & Stratton, Inc. (1948).

Goldstein, S.B., and Lanyon, R.I., Parent-clinicians in the language training of an autistic child. *Journal of Speech and Hearing Disorders*, **36**, 552-560 (1971).

Goodglass, H., and Kaplan, E., *The Assessment of Aphasia and Related Disorders*. Philadelphia: Lea and Febiger (1972).

Goodman, K., Reading: Analysis of oral reading miscues: Applied psycholinguistics. *Reading Research Quarterly*, **5**, 9-30 (1969).

Goodman, K., and Goodman, Y., Learning about psycholinguistic processes by analyzing oral reading. *Harvard Educational Review*, **47**, 317-333 (1977).

Gottsleben, R.H., Tyack, D., and Buschini, G., Three case studies in language training: Applied linguistics. *Journal of Speech and Hearing Disorders*, **39**, 213-224 (1974).

Graham, J., and Graham, L., Language behavior of the mentally retarded: Syntactic characteristics. *American Journal Mental Deficiency*, **75**, 623-629 (1971).

Graham, L.W., Language programming and intervention. In L.L. Lloyd (Ed.), *Communication Assessment and Intervention Strategies*. Baltimore: University Park Press (1976).

Graham, M.D. (Ed.), *Cleft Palate: Middle Ear Disease and Hearing Loss*. Springfield, Ill.: Charles C Thomas, Publisher (1978).

Graham, J.T., and Graham, L.W., Language behavior of the mentally retarded: Syntactic Characteristics. *American Journal of Mental Deficiency,* **75,** 623-629 (1971).

Greene, M.C.L., Speechless and backward at three. *British Journal of Disorders of Communication,* **2,** 134-145 (1967).

Greenfield, P.M., and Smith, J.H., *The Structure of Communication in Early Language Development.* New York: Academic Press, Inc. (1976).

Griswold, L.E., and Commings, J., The expressive vocabulary of preschool deaf children. *American Annals of the Deaf,* **119,** 16-28 (1974).

Groht, M.A., *Natural Language for Deaf Children.* Washington, D.C.: Alexander Graham Bell Association for the Deaf (1958).

Gubbay, S.S., *The Clumsy child: A Study of Developmental Apraxic and Agnostic Ataxia.* London: W. B. Saunders Co. Ltd. (1975).

Guess, D., Sailor, W., and Baer, D.M., To teach language to retarded children. In R.L. Schiefelbusch and L.L. Lloyd (Eds.), *Language Perspectives: Acquisition, Retardation, and Intervention.* Baltimore: University Park Press (1974).

Guess, D., Smith, J.O., and Ensminger, E.E., The role of nonprofessional persons in teaching language skills to mentally retarded children. *Exceptional Children,* **37,** 447-453 (1971).

Guralnick, M.J., A language development program for severely handicapped children. *Exceptional Children,* **39,** 45-49 (1972).

Guralnick, M.J., and Paul-Brown, D., The nature of verbal interactions among handicapped and nonhandicapped preschool children. *Child Development,* **48,** 254-260 (1977).

Guttman, E., Aphasia in children. *Brain,* **65,** 205-219 (1942).

Hadden, W.B., On certain defects of articulation in children with cases illustrating the result of education of the oral system. *Journal of Mental Science,* **37,** 96 (1891).

Hagen, C., Porter, W., and Brink, J., Nonverbal communication: An alternate mode of communication for the child with severe cerebral palsy. *Journal of Speech and Hearing Disorders,* **38,** 448-455 (1973).

Hall, P.K., The occurrence of disfluencies in language-disordered school-age children. *Journal of Speech and Hearing Disorders,* **42,** 364-369 (1977).

Hall, P.K., and Tomblin, J.B., A follow-up study of children with articulation and language disorders. *Journal of Speech and Hearing Disorders,* **43,** 227-241 (1978).

Halliday, M.A.K., *Explorations in the Functions of Language.* New York: Elsevier North-Holland, Inc. (1973).

Halliday, M.A.K., *Explorations in the Functions of Language.* New York: Elsevier North-Holland, Inc. (1977a).

Halliday, M.A.K., *Learning How to Mean: Explorations in the Development of Language.* London: Edward Arnold (1975).

Halliday, M.A.K., *Learning How to Mean: Explorations in the Development of Language.* New York: Elsevier North-Holland, Inc. (1977b).

Hammill, D., and Larsen, S., The effectiveness of psycholinguistic training. *Exceptional Children,* **40,** 5-13 (1974).

Hanson, D.G., and Ulvestad, R.F. (Eds.), Otitis media and child development: Speech, language and education. *The Annals of Otology, Rhinology and Laryngology,* Supplement 60, Vol. 88, No. 5, Part 2 (1979).

Hardy, W.G., On language disorders in young children: A reorganization of thinking. *Journal of Speech and Hearing Disorders,* **30,** 3-16 (1965).

Harrison, S., A review of research in speech and language development of the mentally retarded child. *American Journal of Mental Deficiency,* **63,** 236-240 (1958).

Hartman, D.E., and Hood, S.E., Diagnosing communication deficits in cerebral palsy. *Ohio Journal of Speech and Hearing,* **9,** 41-57 (1973).

Hartung, J.R., A review of procedures to increase verbal imitation skills and functional speech in autistic children. *Journal of Speech and Hearing Disorders,* **35,** 203-217 (1970).

Haskins, J., A phonetically-balanced test of speech discrimination for children. Unpublished Master's thesis. Northwestern University, Evanston, Ill. (1949).

Hauser, S.L., Delong, G.R., and Rosman, N.P., Pneumographic findings in the infantile autism syndrome: A correlation with temporal lobe disease. *Brain,* **98,** 667-688 (1975).

Head, H., *Aphasia and Kindred Disorders of Speech.* (2 vols.) Cambridge University Press (1926). Reprinted by Hafner Publishing Co., Inc., New York (1963).

Healy, J., A study of hyperlexia. Doctoral dissertation. Cleveland: Case Western Reserve University (1980).

Hecaen, H., Acquired aphasia in children and the ontogenesis of hemispheric functional specialization. *Brain and Language,* **3,** 114-134 (1976).

Hegde, M.N., and Gierut, J., The operant training and generalization of pronouns and a verb form in a language delayed child. *Journal of Communication Disorders,* **12,** 23-34 (1979).

Hendrick, D.L., Prather, E.M., and Tobin, A.R., *Sequenced Inventory of Communication Development.* Seattle: University of Washington Press (1975).

Hermelin, B., and Frith, U., Psychological studies of childhood autism: Can autistic children make sense of what they see and hear? *Journal of Special Education,* **5,** 107-117 (1971).

Hetenyi, K.B., Interactions between language-delayed children and their parents—A case study. Paper presented at the Annual Convention of the American Speech-Language and Hearing Association, Las Vegas (1974).

Hier, D.B., LeMay, M., Rosenberger, P.B., and Perlo, V.P., Developmental dyslexia: Evidence for a subgroup with a reversal of cerebral asymmetry. *Archives of Neurology*, **35**, 90-92 (1978).

Hodson, B.W., A preliminary hierarchical model for phonological remediation. *Language, Speech and Hearing Services in Schools*, **9**, 236-240 (1978).

Hodson, B.W., *The Assessment of Phonological Processes*. Danville, Ill.: The Interstate Printers and Publishers (1980).

Holinger, P.H., Johnson, K.C., and Schiller, F., *Annals of Otolaryngology, Rhinology and Laryngology*, 581-606 (1954).

Holland, A.L., Language therapy for children: Some thoughts on context and content. *Journal of Speech and Hearing Disorders*, **40**, 514-523 (1975).

Hopper, R., and Naremore, R.C., *Children's Speech: A Practical Introduction to Communication Development*. New York: Harper & Row, Publishers, Inc. (1973).

Horstmeier, D.S., and MacDonald, J.D., *A Trainer's Manual for Ready, Set, Go and the Environmental Language Intervention Program*. Columbus, Ohio: Charles E. Merrill Publishing Co. (1978).

Horstmeier, D.S., and MacDonald, J.D., *Environmental Prelanguage Battery*. Columbus, Ohio: Charles E. Merrill Publishing Co. (1978).

Horstmeier, D.S., and MacDonald, J.D., *Ready, Set, Go—Talk to Me*. Columbus, Ohio: Charles E. Merrill Publishing Co. (1978).

Hutchinson, B.B., Hanson, M.L., and Mecham, M.J., *Diagnostic Handbook of Speech Pathology*. Baltimore: The Williams & Wilkins Co. (1979).

Hymes, D., Competence and performance in linguistic theory. In R. Huxley and E. Ingram (Eds.), *Language Acquisition: Models and Methods*. New York: Academic Press, Inc. (1971).

Ingram, D., Current issues in child phonology. In D.M. Morehead and A.E. Morehead (Eds.), *Normal and Deficient Child Language*. Baltimore: University Park Press (1976a).

Ingram, D., *Phonological Disability in Children*. New York: Elsevier North-Holland, Inc. (1976b).

Ingram, D., The relationship between comprehension and production. In R.L. Schiefelbusch, and L.L. Lloyd (Eds.), *Language Perspectives—Acquisition, Retardation and Intervention*. Baltimore: University Park Press (1974).

Ingram, D., and Eisenson, J., Therapeutic approaches III: Establishing and developing language in congenitally aphasic children. In J. Eisenson, *Aphasia in Children*. New York: Harper & Row, Publishers, Inc. (1972).

Ingram, T.T.S., and Reid, J.F., Developmental aphasia observed in a department of child psychiatry. *Archives of Disease in Childhood*, **31**, 161-172 (1956).

Irwin, J.V., and Marge, M., (Eds.), *Principles of Childhood Language Disabilities*. New York: Meredith Corp. (1972).

Irwin, O.C., *Communication Variables of Cerebral Palsied and Mentally Retarded Children*. Springfield, Ill., Charles C Thomas, Publisher (1972).

Ivimey, G., The written syntax of an English deaf child: An exploration of method. *British Journal of Disordered Communication*, **2**, 105-120 (1976).

Jaffee, M.B., An investigation of perceptual abilities in developmental apraxia of speech: A comparison with functional articulation disorders. Doctoral dissertation, Pittsburgh: University of Pittsburgh (1979).

Jaffe, M.L., Perceptual abilities in apraxic and articulation-disordered children. Paper presented at the Annual Convention of the American-Speech-Language and Hearing Association, Atlanta (1979).

Jakobson, R., *Child Language, Aphasia, and Phonological Universals*. The Hague: Mouton (1968).

Jansky, J., and deHirsch, K., *Preventing Reading Failure: Prediction, Diagnosis, Intervention*. New York: Harper & Row, Publishers, Inc. (1972).

Jeffree, D., Wheldall, K., and Mittler, P., Facilitating two-word utterances in two Down's Syndrome boys. *American Journal of Mental Deficiency*, **78**, 117-122 (1973).

Johnson, A.F., Newman, C.W., and Glennan-Brethauer, N., Central auditory and language disorders associated with conductive hearing loss. Paper presented at the Annual Convention of the American Speech-Language Hearing Association, Atlanta, Georgia (1979).

Johnson, C.A., and Katz, R.C., Using parents as change agents for their children: A review. *Child Psychology and Psychiatry*, **14**, 181-200 (1973).

Johnson, D.J., and Myklebust, H.R., *Learning Disabilities: Educational Principles and Practices*. New York: Grune & Stratton, Inc. (1967).

Johnson, O.G., *Tests and Measurements in Child Development: Handbook II*. (2 vols.) San Francisco: Jossey-Bass, Inc., Publishers (1976).

Johnson, O.G., and Bommarito, J.W., *Tests and Measurements in Child Development: A Handbook*. San Francisco: Jossey-Bass, Inc., Publishers (1971).

Johnson, W., Darley, F.L., and Spriestersbach, D.C., *Diagnostic Methods in Speech Pathology*. New York: Harper & Row, Publishers, Inc. (1963).

Johnston, J.R., and Schery, T.K., The use of grammatical morphemes of children with communication disorders. In D.M. Morehead, and A.E. Morehead (Eds.), *Normal and Deficient Child Language.* Baltimore: University Park Press (1976).

Jordan, T., Language and mental retardation: A review of the literature. In R. Schiefelbusch, R. Copeland, and J. Smith (Eds.), *Language and Mental Retardation,* New York: Holt, Rinehart & Winston, Inc. (1967).

Kamhi, A.G., Nonlinguistic symbolic and conceptual abilities of language impaired and normally developing children. *Journal of Speech and Hearing Research* **24,** 446-453 (1981).

Kanner, L., Autistic disturbances of affective contact. *Nervous Child,* **2,** 217-250 (1943).

Kanner, L., Irrelevant and metaphorical language in early infantile autism. *American Journal of Psychiatry,* **103,** 242-246 (1946).

Karlin, I.W., Congenital verbal-auditory agnosia. *Pediatrics,* **7,** 60-69 (1951).

Kastein, S., and Gillman, A.E., The interaction of emotional stress and language development: Case studies of three visually impaired children. *Journal of Communication Disorders,* **9,** 135-141 (1976).

Katz, J. (Ed.), *Handbook of Clinical Audiology.* (2nd ed.) Baltimore: The Williams & Wilkins Co. (1978).

Kavanagh, J.F., and Mattingly, I.G., *Language by Ear and Eye: The Relationship Between Speech and Reading.* Cambridge, Mass.: MIT Press (1972).

Keenan, E.O., and Schieffelin, B.B., Topic as a discourse notion: A study of topic in the conversations of children and adults. In C.N. Li (Ed.), *Subject and Topic.* New York: Academic Press, Inc. (1976).

Keith, R. (Ed.), *Central Auditory Dysfunction.* New York: Grune & Stratton, Inc. (1977).

Kemp, J.C., and Dale, P.S., Spontaneous imitation and free speech: A grammatical comparison. Paper presented to the Society for Research in Child Development, Philadelphia (1973).

Kinsbourne, M., The ontogeny of cerebral dominance. In D. Aaronson, and R.W. Rieber (Eds.), Developmental Psycholinguistic and Communication Disorders. *Annals of the New York Academy of Sciences,* **263,** New York: New York Academy of Sciences (1975).

Kinsbourne, M., and Caplan, P.J., *Children's Learning and Attention Problems.* Boston: Little, Brown & Co. (1979).

Kinsbourne, M., and Hiscock, M., Does cerebral dominance develop? In S.J. Segalowitz and F.A. Gruber (Eds.), *Language Development and Neurological Theory.* New York: Academic Press, Inc. (1977).

Kirk, S.A., and Kirk W.D., *Psycholinguistic Learning Disabilities.* Urbana, Ill.: University of Illinois Press (1971).

Kirk, S.A., and McCarthy, J.J., The Illinois test of psycholinguistic abilities—an approach to differential diagnosis. *American Journal of Mental Deficiency,* **66,** 399-412 (1961).

Kirk, S.A., McCarthy, J., and Kirk, W.D., *Illinois Test of Psycholinguistic Abilities.* (Rev. Ed.) Urbana, Ill.: University of Illinois Press (1968).

Klassen, E., *The Syndrome of Specific Dyslexia.* Baltimore: University Park Press (1972).

Kleffner, F.R., The direct teaching approach for children with auditory processing and learning disabilities. *Acta Symbolica,* **6,** 65-93 (1975).

Knight, G., A comment on Muma's "The communication game: Dump and play." Letter to the Editor, *Journal of Speech and Hearing Disorders,* **41,** 277-278 (1976).

Kogan, K.L., Wimberger, H.C., and Bobbitt, R.A., Analysis of mother-child interaction in young mental retardates. *Child Development,* **4,** 799-812 (1969).

Kohn, B., Right hemisphere speech representation and comprehension of syntax after left cerebral injury. *Brain and Language,* **9,** 350-361 (1980).

Kolers, E., Experiments in reading. *Scientific American,* 227, 84-91, (1972).

Konkle, D., Freeman, B., Riggs, D., et al., Calibration procedures for time-compressed/expanded speech. In E. Foulke (Ed.), *Proceedings of the Third Louisville Conference on Time-Compressed Speech.* Louisville: University of Louisville (1977).

Krashen, S.D., The critical period for language acquisition and its possible bases. In D. Aaronson and R.W. Rieber (Eds.), Developmental Psycholinguistics and Communication Disorders. *Annals of the New York Academy of Sciences,* 263, New York: New York Academy of Sciences (1975).

Kuhl, P.K., and Miller, J.D., Speech perception by the chinchilla: Voice-voiceless distinction in alveolar plosive consonants. *Science,* **190,** 69-72 (1975).

Kurdziel, S.A., Noffsinger, D., and Olson, W., Performance by cortical lesion patients on 40 and 60% time-compressed materials. *Journal of the American Audiological Society,* **2,** 3-7 (1976).

Kurdziel, S.A., Rintelmann, W.F., and Beasley, D., Performance of noise-induced hearing-impaired listeners on time-compressed CNC monosyllables. *Journal of the American Audiological Society,* **1,** 54-60 (1975).

Lackner, J., A developmental study of language behavior in retarded children. *Neuropsychologia,* **6,** 301-320 (1968).

Landau, W., Goldstein, R., and Kleffner, F.R., Congenital aphasia: A clinicopathologic study. *Neurology,* **10,** 915-921 (1960).

Landau, W.U., and Kleffner, F.R., Syndrome of acquired

aphasia with convulsive disorder in children. *Neurology*, **7**, 523-530 (1957).

Lasky, E.Z., and Tobin, H., Linguistic and nonlinguistic competing message effects. *Journal of Learning Disabilities*, **6**, 243-250 (1973).

Lee, F.F., Time compression of speech by the sampling method. *Journal of Audiological Engineering Society*, **20**, 738-742 (1972).

Lee, L.L., A screening test for syntax development. *Journal of Speech and Hearing Disorders*, **35**, 103-112 (1970).

Lee, L.L., *Developmental Sentence Analysis*. Evanston, Ill: Northwestern University Press (1974).

Lee, L.L., *Developmental Sentence Analysis: A Grammatical Assessment Procedure for Speech and Language Clinicians*. Evanston, Ill.: Northwestern University Press (1974).

Lee, L.L., Developmental sentence types: A method for comparing normal and deviant syntactic development. *Journal of Speech and Hearing Disorders*, **31**, 311-330 (1966).

Lee, L.L., *The Northwestern Syntax Screening Test*. Evanston, Ill.: Northwestern University Press (1969).

Lee, L.L., and Canter, S.M., Developmental sentence scoring: A clinical procedure for estimating syntactic development in children's spontaneous speech. *Journal of Speech and Hearing Disorders*, **36**, 315-340 (1971).

Lee, L.L., Koenigsknecht, R.A., and Mulhern, S.T., *Interactive Language Development Teaching: The Clinical Presentation of Grammatical Structure*. Evanston, Ill.: Northwestern University Press (1975).

LeMay, M., and Geschwind, N., Asymmetries of the human cerebral hemispheres. In A. Caramazza, and E.B. Zurif (Eds.), *Language Acquisition and Language Breakdown*. Baltimore: Johns Hopkins Press (1978).

Lenneberg, E.H., *Biological Foundations of Language*. New York: John Wiley & Sons, Inc. (1967).

Lenneberg, E.H., Understanding language without the ability to speak. *Journal of Abnormal and Social Psychology*, **65**, 419-425 (1962).

Leonard, L.B., A preliminary view of generalization in language training. *Journal of Speech and Hearing Disorders*, **39**, 429-436 (1974).

Leonard, L.B., Language impairment in children. *Merrill-Palmer Quarterly*, **25**, 205-232 (1979).

Leonard, L.B., *Meaning in Child Language: Issues in the Study of Early Semantic Development*. New York: Grune & Stratton, Inc. (1976).

Leonard, L.B., Relational meaning and the facilitation of slow-learning children's language. *American Journal of Mental Deficiency*, **80**, 180-185 (1975).

Leonard, L.B., Teaching by the rules. *Journal of Speech and Hearing Disorders*, **38**, 174-183 (1973).

Leonard, L.B., What is deviant language? *Journal of Speech and Hearing Disorders*, **37**, 427-446 (1972).

Leonard, L.B., Bolders, J.G., and Miller, J.A., An examination of the semantic relations reflected in the language usage of normal and language disordered children. *Journal of Speech and Hearing Research*, **19**, 371-392 (1976).

Leonard, L.B., and Holland, A., What child language interventionists can teach adult aphasiologists or vice versa. Miniseminar presented at the Annual Convention of the American Speech-Language and Hearing Association, Detroit (1980).

Leonard, L.B., Prutting, C.A., Perozzi, J.A., and Berkley, R.K., Nonstandardized approaches to the assessment of language behaviors. *Asha*, **20**, 371-379 (1978).

Lerman, J., Ross, M., and McLaughlin, R., A picture-identification test for hearing-impaired children. *Journal of Auditory Research*, **5**, 273-278 (1965).

Lesser, R., *Linguistic Investigation of Aphasia*. New York: Elsevier North-Holland, Inc. (1978).

Liberman, A.M., Cooper, F.S., Harris, K.S., MacNeilage, P.F., and Studdert-Kennedy, M.G., Some observations on a model for speech perception. In W. Wathen-Dunn (Ed.), *Models for the Perception of Speech and Visual Form*. Cambridge, Mass.: MIT Press (1967a).

Liberman, A.M., Cooper, F.S., Shankweiler, D.P., and Studdert-Kennedy, M.G., Perception of the speech code. *Psychological Reivew*, **74**, 431-461 (1967b).

Lieberman, P., Speech acoustics and perception. In H. Halpern (Ed.), *Studies in Communicative Disorders Series*. Indianapolis: The Bobbs-Merrill Co., Inc. (1972).

Liles, B.Z., Shulman, M.D., and Bartlett, S., Judgments of grammaticality by normal and language-disordered children. *Journal of Speech and Hearing Disorders*, **42**, 199-209 (1977).

Ling, D., *Speech and the Hearing-Impaired Child: Theory and Practice*. Washington, D.C.: The Alexander Graham Bell Association for the Deaf, Inc. (1976).

Ling, D., and Ling, A.H., *Aural Habilitation: The Foundations of Verbal Learning in Hearing-Impaired Children*. Washington, D.C.: The Alexander Graham Bell Association for the Deaf, Inc. (1978).

Lloyd, L.L. (Ed.), *Communication Assessment and Intervention Strategies*. Baltimore: University Park Press (1976).

Locke, J.L., The inference of speech perception in the phonologically disordered child. Part I: A rationale, some criteria, the conventional tests. *Journal of Speech and Hearing Disorders*, **45**, 431-444 (1980a).

Locke, J.L., The inference of speech perception in the phonologically disordered child. Part II: Some clinically novel procedures, their use, some findings. *Journal of Speech and Hearing Disorders*, **45**, 445-468 (1980b).

Logue, R., and McClumpha, S., Apraxia of speech in children: A case description. Paper presented at the Annual Convention of the American Speech-Language and Hearing Association, New York (1970).

Lovaas, O.I., *The Autistic Child*. New York: Halstead Press (1977).

Love, R.J., Oral language behavior of older cerebral palsied children. *Journal of Speech and Hearing Research*, **7**, 349-359 (1964).

Lowe, A.D., and Campbell, R.A., Temporal discrimination in aphasoid and normal children. *Journal of Speech and Hearing Research*, **8**, 313-314 (1965).

Lowell, E.L., and Pollack, D.B., Remedial practices with the hearing impaired. In S. Dickson (Ed.), *Communication Disorders: Remedial Principles and Practices*. Glenview, Illinois: Scott, Foresman & Co. (1974).

Lozar, B., Wepman, J.M., and Haas, W., Syntactic indices of language use of mentally retarded and normal children. *Language and Speech*, **16**, 22-33 (1973).

Ludlow, C.L., Children's language disorders: Recent research advances. *Annals of Neurology*, **7**, 497-507 (1980).

Macaluso-Haynes, S., Developmental apraxia of speech: Symptoms and Treatment. In D.F. Johns (Ed.), *Clinical Management of Neurogenic Communication Disorders*. Boston: Little, Brown & Co. (1978).

Maccoby, E.E., and Jacklin, C.N., *The Psychology of Sex Differences*. Stanford, Calif.: Stanford University Press (1974).

MacDonald, J.D., *Environmental Language Inventory*. Columbus, Ohio: Charles E. Merrill Publishing Co. (1978).

MacDonald, J.D., and Blott, J.P., Environmental language intervention: A rationale for diagnostic and training strategy through rules, context and generalization. *Journal of Speech and Hearing Disorders*, **39**, 395-415 (1974).

MacDonald, J.D., Blott, J.P., Gordon, K., Spiegel, B., and Hartmann, M., An experimental parent-assisted treatment program for preschool language-delayed children. *Journal of Speech and Hearing Disorders*, **39**, 379-394 (1974).

MacNamara, J., The cognitive basis of learning in infants. *Psychological Review*, **79**, 1-13 (1972).

Maki, J.E., Beasley, D., Shoup. J., et. al., Speech discrimination and response latency of normal-hearing and hearing-impaired children as a function of time compression. Paper presented at American Speech-Language and Hearing Association Convention, Houston (1976).

Manning, W.H., Johnston, K.L., and Beasley, D.S., The performance of children with auditory perceptual disorders on a time-compressed speech discrimination measure. *Journal of Speech and Hearing Disorders*, **42**, 77-84 (1977).

Marge, M., The general problem of language disabilities in children. In M. Marge, and J.V. Irwin (Eds.), *Principles of Childhood Language Disabilities*. Englewood Cliffs, N.J.: Prentice-Hall, Inc. (1972).

Marge, M., and Irwin, J.V. (Eds.), *Principles of Childhood Language Disabilities*. Englewood Cliffs, N.J.: Prentice-Hall, Inc. (1972).

Marquardt, T.P., and Saxman, J.H., Language comprehension and auditory discrimination in articulation deficient kindergarten children. *Journal of Speech and Hearing Research*, **15**, 382-389 (1972).

Marshall, N.R., and Hegrenes, J., The use of written language as a communication system for an autistic child. *Journal of Speech and Hearing Disorders*, **37**, 258-261 (1972).

Marshall, N.R., Hegrenes, J.R., and Goldstein, S., Verbal interactions: Mothers and their retarded children vs. mothers and their nonretarded children. *American Journal of Mental Deficiency*, **77**, 415-419 (1973).

Martin, A.D., Some objections to the term of apraxia of speech. *Journal of Speech and Hearing Disorders*, **39**, 53-64 (1974).

Martin, A.D., and Rigrodsky, S., An investigation of phonological impairment in aphasia. Part I and II. *Cortex*, **10**, 317-328, 329-349 (1974).

Martin, F.N. (Ed.), *Pediatric Audiology*, Englewood Cliffs, N.J.: Prentice-Hall, Inc. (1978).

Massaro, D.W. (Ed.), *Understanding Language*. New York: Academic Press, Inc. (1975).

Massengill, R., Certain speech characteristics of mentally retarded children. *Folia Phoniatrica*, **22**, 139-142 (1970).

Mattingly, I.G., Reading, the linguistic process, and linguistic awareness. In J.E. Kavanagh and I.G. Mattingly (Eds.), *Eye: Language by Ear and By Eye*. Cambridge, Mass.: MIT Press (1972).

McClumpha, S., and Logue, R., Approaches to children with motor programming disorders of speech. Paper presented to the American Speech-Language and Hearing Convention, San Francisco (1972).

McDonald, E.T., and Chance, B., *Cerebral Palsy*. Englewood Cliffs: Prentice-Hall, Inc. (1964).

McDonald, E.T., and Schultz, A.R., Communication boards for cerebral-palsied children. *Journal of Speech and Hearing Disorders*, **38**, 73-88 (1973).

McFie, J., Intellectual impairment in children with localized post-infantile cerebral lesions. *Journal of Neurology, Neurosurgery and Psychiatry*, 361-365 (1961).

McGinnis, M.A., *Aphasic Children: Identification and Education by the Association Method*. Washington, D.C.: Alexander Graham Bell Association for the Deaf (1963).

McGinnis, M.A., Kleffner, F.R., and Goldstein, R., Teaching aphasic children. *Volta Review*, **58**, 239-244 (1956).

McGrady, H.J., Language pathology and learning disabilities. In H.R. Myklebust (Ed.), *Progress in Learning Disabilities*. (Vol. I) New York: Grune & Stratton, Inc. (1968).

McGrady, H.J., and Olson, D.A., Visual and auditory learning processes in normal children with learning disabilities. *Exceptional Children*, **36**, 581-589 (1970).

McLean, L.P., and McLean, J.E., A language training program for nonverbal autistic children. *Journal of Speech and Hearing Disorders*, **39**, 186-193 (1974).

McLean, J.E., and Snyder-McLean, L.K., *A Transactional Approach to Early Language Training*. Columbus, Ohio: Charles E. Merrill Publishing Co. (1978).

McNeill, D., Developmental psycholinguistics. In F. Smith and G.A. Miller (Eds.), *The Genesis of Language*. Cambridge, Mass.: MIT Press (1966).

McNeill, D., Developmental psycholinguistics. Paper to appear in Proceedings of Conference on Language Development in Children, Old Point Comfort, Va. (April 1965).

McNeill, D., *The Acquisition of Language: The Study of Developmental Psycholinguistics*. New York: Harper & Row, Publishers, Inc. (1970).

McReynolds, L.V. (Ed.), Developing systematic procedures for training children's language. *ASHA Monographs*, **18**, American Speech and Hearing Association. (1974).

McReynolds, L.V., Operant conditioning for investigating speech sound discrimination in aphasic children. *Journal of Speech and Hearing Research*, **9**, 519-528 (1966).

McReynolds, L.V., and Engmann, D.L., *Distinctive Feature Analysis of Misarticulations*. Baltimore: University Park Press (1975).

McReynolds, L.V., and Huston, D.A., A distinctive feature analysis of children's misarticulations. *Journal of Speech and Hearing Disorders*, **36**, 155-166 (1971).

Mecham, M.J., Berko, M.J., Berko, F.G., and Palmer, M.F., *Communication Training in Childhood Brain Damage*. Springfield, Ill.: Charles C Thomas, Publisher (1966).

Mecham, M., Jex, J., and Jones, J., *Utah Test of Language Development*. Salt Lake City: Communication Research Associates (1967).

Mecham, M.J., Jex, J.L., and Jones, J.D., *Utah Test of Language Development*. (Rev. Ed.) Salt Lake City, Utah: Communication Research Association (1967).

Meier, J.H., Prevalance and characteristics of learning disabilities found in second grade children. *Journal of Learning Disabilities*, **4**, 1-16 (1971).

Menyuk, P., Alternation of rules in children's grammar. *Journal of Verbal Learning and Verbal Behavior*, **8**, 480-488 (1964a).

Menyuk, P., A preliminary evaluation of grammatical capacity in children. *Journal of Verbal Learning and Verbal Behavior*, **2**, 429-439 (1963).

Menyuk, P., Comparison of grammar of children with functionally deviant and normal speech. *Journal of Speech and Hearing Research*, **8**, 109-121 (1964).

Menyuk, P., *Language and Maturation*. Cambridge, Mass.: MIT Press (1977).

Menyuk, P., Linguistic problems in children with developmental dysphasia. In M.A. Wyke (Ed.), *Developmental Dysphasia*. New York: Academic Press, Inc. (1978).

Menyuk, P., *Sentences Children Use*. Cambridge, Mass.: MIT Press (1969).

Menyuk, P., Syntactic rules used by children from preschool through first grade. *Journal of Child Development*, **35**, 533-546 (1964c).

Menyuk, P., *The Acquisition and Development of Language*. Englewood Cliffs, N.J.: Prentice-Hall, Inc. (1971).

Menyuk, P., The role of distinctive features in children's acquisition of phonology. *Journal of Speech and Hearing Research*, **11**, 138-146 (1968).

Menyuk, P., and Anderson, S., Children's identification and reproduction of /w/, /r/, and /l/. *Journal of Speech and Hearing Research*, **12**, 39-52 (1969).

Menyuk, P., and Looney, P., A problem of language disorder: Length versus structure. *Journal of Speech and Hearing Research*, **15**, 264-279 (1972a).

Menyuk, P., and Looney, P., Relationships among components of the grammar in language disorder. *Journal of Speech and Hearing Research*, **15**, 395-406 (1972b).

Miller, A., and Miller, E.E., Cognitive developmental training with elevated boards and sign language. *Journal of Autism and Childhood Schizophrenia*, **3**, 65-85 (1973).

Miller, J.F., Assessing children's language behavior: A developmental process approach. In R.L. Schiefelbusch (Ed.), *Bases of Language Intervention*. Baltimore: University Park Press (1978).

Miller, J.F., and Yoder, D.E., An ontogenetic language teaching strategy for retarded children. In R.L. Schiefelbusch, and L.L. Lloyd (Eds.), *Language Perspectives—Acquisition, Retardation, and Intervention*. Baltimore: University Park Press (1974).

Miller, J.F., and Yoder, D.E., A syntax teaching program. In J.E. McLean, D.E. Yoder, and R.L. Schiefelbusch (Eds.), *Language Intervention with the Retarded*. Baltimore: University Park Press (1972).

Miller, L., Pragmatics and early childhood language disorders: Communicative interactions in a half-hour sample. *Journal of Speech and Hearing Disorders*, **43,** 419-436 (1978).

Miller, W., and Ervin, S., The development of grammar in child language. *Child Development Monographs*, **29,** 9-34 (1964).

Milner, B., Disorders of learning and memory after temporal lobe lesions in man. *Clinical Neurosurgery*, **19,** 421-446 (1972).

Miner, L.E., Scoring procedures for the length-complexity index: A preliminary report. *Journal of Communication Disorders*, **2,** 224-240 (1969).

Minski, L., and Shepperd, M.J., *Non-Communicating Children*. New York: Appleton-Century-Crofts (1970).

Moerk, E.L., Changes in verbal child-mother interactions with increasing language skills of the child. *Journal of Psycholinguistic Research*, **3,** 101-116 (1974).

Moerk, E.L., *Pragmatic and Semantic Aspects of Early Language Development*. Baltimore: University Park Press (1977).

Moerk, E.L., Verbal interactions between children and their mothers during the preschool years. *Developmental Psychology*, **11,** 788-794 (1975).

Moffitt, A.R., Consonant cue perception by twenty- to twenty-four-week-old infants. *Child Development*, **42,** 717-731 (1971).

Molfese, D.L., Cortical involvement in the semantic processing of coarticulated speech cues. *Brain and Language*, **7,** 86-100 (1979).

Molfese, D.L., Infant cerebral asymmetry, In S.J. Segalowitz and F.A. Gruber (Eds.), *Language Development and Neurological Theory*. New York: Academic Press, Inc. (1977).

Monsees, E.K., Aphasia in children. *Journal of Speech and Hearing Disorders*. **26,** 83-86 (1961).

Moore, M.V., Speech, hearing and language in DeLange syndrome. *Journal of Speech and Hearing Disorders*, **35,** 60-69 (1970).

Moran, M.R., and Byrne, M.C., Mastery of verb tense markers by normal and learning-disabled children. *Journal of Speech and Hearing Research*, **20,** 529-542 (1977).

Morehead, D.M., The study of linguistically deficient children. In S. Singh (Ed.), *Measurement Procedures in Speech, Hearing, and Language*. Baltimore: University Park Press (1975).

Morehead, D.M., and Ingram, D., The development of base syntax in normal and linguistically deviant children. *Journal of Speech and Hearing Research*, **16,** 330-352 (1973).

Morehead, D.M., and Morehead, A., From signal to sign: A Piagetian view of thought and language during the first two years. In R.L. Schiefelbusch, and L.L. Lloyd (Eds.), *Language Perspectives—Acquisition, Retardation, and Intervention*. Baltimore: University Park Press (1974).

Morley, M.E., *The Development and Disorders of Speech in Childhood*. Edinburgh: E. & S. Livingstone Ltd. (1957).

Morley, M.E., *The Development and Disorders of Speech in Childhood*. (2nd ed.) Baltimore: The Williams & Wilkins Co. (1965).

Morley, M.E., *The Development and Disorders of Speech in Childhood*. (2nd ed.) Baltimore: The Williams & Wilkins Co. (1967).

Morley, M.E., *The Development and Disorders of Speech in Childhood*. (3rd ed.) Edinburgh: Churchill Livingstone (1972).

Morley, M.E., Receptive/expressive developmental aphasia. *British Journal of Disorders of Communication*, **8,** 21 (1973).

Morris, H., Communication skills of children with cleft lip and palate. *Journal of Speech and Hearing Research*, **5,** 79-90 (1962).

Morse, P.A., Infant speech perception. In D.A. Sanders (Ed.), *Auditory Perception of Speech: An Introduction to Principles and Problems*. Englewood Cliffs, N.J.: Prentice-Hall, Inc. (1977).

Morse, P.A., Infant speech perception: A preliminary model and review of the literature. In R.L. Schiefelbusch and L.L. Lloyd (Eds.), *Language Perspectives— Acquisition, Retardation and Intervention*. Baltimore: University Park Press (1974).

Morse, P.A., and Snowdon, C.T., An investigation of categorical speech discrimination by rhesus monkeys. *Perception and Psychophysics*, **17,** 9-16 (1975).

Moscovitch, M., The development of lateralization of language functions and its relation to cognitive and linguistic development: A review and some theoretical speculations. In S.J. Segalowitz, and F.A. Gruber (Eds.), *Language Development and Neurological Theory*. New York: Academic Press, Inc. (1977).

Mulac, A., and Tomlinson, C.N., Generalization of an operant remediation program for syntax with language delayed children. *Journal of Communication Disorders*, **10,** 231-243 (1977).

Muma, J.R., *Language Handbook: Concepts, Assessment, Intervention*. Englewood Cliffs, N.J.: Prentice-Hall, Inc. (1978).

Muma, J.R., *Muma Assessment Program: Descriptive Assessment Procedures: Cognitive-Linguistic-Communicative Systems*. Lubbock, Texas: Natural Child Publishing Co. (1979).

Muma, J.R., *Parent-Child Development Center: Conceptualization, Program, Evaluation*. Birmingham, Ala.: Parent-Child Development Center (1971).

Muma, J.R., Reply to Knight's comment on "The communication game: Dump and play." Letter to the Editor, *Journal of Speech and Hearing Disorders*, **41**, 278-280 (1976).

Muma, J.R., Syntax of preschool fluent and disfluent speech: A transformational analysis. *Journal of Speech and Hearing Research*, **14**, 428-441 (1971).

Muma, J.R., The communication game: Dump and play. *Journal of Speech and Hearing Disorders*, **40**, 296-309 (1975).

Myers, P., A study of language disabilities in cerebral palsied children. *Journal of Speech and Hearing Research*, **8**, 129-136 (1965).

Myklebust, H.R., *Auditory Disorders in Children: A Manual for Differential Diagnosis*. New York: Grune & Stratton, Inc. (1954).

Myklebust, H.R., *The Psychology of Deafness*. New York: Grune & Stratton, Inc. (1964).

Myklebust, H.R., Training aphasic children: Suggestions for parents and teachers. *Volta Review*, **57**, 149-157 (1955).

Mysak, E.D., *Neuroevolutional Approach to Cerebral Palsy and Speech*. New York: Teachers College Press (1968).

Mysak, E.D., *Speech Pathology and Feedback Theory*. Springfield, Ill.: Charles C Thomas, Publisher (1966).

Naremore, R.C., and Dever, R.B., Language performance of educable mentally retarded and normal children at five age levels. *Journal of Speech and Hearing Research*, **18**, 82-95 (1975).

Nation, J.E., A vocabulary usage test. *Journal of Psycholinguistic Research*, **1**, 221-231 (1972).

Nation, J.E., Determinants of vocabulary development of preschool cleft palate children. *Cleft Palate Journal*, **7**, 645-651 (1970).

Nation, J.E., Management of speech and language disorders. In N.J. Lass, J.L. Northern, D.E. Yoder, and L.V. McReynolds (Eds.), *Speech, Language and Hearing*. Philadelphia: W.B. Saunders Co. (1982).

Nation, J.E., Vocabulary comprehension and usage of preschool cleft palate and normal children. *Cleft Palate Journal*, **7**, 639-644 (1970).

Nation, J.E., and Aram, D.M., *Diagnosis of Speech and Language Disorders*. St. Louis: The C.V. Mosby Co. (1977).

Nation, J.E., and Aram, D.M., The diagnostic process. In N.J. Lass, J.L. Northern, D.E. Yoder, and L.V. McReynolds (Eds.), *Speech, Language and Hearing*. Philadelphia: W. B. Saunders Co. (1982).

National Advisory Committee on Handicapped Children, January, 1968. First Annual Report, "Special Education for Handicapped Children". National Advisory Neurological Diseases and Stroke Council. *Human Communication and Its Disorders—An Overview*. NIH: Bethesda, Md. (1969).

Nelson, K., Structure and strategy in learning to talk. *Monographs of the Society for Research in Child Development*, **38**, (1973).

Newfield, M., and Schlanger, B., The acquisition of English morphology by normal and educable mentally retarded children. *Journal of Speech and Hearing Research*, **11**, 693-706 (1968).

Nice, M., A child who would not talk. *Pedagogical Seminary* **32**, 105-144 (1925).

Ninio, A., and Bruner, J.S., The achievement and antecedents of labelling. *Journal of Child Language*, **5**, 1-16 (1978).

Northern, J.L., and Downs, M.P., *Hearing in Children*. (2nd ed.) Baltimore: The Williams & Wilkins Co. (1978).

Novakovich, H., Smith, J., and Teegarden, C., *Target on Language*. Bethesda, Md.: Christ Church Child Center (1973, 1977).

Oelschlaeger, M.L., and Orchik, D., Time-compressed speech discrimination in central auditory disorder: A pediatric case study. *Journal of Speech and Hearing Disorders*, **42**, 483-486 (1977).

Oelschlaeger, M.L., and Scarborough, J., Traumatic aphasia in children: A case study. *Journal of Communication Disorders*, **9**, 281-288 (1976).

Oldfield, R.C., and Wingfield, A., *A Series of Pictures for Use in Object Naming*. M.R.C. Psycholinguistic Research Unit Special Report No. PLU/65/19 (1965).

Oller, D.K., Regularities in abnormal child phonology. *Journal of Speech and Hearing Disorders*, **38**, 36-47 (1973).

Oller, D.K., Jensen, H.T., and Lafayette, R.H., The relatedness of phonological processes of a hearing-impaired child. *Journal of Communication Disorders*, **11**, 97-105 (1978).

Olmsted, D., *Out of the Mouth of Babes*. The Hague: Mouton (1971).

Olson, G.M., Memory development and language acquisition. In T.E. Moore (Ed.), *Cognitive Development and the Acquisition of Language*. New York: Academic Press, Inc., 145-157 (1973).

Olson, J.L., Differential diagnosis: Deaf and sensory aphasic children. *Exceptional Child*, **28**, 422-424 (1961).

Olswang, L.B., and Carpenter, R.L., Elicitory effects on the language obtained from young language-impaired children. *Journal of Speech and Hearing Disorders*, **43**, 76-88 (1978).

Orton, S.T., *Reading, Writing and Speech Problems in Children: A Presentation of Certain Types of Disorders in the Development of the Language Faculty*. New York: W.W. Norton & Co., Inc. (1937).

Osgood, C.E., Motivational dynamics of language behavior. In M. Jones (Ed.), *Nebraska Symposium on Motivation.* Lincoln, Neb.: University of Nebraska Press (1957).

Paden, E., Whatever happened to functional articulation disorders: Phonological disorders. Paper presented at the Annual Convention of the American Speech-Language and Hearing Association, Detroit (1980).

Panagos, J.M., Abstract phonology, grammatical reduction and delayed speech development. *Acta Symbolica,* **7,** 1-12 (1978).

Panagos, J.M., Persistence of the open syllable reinterpreted as a symptom of language disorder. *Journal of Speech and Hearing Disorders,* **39,** 23-31 (1974).

Panagos, J.M., Quine, M.E., and Klich, R.J., Syntactic and phonological influences on children's articulation. *Journal of Speech and Hearing Research,* **22,** 841-848 (1979).

Pannbacker, M., Oral language skills of adult cleft palate speakers. *Cleft Palate Journal,* **12,** 95-106 (1975).

Papania, N., A qualitative analysis of vocabulary responses of institutionalized mentally retarded children. *Journal of Clinical Pathology,* **10,** 361-365 (1954).

Paradise, J.L., Bluestone, C.D., and Felder, H., The universality of otitis media in fifty infants with cleft palate. *Pediatrics,* **44,** 35-42 (1969).

Peins, M., Client-centered communication therapy for mentally retarded delinquents. *Journal of Speech and Hearing Disorders,* **32,** 154-161 (1967).

Perkins, W.H., *Human Perspectives in Speech and Language Disorders.* St. Louis: The C.V. Mosby Co. (1978).

Perkins, W.H., *Speech Pathology: An Applied Behavioral Science.* (2nd ed.) St. Louis: The C.V. Mosby Co. (1977).

Petrie, I., Characteristics and progress of a group of language-disordered children with severe receptive difficulties. *British Journal of Disorders of Communication,* **10,** 123-127, (1975).

Philips, B.J., and Harrison, R., Language skills of preschool cleft palate children. *Cleft Palate Journal,* **6,** 108-119 (1969).

Phillips, J.F., Syntax and vocabulary of mother's speech to young children: Age and sex comparisons. *Child Development,* **44,** 182-185 (1973).

Piaget, J., *Language and Thought of the Child.* New York: Harcourt & Brace (1926).

Piaget, J., *The Language and Thought of the Child.* New York: Meridian (1955).

Pierce, S., and Bartolucci, G., A syntactic investigation of verbal, autistic, mentally retarded and normal children. *Journal of Autism and Childhood Schizophrenia,* **7,** 121-133 (1977).

Pisoni, D.B., Mechanisms of auditory discrimination and coding of linguistic information. *Acta Symbolica,* **5,** 65-111 (1975).

Pollack, E., and Rees, N., Disorders of articulation: Some clinical applications of distinctive feature theory. *Journal of Speech and Hearing Disorders,* **37,** 451-461 (1972).

Poppen, R., Stark, J., Eisenson, J., Forrest, T., and Wertheim, G., Visual sequencing performance of aphasic children. *Journal of Speech and Hearing Research,* **12,** 288-300 (1969).

Prichard, C.L., Tekieli, M.E., and Kozup, J.M., Developmental dyspraxia: Diagnostic considerations. *Journal of Communication Disorders,* **12,** 337-348 (1979).

Prizant, B.M., and Ferraro, B.C., Analysis of the functions of immediate echolalia in autistic children. Miniseminar presented at the Annual Convention of the American Speech-Language and Hearing Association, Atlanta (1979).

Pronovost, W., *Boston University Speech Discrimination Test.* Cedar Falls, Iowa: Go-Mo Products (1953).

Pronovost, W., The speech behavior and language comprehension of autistic children. *Journal of Chronic Disorders,* **13,** 228-233 (1961).

Prutting, C.A., Process /pra/,ses/ n: The action of moving forward progressively from one point to another on the way to completion. *Journal of Speech and Hearing Disorders,* **44,** 3-30 (1979).

Prutting, C.A., and Connolly, J.E., Imitation: A closer look. *Journal of Speech and Hearing Disorders,* **41,** 412-422 (1976).

Prutting, C.A., Gallagher, T.M., and Mulac, A., The expressive portion of the NSST compared to a spontaneous language sample. *Journal of Speech and Hearing Disorders,* **40,** 40-48 (1975).

Quigley, S.P., Power, D.J., and Steinkamp, M.W., The language structure of deaf children. *Volta Review,* **79,** 73-84 (1977).

Ramer, A.L.H., The function of imitation in child language. *Journal of Speech and Hearing Research,* **19,** 700-717 (1976).

Rankin, J.M., Aram, D.M., and Horwitz, S.J., Language ability in right and left hemiplegic children. Submitted to *Brain and Language* (May, 1980).

Rapin, I., and Allen, D.A., Developmental language disorders—nosologic considerations. New York: Albert Einstein College of Medicine (working paper).

Rapin, I., and Wilson, B.C., Children with developmental language disability: Neurological aspects and assessment. In M. Wyke (Ed.), *Developmental Dysphasia.* New York: Academic Press, Inc. (1978).

Rasmussen, T., and Milner, B., The role of early left-brain injury in determining lateralization of cerebral speech functions. In S.J. Diamong and D.A. Blizard (Eds.), *Evolution and Lateralization of the Brain.* Annals of the New York Academy of Sciences, **299** (1977).

Ratner, N., and Bruner, J.S., Games, social exchange and the acquisition of language. *Journal of Child Language,* **5,** 391-402 (1978).

Ratusnik, C.M., and Ratusnik, D.L., A therapeutic milieu for establishing and expanding communicative behaviors in psychotic children. *Journal of Speech and Hearing Disorders,* **41,** 70-92 (1976).

Rees, N.S., Art and science of diagnosis in hearing, language, and speech. In S. Singh and J. Lynch (Eds.), *Diagnostic Procedures in Hearing, Language, and Speech.* Baltimore: University Park Press (1978).

Rees, N.S., Auditory processing factors in language disorders: The view from Procruste's bed. *Journal of Speech and Hearing Disorders,* **38,** 304-315 (1973).

Rees, N.S., Bases of decision in language training. *Journal of Speech and Hearing Disorders,* **37,** 283-304 (1972).

Rees, N.S., Imitation and language development: Issues and clinical implications. *Journal of Speech and Hearing Disorders,* **40,** 339-350 (1975).

Rees, N.S., and Shulman, M., I don't understand what you mean by comprehension. *Journal of Speech and Hearing Disorders,* **43,** 208-219 (1978).

Ricks, N., Sustained attention and the effects of distraction in under-achieving second grade children. Unpublished doctoral dissertation, Boston University (1974).

Rieber, R.W., and Brubaker, R.S., *Speech Pathology.* Philadelphia: J.B. Lippincott Co. (1966).

Roeser, P.J., Campbell, J.C., and Daly, D.D., Recovery of auditory function following meningitic deafness. *Journal of Speech and Hearing Disorders,* **40,** 405-411 (1975).

Rosch, E.H., On the internal structure of perceptual and semantic categories. In T.E. Moore (Ed.), *Cognitive Development and the Acquisition of Language.* New York: Academic Press, Inc. (1973).

Rose, D.E., *Audiological Assessment.* Englewood Cliffs, N.J.: Prentice-Hall, Inc. (1971).

Rosenbek, J., Hansen, R., Baughman, C., and Lemme, M., Treatment of developmental apraxia of speech: A case report. *Language, Speech and Hearing Services in Schools,* **5,** 13-22 (1974).

Rosenbek, J., and Wertz, R., A review of 50 cases of developmental apraxia of speech. *Language, Speech and Hearing Services in Schools,* **3,** 23-33 (1972).

Ross, M., and Lerman, J., A picture identification test for hearing-impaired children. *Journal of Speech and Hearing Research,* **13,** 44-53 (1970).

Ross, M., and Lerman, J., *Word Intelligibility By Picture Identification.* Pittsburgh: Stanwix House, Inc. (1971).

Ruben, R.J., and Hanson, D.G., Summary of discussion and recommendations made during the workshop on otitis media and development. *The Annals of Otology Rhinology and Laryngology,* Supplement 60, Vol. 88 No. 5, Part 2, 107-111 (1979).

Rudel, R.G., Tueber, H.L., and Twitchell, T.E., Levels of impairment of sensori-motor functions in children with early brain damage. *Neuropsychologia,* **12,** 95-108 (1974).

Ruder, K.F., and Smith, M.D., Issues in language training. In R.L. Schiefelbusch, and L.L. Lloyd (Eds.), *Language Perspectives: Acquisition, Retardation and Intervention.* Baltimore: University Park Press (1974).

Russell, W.K., Quigley, S.P., and Power, D.J., *Linguistics and Deaf Children: Transformational Syntax and Its Application.* Washington, D.C.: Alexander Graham Bell Association for the Deaf (1976).

Rutter, M., Concepts of autism. *Journal of Child Psychology and Psychiatry,* **9,** 1-25 (1968).

Rutter, M., and Schopler, E. (Eds.), *Autism: A Reappraisal of Concepts and Treatment.* New York: Plenum Press (1978).

Sachs, J., and Devin, J., Young children's use of age-appropriate speech styles in social interaction and role playing. *Journal of Child Language,* **3,** 81-98 (1976).

Saleeby, M.C., Hadjian, S., Martinkosky, S.J., and Swift, M.R., Familial verbal dyspraxia: A clinical study. Paper presented at the Annual Convention of the American Speech-Language and Hearing Association, San Francisco (1978).

Sameroff, A.J., Early influences on development: Fact or fancy? *Merrill-Palmer Quarterly of Behavior and Development,* **21,** 3-33 (1975).

Sanders, D.A., *Auditory Perception of Speech: An Introduction to Principles and Problems.* Englewood Cliffs, N.J.: Prentice-Hall, Inc. (1977).

Saxman, J.H., and Miller, J.F., Short-term memory and language skills in articulation-deficit children. *Journal of Speech and Hearing Research,* **16,** 721-730 (1973).

Schachter, F.F., Fosha, D., Stemp, S., Brotman, N., and Ganger, S., Everyday caretaker talk to toddlers vs. threes and fours. *Journal of Child Language,* **3,** 221-245 (1976).

Schane, S., *Generative Phonology.* Englewood Cliffs, N.J.: Prentice-Hall, Inc. (1973).

Schell, R.E., Stark, J., and Giddan, J.J., Development of language behavior in an autistic child. *Journal of Speech and Hearing Disorders,* **32,** 51-64 (1967).

Schiefelbusch, R.L., and Lloyd, L.L. (Eds.), *Language Perspectives—Acquisition, Retardation, and Intervention.* Baltimore: University Park Press (1974).

Schiff, N.B., The influence of deviant maternal input on the development of language during the preschool years. *Journal of Speech and Hearing Research,* **22,** 581-603 (1979).

Schiff, N.B., and Ventry, I.M., Communication problems in hearing children of deaf parents. *Journal of Speech and Hearing Disorders,* **41,** 348-358, (1976).

Schuler, A.L., Echolalia: Issues and clinical applications. *Journal of Speech and Hearing Disorders,* **44,** 441-434 (1979).

Schwartz, A.H., and Goldman, R., Variables influencing performance on speech-sound discrimination test. *Journal of Speech and Hearing Research,* **17,** 25-32 (1974).

Schwartz, E.R., Characteristics of speech and language development in the child with myelomeningocele and hydrocephalus. *Journal of Speech and Hearing Disorders,* **39,** 465-468 (1974).

Searle, J.R., *Speech Acts: An Essay in the Philosophy of Language.* Cambridge, England: Cambridge University Press (1969).

Segalowitz, S.J., and Gruber, F.A. (Eds.), *Language Development and Neurological Theory.* New York: Academic Press, Inc. (1977).

Seitz, S., and Marcus, S., Mother-child interactions: A foundation for language development. *Exceptional Child,* 445-449 (1976).

Semel, E.M., and Wiig, E.H., Comprehension of syntactic structures and critical verbal elements by children with learning disabilities. *Journal of Learning Disabilities,* **8,** 53-58 (1975).

Shames, G.H., and Egolf, D.B., *Operant Conditioning and the Management of Stuttering.* Englewood Cliffs, N.J.: Prentice-Hall, Inc. (1976).

Shatz, M., and Gelman, R., The development of communication skills: Modification in the speech of young children as a function of listener. *Monographs of the Society for Research in Child Development,* **38** (1973).

Shriberg, L., and Kwiatkowski, J., *Natural Process Analysis (NPA): A Procedure for Phonological Analysis of Continuous Speech Samples.* New York: John Wiley & Sons, Inc. (1980).

Shriner, T.H., Holloway, M.S., and Daniloff, R.G., The relationship between articulatory deficits and syntax in speech defective children. *Journal of Speech and Hearing Research,* **12,** 319-325 (1969).

Shoumaker, R.D., Bennett, D.R., Bray, R.F., and Curless, R., Clinical and EEG manifestations of an unusual aphasic syndrome in children. *Neurology,* **24,** 10-16 (1974).

Silverman, F.H., *Communication for the Speechless.* Englewood Cliffs, N.J.: Prentice-Hall, Inc. (1980).

Silverman, S.R., From Aristotle to Bell. In H. Davis, and S.R. Silverman (Eds.), *Hearing and Deafness.* New York: Holt, Rinehart & Winston, Inc., 405-412 (1961).

Simmons, F.B., and Russ, F., Automated newborn hearing screening, the Crib-O-Gram. *Archives of Otolaryngology,* **100,** 1-7 (1974).

Simon, N., Echolalic speech in childhood autism: Consideration of possible underlying loci of brain damage. *Archives of General Psychiatry,* **32,** 1439-1446 (1975).

Sinclair, H., Developmental psycholinguistics. In D. Elkind, and J. Flavell, (Eds.), *Studies in Cognitive Development.* New York: Oxford University Press (1969).

Sinclair, H., Sensorimotor action patterns as a condition for the acquisition of syntax. In R. Huxley, and E. Ingram (Eds.), *Language Acquisition: Models and Methods.* New York: Academic Press, Inc. (1971).

Singh, S., *Distinctive Features: Theory and Validation.* Baltimore: University Park Press (1976).

Skinner, B.F., *Verbal Behavior.* New York: Appleton-Century-Crofts (1957).

Slobin, D.I., Studies of imitation and comprehension. In C. Ferguson and D. Slobin (Eds.), *Studies of Child Language Development.* New York: Holt, Rinehart & Winston, Inc. (1973).

Slobin, D.Z., Developmental psycholinguistics. In W. Dingwall (Ed.), *A Survey of Linguistic Science.* (2nd ed.) Stamford, Conn.: Greylock Publishers (1978).

Smith, C.S., An experimental approach to children's linguistic competence. In J.R. Hayes (Ed.), *Cognition and the Development of Language.* New York: John Wiley & Sons, Inc. (1970).

Smith, F., *Understanding Reading: A Psycholinguistic Analysis of Reading and Learning to Read.* New York: Holt, Rinehart, & Winston, Inc. (1971).

Smith, N.V., *The Acquisition of Phonology: A Case Study.* Cambridge, England: Cambridge University Press (1973).

Smith, R., and McWilliams, B.J., Psycholinguistic abilities of children with clefts. *Cleft Palate Journal,* **3,** 375-383 (1968).

Snow, C.E., Mothers' speech to children learning language. *Child Development,* **43,** 549-565 (1972).

Snow, C.E., and Ferguson, C.A. (Eds.), *Talking to Children: Language Input and Acquisition.* Cambridge, England: Cambridge University Press (1977).

Snow, J., Rintelmann, W., Miller, J., et. al., Central auditory imperception. Eastern Section of American Laryngological, Rhinological and Otological Society, Hamilton, Bermuda (1977).

Snyder, L.K., Lovitt, T.C., and Smith, J.O., Language training for the severely retarded: Five years of behavior analysis research. *Exceptional Children,* **42,** 7-14 (1975).

Snyder, L.S., and Johnston, J.R., Language, cognition and reading in language/learning disabled children. Short course presented at the Annual Convention of the American Speech-Language and Hearing Association, Detroit (1980).

Soderberg, G.A., Linguistic factors in stuttering. *Journal of Speech and Hearing Research,* **10,** 801-810 (1967).

Sommers, R.K., Factors in the effectiveness of articulation therapy with educable retarded children. *Journal of Speech and Hearing Research,* **13,** 304-316 (1970).

Sommers, R.K., Cox, S., and West, C., Articulatory effectiveness, stimulability and children's performance on perceptual and memory tasks. *Journal of Speech and Hearing Research,* **15,** 579-589 (1972).

Sperber, R.D., Ragain, R.D., and McCauley, C., Reassessment of category knowledge in retarded individuals. *Journal of Mental Deficiency,* **81,** 227-234 (1976).

Spradlin, J.E., Assessment of speech and language of retarded children. The Parsons language sample. *Journal of Speech and Hearing Disorders,* Monograph Supplement 10, 8-31 (1963).

Spreen, O., Language functions in mental retardation: A review. *American Journal of Mental Deficiency,* **69,** 482-494 (1965).

Spriestersbach, D., Darley, F., and Morris, H., Language skills in children with cleft palates. *Journal of Speech and Hearing Research,* **1,** 279-283 (1958).

Stampe, E., The acquisition of phonetic representation. *Papers from the Fifth Regional Meeting, Chicago Linguistic Society,* 433-44 (1969).

Stark, J., A comparison of aphasic children on three sequencing tasks. *Journal of Communication Disorders,* **1,** 31-34 (1967).

Stark, J., Reading failure: A language-based problem. *Asha,* **17,** 832-834 (1975).

Stark, J., Giddan, J.J., and Meisel, J., Increasing verbal behavior in an autistic child. *Journal of Speech and Hearing Disorders,* **33,** 42-47 (1968).

Steckol, K.F., and Leonard, L.B., The use of grammatical morphemes by normal and language-impaired children. *Journal of Communication Disorders,* **12,** 291-301 (1979).

Stein, L.K., and Curry, F.K.W., Childhood auditory agnosia. *Journal of Speech and Hearing Disorders,* **33,** 361-370 (1968).

Stephens, M.I., The problem of subject specification in studies of language impaired children. Paper presented at the Annual Convention of the American Speech-Language and Hearing Association, Atlanta (1979).

Stern, D.N., Jaffe, J., Beebe, B., and Bennett, S.L., Vocalizing in unison and in alternation: Two modes of communication within the mother-infant dyad. *Annals of the New York Academy of Sciences,* **263,** 89-100 (1975).

Stevens, K.N., Segments, features and analysis-by-synthesis. In J.F. Kavanagh and I.G. Mattingly (Eds.), *Language by Eye and Ear.* Cambridge, Mass.: MIT Press (1972).

Stevens, K.N., and Halle, M., Remarks on analysis-by-synthesis and distinctive features. In W. Wathen-Dunn (Ed.), *Models for the Perception of Speech and Visual Form.* Cambridge, Mass.: MIT Press (1967).

Stevens-Long, J., and Rasmussen, M., The acquisition of simple and compound sentence structure in an autistic child. *Journal of Applied Behavior Analysis,* **7,** 473-479 (1974).

St. Louis, K.O., Linguistic and motor aspects of stuttering. In N.J. Lass (Ed.), *Speech and Language: Advances in Basic Research and Practice.* (Vol. 1) New York: Academic Press, Inc. (1979).

Strauss, A.A., Aphasia in children. *American Journal of Physical Medicine,* **33,** 93-99 (1954).

Strauss, A.A., and Kephart, N.C., *Psychopathology and Education of the Brain-Injured Child: Progress in Theory and Clinic.* (Vol. II) New York: Grune & Stratton, Inc. (1955).

Strauss, A.A., and Lehtinen, L.E., *Psychopathology and Education of the Brain Injured Child.* New York: Grune & Stratton, Inc. (1947).

Streeter, L.A., Language perception of 2-month-old infants shows effects of both innate mechanisms and experience. *Nature,* **259,** 39-41 (1976).

Streissguth, A.P., Herman, C.S., and Smith, D.W., Intelligence, behavior, and dysmorphogenesis in the fetal alcohol syndrome: A report of 20 patients. *The Journal of Pediatrics,* **92,** 363-367 (1978).

Sulzbacher, S.E., and Costello, J.M., A behavioral strategy for language training of a child with autistic behaviors. *Journal of Speech and Hearing Disorders,* **35,** 256-277 (1970).

Summers, J., The use of the electrolarynx in patients with temporary tracheotomies. *Journal of Speech and Hearing Disorders,* **38,** 335-338 (1973).

Swoboda, P.J., Morse, P.A., and Leavitt, L.A., A continuous vowel discrimination in normal and at risk infants. *Child Development,* **47,** 549-565 (1976).

Swope, S., and Liebergott, J., Developmental language teaching workshop. American Speech and Hearing Association Convention, San Francisco (1977).

Tallal, P., A response to Manning, Johnson and Beasley. *Journal of Speech and Hearing Disorders,* **44,** 136-137 (1979).

Tallal, P., Perceptual and linguistic factors in the language impairment of developmental dysphasics: An experimental investigation with the Token Test. *Cortex,* **9,** 196-205 (1975).

Tallal, P., Rapid auditory processing in normal and disordered language development. *Journal of Speech and Hearing Research,* **19,** 561-571 (1976).

Tallal, P., and Piercy, M., Defects of auditory perception in children with developmental dysphasia. In M. Wyke (Ed.), *Developmental Dysphasia.* New York: Academic Press, Inc. (1978).

Tallal, P., and Piercy, M., Defects of nonverbal auditory perception in children with developmental dysphasia. *Nature,* **241,** 468-499 (1973a).

Tallal, P., and Piercy, M., Developmental aphasia: Impaired rate of nonverbal processing as a function of sensory modality. *Neuropsychologia,* **11,** 389-398 (1973b).

Tallal, P., and Piercy, M., Developmental aphasia: Rate of auditory processing and selective impairment of consonant perception. *Neuropsychologia,* **12,** 83-93 (1974).

Tallal, P., and Piercy, M., Developmental aphasia: The perception of brief vowels and extended stop consonants. *Neuropsychologia,* **13,** 69-74 (1975).

Tallal, P., and Stark, R., The Relation Between Lower-Level Linguistic Analysis in Developmental Dysphasics. New York: The International Neuropsychology Society Meetings (1979).

Tallal, P., Stark, R., and Curtiss, B., The relation between speech perception impairment and speech production impairment in children with developmental dysphasia. *Brain and Language,* **3,** 305-317 (1976).

Taylor, A.M., Thurlow, M.L., and Turner, J.E., Vocabulary development of educable retarded children. *Exceptional Children,* **43,** 444-450 (1977).

Templin, M.C., *Certain Language Skills in Children, Their Development and Interrelationships.* Institute of Child Welfare, Monograph Series No. 26. Minneapolis: University of Minnesota Press (1957).

Thies, T.L., and Thies, H.H., Responses to distorted speech and competing messages of children with severe language disorders. Presented at the American Speech and Hearing Association Convention, San Francisco (1972).

Thomas, A., Chess, S., and Birch, H.G., *Temperament and Behavior Disorders in Children.* New York: New York University Press (1968).

Tobey, E.A., Cullen, J.K., Rampp, D.L., and Fleischer-Gallagher, A.M., Effects of stimulus-onset asynchrony on the dichotic performance of children with auditory processing disorders. *Journal of Speech and Hearing Research,* **22,** 197-211 (1979).

Town, C.H., Congenital aphasia. *Psychological Clinics,* **6** (1911).

Trantham, C.R., and Pederson, J.K., *Normal Language Development: The Key to Diagnosis and Therapy for Language-Disordered Children.* Baltimore: The Williams & Wilkins Co. (1976).

Trehub, S.E., Infant's sensitivity to vowel and tonal contrasts. *Developmental Psychology,* **9,** 91-96 (1973).

Tweney, R.D., Hoemann, H.W., and Andrews, C.E., Semantic organization in deaf and hearing subjects. *Journal of Psycholinguistic Research,* **4,** 61-73 (1975).

Tyack, D., and Gottsleben, R., *Language Sampling, Analysis and Training: A Handbook for Teachers and Clinicians.* Palo Alto, Calif.: Consulting Psychological Press (1974).

Uzgiris, I.C., and Hunt, J. McV., *Assessment in Infancy.* Urbana, Ill.: University of Illinois Press (1975).

Vahcic, B., Nation, J.E., and Sugarman, M.D., An adult speech sound disorder: Phonology or articulation? In J.R. Andrews and M.S. Burns (Eds.), *Selected Papers in Language and Phonology.* (Vol. III) *Phonological Deviance.* Evanston, Ill.: Institute for Continuing Professional Education (1977).

Vandemark, A.H., and Mann, M.B., Oral language skills of children with defective articulation. *Journal of Speech and Hearing Research,* **8,** 409-414 (1965).

Van Kleeck, A., and Carpenter, R.L., The effects of children's language comprehension level on adults' child-directed talk. *Journal of Speech and Hearing Research,* **23,** 546-569 (1980).

Van Riper, C., *Speech Correction: Principles and Methods.* (3rd Ed.) Englewood Cliffs, N.J.: Prentice-Hall, Inc. (1954).

Vellutino, F.R., Alternative conceptualizations of dyslexia: Evidence in support of a verbal-deficit hypothesis. *Harvard Educational Review,* **47,** 334-354 (1977).

Vellutino, F.R., *Dyslexia: Theory and Research.* Cambridge, Mass.: MIT Press (1978).

Vellutino, F.R., DeSetto, L., and Steger, J.A., Categorical judgement and the Wepman Test of Auditory Discrimination. *Journal of Speech and Hearing Disorders,* **37,** 252-257 (1972).

Ventry, I.M., Effects of conductive hearing loss: Fact or fiction. *Journal of Speech and Hearing Disorders,* **45,** 143-156 (1980).

Vernon, M., Meningitis and deafness: The problem, its physical, audiological, psychological, and educational manifestations in deaf children. *Laryngoscope,* **77,** 1856-1874 (1967).

Vetter, H., *Language Behavior and Psychopathology.* Chicago: Rand McNally & Co. (1969).

Warrington, E.K., and Kinsbourne, M., The incidence of verbal disability associated with reading retardation. *Neuropsychologia,* **5,** 175-180 (1967).

Waters, R.S., and Wilson, W.A., Jr., Speech perception by rhesus monkeys: The voicing distinction in synthesized labial and velar stop consonants. *Perception and Psychophysics,* **19,** 285-289 (1976).

Waterson, N., and Snow, C. (Eds.), *The Development of Communication.* New York: John Wiley & Sons, Inc. (1978).

Watzlawick, P., Beavin, J.H., Helmick, A.B., and Jackson, D.D., *Pragmatics of Human Communication: A Study of Interactional Patterns, Pathologies, and Paradoxes.* New York: W.W. Norton & Co., Inc. (1967).

Wechsler, D., *Manual for the Weschler Adult Intelligence Scale,* New York: The Psychological Corporation (1955).

Weeks, T., *The Slow Speech Development of a Bright Child.* Lexington, Mass.: D.C. Heath & Co. (1974).

Weener, P.D., Toward a developmental model of auditory processes. *Acta Symbolica,* **5,** 85-104 (1974).

Weiner, F., *Phonological Process Analysis.* Baltimore: University Park Press (1970).

Weiner, P.S., A language-delayed child at adolescence. *Journal of Speech and Hearing Disorders,* **39,** 202-212 (1974).

Weiner, P.S., Auditory discrimination and articulation. *Journal of Speech and Hearing Disorders,* **32,** 19-28 (1967).

Weiner, P.S., The perceptual level functioning of dysphasic children. A follow-up study. *Journal of Speech and Hearing Research,* **15,** 423-438 (1972).

Weisenburg, T., and McBride, K.E., *Aphasia: A Clinical and Psychological Study.* The Commonwealth Fund, Division of Publications (1935) and New York: Hafner Publishing Co. (1964).

Weiss, D.A., *Cluttering.* Englewood Cliffs, N.J.: Prentice-Hall, Inc. (1964).

Wepman, J., *Auditory Discrimination Test.* Chicago: Language Research Associates (1958).

Wernicke, K., The symptom-complex of aphasia (1874). In A. Church (Ed.), *Diseases of the Nervous System.* New York: Appleton-Century-Crofts (1908).

West, R., (Ed.), *Childhood Aphasia.* Proceedings of the Institute on Childhood Aphasia. San Francisco: California Society for Crippled Children and Adults (1962).

West, R., Kennedy, L., and Carr, A., *The Rehabilitation of Speech.* (Rev. ed.) New York: Harper & Brothers (1947).

West and Weber, A linguistic analysis of the morphophonemic and syntactic structures of a hard-of-hearing child. *Language and Speech,* **17,** 68-79 (1974).

Westlake, H., and Rutherford, D., *Speech Therapy for the Cerebral Palsied.* Chicago: National Society for Crippled Children and Adults (1961).

Whitaker, H., A model for neurolinguistics. *Occasional Papers 10,* Language Centre, Colchester, England: University of Essex (1970).

Whitaker, H.A., Neurolinguistics. In W.O. Dingwall (Ed.), *A Survey of Linguistic Science.* College Park, Md.: Linguistic Program, University of Maryland (1971).

Whitehurst, G.J., Novak, G., and Zorn, G.A., Delayed speech studied in the home. *Developmental Psychology,* **7,** 169-177 (1971).

Wiig, E.H., and Semel, E.M., Comprehension of linguistic concepts requiring logical operations by learning-disabled children. *Journal of Speech and Hearing Research,* **16,** 627-636 (1973).

Wiig, E.H., and Semel, E.M., *Language Assessment and Intervention for the Learning Disabled.* Columbus, Ohio: Charles E. Merrill Publishing Co. (1980).

Wiig, E.H., and Semel, E.M., *Language Disabilities in Children and Adolescents.* Columbus, Ohio: Charles E. Merrill Publishing Co. (1976).

Wiig, E.H., and Semel, E.M., Production language abilities in learning disabled adolescents. *Journal of Learning Disabilities,* **8,** 578-586 (1975).

Wilcox, M.J., and Leonard, L.B., Experimental acquisition of WH-questions in language disordered children. *Journal of Speech and Hearing Research,* **21,** 220-239 (1978).

Wilson, F.B., Efficacy of speech therapy with educable mentally retarded children. *Journal of Speech and Hearing Research,* **9,** 423-433 (1966).

Wilson, L.F., Doehring, D.G., and Hirsch, I.J., Auditory discrimination learning by aphasic and non-aphasic children. *Journal of Speech and Hearing Research,* **3,** 130-137 (1960).

Winitz, H., *Articulatory Acquisition and Behavior.* New York: Appleton-Century-Crofts (1969).

Winters, J.J., and Brzoska, M.A., Development of lexicon in normal and retarded persons. *Psychological Reports,* **37,** 391-402 (1975).

Witelson, S.F., Developmental dyslexia: Two right hemispheres and none left. *Science,* **195,** 309-311 (1977a).

Witelson, S.F., Early hemisphere specialization and interhemisphere plasticity: An empirical and theoretical review. In S.J. Segalowitz, and F.A. Gruber (Eds.), *Language Development and Neurological Theory.* New York: Academic Press, Inc. (1977b).

Witelson, S.F., Sex and the single hemisphere: Specialization of the right hemisphere for spatial processing. *Science,* **193,** 425-427 (1976).

Witelson, S.F., and Pallie, W., Left-hemisphere specialization for language in the newborn: Neuroanatomical evidence of asymmetry. *Brain,* **96,** 641-646 (1973).

Wolfus, B., Moscovitch, M., and Kinsbourne, M., Subgroups of developmental language impairment. *Brain and Language,* **9,** 152-171 (1980).

Wolpaw, T., Nation, J.E., and Aram, D.M., Developmental language disorders: A follow-up study. *Selected Papers in Language and Phonology: Vol. 1: Identification and Diagnosis of Language Disorders.* Evanston, Illinois: Institute for Continuing Professional Education (1977).

Wood, B.S., *Children and Communication: Verbal and Nonverbal Language Development.* Englewood Cliffs, N.J.: Prentice-Hall, Inc. (1976).

Wood, N.E., *Delayed Speech and Language Development*. Englewood Cliffs, N.J.: Prentice-Hall, Inc. (1964).

Worster-Drought, C., An unusual form of acquired aphasia in children. *Develop. Med. Child Neurology.*, **13,** 563-571 (1971).

Worster-Drought, C., Congenital auditory imperception (congenital word-deafness) and its relation to idioglossia and allied speech defects. *Medical Press and Circular,* **210,** 411-417 (1943).

Worster-Drought, C., and Allen, I.M., Congenital auditory imperception (congenital word-deafness): With report of a case. *Journal of Neurology and Psychopathology,* **9,** 193-208 (1929).

Worthley, W.J., *Sourcebook of Language Learning Activities*. Boston: Little, Brown & Co. (1978).

Wulbert, M., Inglis, S., Kriegsmann, E., and Mills, B., Language delay and associated mother-child interactions. *Developmental Psychology,* **2,** 61-70 (1975).

Yeni-Komshian, G.H., Speech perception in brain injured children. Conference on the Biological Bases of Delayed Language Development, New York (1977).

Yoder, D., and Miller, J., What we may know and what we can do: Input towards a system. In J. McLean, D. Yoder, and R. Schiefelbusch (Eds.), *Language Intervention with the Retarded: Developing Strategies*. Baltimore: University Park Press (1972).

Yoss, K.A., Therapy in developmental apraxia of speech. *Language, Speech and Hearing Services in Schools,* **5,** 23-31 (1974).

Yoss, K.A., and Darley, F., Developmental apraxia of speech in children with defective articulation. *Journal of Speech and Hearing Research,* **17,** 399-416 (1974).

Yost, W.A., and Nielsen, D.W., *Fundamentals of Hearing: An Introduction*. New York: Holt, Rinehart & Winston, Inc. (1977).

INDEXES

Author index

Subject index